# Invasive Outpatient Procedures in Reproductive Medicine

# Invasive Outpatient Procedures in Reproductive Medicine

Mark I. Evans, MD
Professor, Vice Chairman, and Vice Chief of Obstetrics and Gynecology
Professor of Molecular Medicine & Genetics
Professor of Pathology
Director, Division of Reproductive Genetics
Director, Center for Fetal Diagnosis and Therapy
Wayne State University/Hutzel Hospital
Detroit, Michigan

Mark P. Johnson, MD
Associate Director, Division of Reproductive Genetics
Associate Director, Center for Fetal Diagnosis and Therapy
Associate Professor, Departments of Obstetrics & Gynecology,
Molecular Medicine & Genetics, and Pathology
Wayne State University/Hutzel Hospital
Detroit, Michigan

Kamran S. Moghissi, MD
Professor of Obstetrics and Gynecology
Division of Reproductive Endocrinology and Infertility
Wayne State University/Hutzel Hospital
Detroit, Michigan

With 28 additional contributors

Illustrations by Harry Oliver Burdett

Lippincott - Raven
PUBLISHERS
Philadelphia • New York

Acquisitions Editor: R. Craig Percy
Senior Production Editor: Virginia Barishek
Production Service: Caslon, Inc.
Compositor: Maryland Composition Company
Printer/Binder: Courier Book Company/Westford
Cover Designer: Robert Freese Design



**Library of Congress Cataloging-in-Publication Data**

Invasive outpatient procedures in reproductive medicine / [edited by]
Mark I. Evans, Mark P. Johnson, Kamran S. Moghissi ; with 28
additional contributors ; illustrations by Harry Oliver Burdett.
p. cm.
Includes bibliographical references and index.
ISBN 0-7817-0283-6
1. Generative organs, Female—Endoscopic surgery. 2. Ambulatory
surgery. 3. Generative organs, Female—Surgery. I. Evans, Mark
I. II. Johnson, Mark P. III. Moghissi, Kamran S., 1925– .
[DNLM: 1. Surgery, Minimally Invasive. 2. Reproductive Medicine.
3. Ambulatory Surgery. WQ 400 I62 1997]
RG104.7.I56 1997
618—dc20
DNLM/DLC
for Library of Congress 96-34375
CIP



9 8 7 6 5 4 3 2 1

To our wives and children: Wendy, Shara, Kiera, Harry, Rufus
Christine, Jennifer, Eric, Rolf
Edie, Diana, Soraya

# Contributors

**David F. Archer, MD**
Professor of Obstetrics and Gynecology
Department of Obstetrics and Gynecology
Eastern Virginia Medical School
601 Colley Avenue
Norfolk, Virginia 23507

**Stanley M. Berry, MD**
Assistant Professor of Obstetrics and Gynecology
Wayne State University
Hutzel Hospital
4707 St. Antoine Boulevard
Detroit, Michigan 48201

**Charla M. Blacker, MD**
Assistant Professor of Obstetrics and Gynecology
Wayne State University
Hutzel Hospital
4707 St. Antoine Boulevard
Detroit, Michigan 48201

**Elizabeth B. Connell, MD**
Professor Emeritus of Obstetrics and Gynecology
Emory University School of Medicine
1440 Clifton Road NE
Atlanta, Georgia 30322

**Marc Dommergues, MD**
Associate Professor of Obstetrics and Gynecology
Groupe Hospitalier Cochin
Clinique Universitaire Port-Royal
123 Boulevard Port-Royal
Paris 75014
France

**Arie Drugan, MD**
Vice Chairman
Department of Obstetrics and Gynecology
Rambam Medical Center
P.O. Box 9602
Haifa 31096, Israel

**Bruce H. Drukker, MD**
Professor and Chair
Department of Obstetrics, Gynecology, and Reproductive Biology
Michigan State University
College of Human Medicine
B316 Clinical Center
East Lansing, Michigan 48824

**Yves Dumez, MD**
Professor of Obstetrics and Gynecology
Groupe Hospitalier Cochin
Clinique Universitaire Port-Royal
123 Boulevard Port-Royal
Paris 75014
France

**Mark I. Evans, MD**
Professor, Vice Chairman, and Vice Chief of Obstetrics and Gynecology
Professor of Molecular Medicine and Genetics
Professor of Pathology
Director, Division of Reproductive Genetics
Director, Center for Fetal Diagnosis and Therapy
Wayne State University
Hutzel Hospital
4707 St. Antoine Boulevard
Detroit, Michigan 48201

**Alan Flake, MD**
Associate Professor of Pediatric Surgery, and Obstetrics and Gynecology
Wayne State University
Children's Hospital of Michigan
3901 Beaubien
Detroit, Michigan 48201

**Kenneth Ginsburg, MD**
Associate Professor of Obstetrics and Gynecology
Wayne State University
Hutzel Hospital
4707 St. Antoine Boulevard
Detroit, Michigan 48201

**Jeanne Grager, RDMS**
Department of Obstetrics and Gynecology
Division of Diagnostic Ultrasound
Wayne State University
Hutzel Hospital
4707 St. Antoine Boulevard
Detroit, Michigan 48201

**Roderick F. Hume, Jr., MD, FACOG, LTC, MC, USA**
Chief, Obstetrics Service
Director, Maternal Fetal Medicine Program
Madigan Army Medical Center
MCHJ-OG (ADC)
Tacoma, Washington 98431

**Nelson B. Isada, MD**
Department of Reproductive Genetics of Alaska
3340 Providence Drive, Suite 366
Anchorage, Alaska 99508

**Mark P. Johnson, MD**
Associate Director, Division of Reproductive Genetics
Associate Director, Center for Fetal Diagnosis and Therapy
Associate Professor, Departments of Obstetrics and Gynecology; Molecular Medicine and Genetics; and Pathology
Wayne State University
Hutzel Hospital
4707 St. Antoine Boulevard
Detroit, Michigan 48201

**Raymond H. Kaufman, MD**
Professor and Emeritus Chairman
Department of Obstetrics and Gynecology
Professor of Pathology
Baylor College of Medicine
One Baylor Plaza
Houston, Texas 77030

**Richard E. Leach, MD**
Assistant Professor
Department of Obstetrics and Gynecology
Wayne State University
Hutzel Hospital
4707 St. Antoine Boulevard
Detroit, Michigan 48201

**Laura Blessed, RDMS**
Department of Obstetrics and Gynecology
Division of Diagnostic Ultrasound
Wayne State University
Hutzel Hospital
4707 St. Antoine Boulevard
Detroit, Michigan 48201

**Linda Littmann, RDMS**
Department of Obstetrics and Gynecology
Division of Diagnostic Ultrasound
Wayne State University
Hutzel Hospital
4707 St. Antoine Boulevard
Detroit, Michigan 48201

**John M. Malone, Jr., MD**
Associate Professor
Department of Obstetrics and Gynecology
Wayne State University
Hutzel Hospital
4707 St. Antoine Boulevard
Detroit, Michigan 48201

**Kamran S. Moghissi, MD**
Professor, Obstetrics and Gynecology
Division of Reproductive Endocrinology and Infertility
Wayne State University
Hutzel Hospital
4707 St. Antoine Boulevard
Detroit, Michigan 48201

**Jean-Francois Oury, MD**
Professor
Department of Obstetrics and Gynecology
Robert Debré Hospital
48 Boulevard Servrier
Paris, 75019
France

**Ruben A. Quintero, MD**
Assistant Professor
Department of Obstetrics and Gynecology
Wayne State University
Hutzel Hospital
4707 St. Antoine Boulevard
Detroit, Michigan 48201

**Nilsa C. Ramirez, MD**
Assistant Professor
Department of Pathology
Wayne State University
Hutzel Hospital
4707 St. Antoine Boulevard
Detroit, Michigan 48201

**Avihai Reichler, MD**
Assistant Professor of Obstetrics and Gynecology
Department of Obstetrics and Gynecology
Albert Einstein College of Medicine
Weiler Hospital
1825 Eastchester Road
Bronx, New York 10461

**Ralph Richert, MD**
Professor of Pathology
Director, Division of Ob/Gyn Pathology
Memorial Sloan Kettering Medical Center
1275 York Avenue
New York, New York 10021

**Alvin M. Siegler, MD**
Professor of Obstetrics and Gynecology
State University of New York
Health Science Center at Brooklyn College of Medicine
450 Clarkson Avenue, Box 97
Brooklyn, New York 11203

**Lori St. Louis, RDMS**
Department of Obstetrics and Gynecology
Wayne State University
Hutzel Hospital
4707 St. Antoine Boulevard
Detroit, Michigan 48201

**Howard J. Tatum, MD**
Professor Emeritus
Emory University School of Medicine
1440 Clifton Road NE
Atlanta, Georgia 30322

**Thomas C. Wright, Jr., MD**
Assistant Professor of Pathology
Columbia University College of Physicians and Surgeons
The Sloane Hospital for Women
630 West 168th Street
New York, New York 10032

**Ivan Zador, PhD**
Director, Computer Support
Department of Obstetrics and Gynecology
Wayne State University
Hutzel Hospital
4707 St. Antoine Boulevard
Detroit, Michigan 48201

# Preface

The rapid pace of change in the practice of medicine mostly necessitated by economic and political agendas has profoundly altered the way in which physicians treat patients. Many procedures that previously were considered as exclusively inpatient are now routinely done on an outpatient basis. With the change to managed care, and the disincentives to refer patients to tertiary subspecialists, many physicians are now performing new procedures in their own office that they would not have done previously.

The introduction of medical technology and procedures into common practice follows two phases: (1) a phase of development, and (2) a phase of diffusion. In the former, a few highly specialized and skilled physicians develop a new technology, work it out under research protocol, try to get the kinks out of the system, and eventually publish their results for presentation to the scientific and medical community. However, such a small cadre of physicians cannot handle the patient demand for these new services once the technology has become established. Therefore the technology enters a phase of ''diffusion'' in which more and more physicians learn how to apply the newer techniques. When such developments occur, residents certainly can be taught the new technologies within the confines of their training program; older, established physicians often find it more difficult to find appropriate ways to learn new procedures. The purpose of this book is to present, in a very detailed fashion, the techniques for a number of increasingly common procedures that are being performed on an outpatient basis. Some of these procedures will be done by virtually all health care providers for women, and others will remain relatively more specialized. The determination of those that are done routinely and those that will still be specialized will be dictated by practice location. Certainly no single physician would be expected to be expert at all of these procedures. We hope this book will be a teaching guide for those people specifically learning how to do some of these procedures, and a more general reference guide for all physicans who need to know how they are done.

Mark I. Evans, MD
Mark P. Johnson, MD
Kamran S. Moghissi, MD

# Acknowledgments

The editors wish to express their sincere appreciation to Craig Percy of Lippincott–Raven Publishers for his help throughout the development of this text, and to Monica Hoopingarner, for her help in coordinating the manuscripts.

# Contents

# I OBSTETRIC PROCEDURES

*Invasive Outpatient Procedures in Reproductive Medicine,* edited by Mark I. Evans, et al. Lippincott–Raven Publishers, Philadelphia © 1997.

# 1 Amniocentesis

Arie Drugan, Mark P. Johnson, Roderick F. Hume Jr, Mark I. Evans

Analysis of amniotic fluid for the diagnosis of genetic disorders was first introduced in the early 1960s. The first diagnoses of fetal chromosomal anomalies made on amniotic fluid specimens[1,2] were shortly followed by enzymatic assays performed on amniocytes for prenatal diagnosis of metabolic disorders.[3] The diagnostic accuracy and the relatively low risk of amniocentesis established it as the basic procedure in modern prenatal diagnosis.[4,5] Amniocentesis is generally considered the "gold standard" to which other methods for prenatal diagnosis are compared.

## INDICATIONS

The most common indication for amniocentesis is advanced maternal age. The association of advanced maternal age with an increased risk of chromosomally abnormal conceptions has been well documented.[6,7] To offer prenatal diagnosis to women aged 35 years or more at delivery is, and has been for many years, the accepted standard of care.[7] Almost all chromosomal abnormalities increase in incidence with advanced maternal age, but the most common in liveborns is trisomy 21, which represents approximately 50% of all chromosomal anomalies.

Other indications for genetic amniocentesis are summarized in Table 1–1. A previous aneuploid offspring born to a woman younger than 30 years confers a 1% risk of recurrence in future pregnancies.[8] A balanced structural rearrangement of parental chromosomes, as encountered in 2–4% of couples investigated for repeated spontaneous abortions, is associated with an increased risk of unbalanced offspring, which may be as high as 2–15%.[9] Recurrent pregnancy loss in itself may be associated with an increased risk of chromosomally abnormal conceptions, even if the parents have normal karyotypes[10,11] and, in our opinion, prenatal diagnosis should be considered in these cases.

Chromosomal anomalies are detected in 30–35% of amniocenteses performed for ultrasound diagnosis of major fetal malformations.[12,13] Even minor ultrasound findings (e.g., fetal choroid plexus cysts, nonseptated cervical cystic hygromas or pyelectasis) may confer a risk of aneuploidy between 1–3%.[14,15]

Abnormally low levels of alpha fetoprotein (AFP), high levels of human chorionic gonadotrophin (HCG), and arguably low levels of unconjugated estriol (uE3) in maternal serum are also associated with increased risk of a chromosomally abnormal pregnancy. Genetic counseling and amniocentesis should be offered when the combined risk of serum biochemical markers and maternal age equals or is higher than the risk of aneuploidy in the gestation of a 35-year-old. The prevalence of chromosomal anomalies diagnosed by amniocentesis performed according to these criteria is 1.1% by AFP alone, and about 2% with HCG; *only half of the anomalies diagnosed are trisomy 21.* Other chromosomal anomalies diagnosed include triploidy, trisomies 13 and 18, unbalanced translocations, and sex chromosome anomalies.[16] In amniocenteses performed for "maternal anxiety" in women without serum screening, the risk

**TABLE 1–1. INDICATIONS FOR AMNIOCENTESIS AND RISK OF GENETIC DISORDERS**

| Indications | Risk of Anomaly |
|---|---|
| A. Increased risk for chromosomal anomalies | |
| 1. Advanced maternal age | >0.5% |
| 2. Previous aneuploid offspring | 1% |
| 3. Parental balanced structural rearrangement | |
| a: Reciprocal translocations | 12–15% |
| b: Robertsonian translocations | 1–3% |
| c: Inversions | 6% |
| 4. Maternal abnormal serum screening | 1% |
| 5. Ultrasound diagnosis of anomalies | |
| a: Major malformations* | 25–30% |
| b: Minor anomalies** | 1–3% |
| B. Previous offspring with neural tube defect (NTD) | 3% |
| C. Parents carriers of Mendelian traits | 25–50% |

* omphalocele, duodenal atresia, atrio-ventricular septal defects, horseshoe kidneys, septated cystic hygroma.

** fetal pyelectasis, increased nuchal thickness, choroid plexus cyst, non-septated cystic hygroma.

of chromosomal anomalies is apparently similar to that observed when the procedure was indicated for low alpha fetoprotein in maternal serum.[17]

Maternal serum AFP levels higher than 2.5 MOM are observed in approximately 3% of screened pregnancies; after excluding wrong dates or multiple gestation, half of these cases will remain without a benign explanation for the abnormal results. In the latter, the risk for fetal anomalies is 5–10% and amniocentesis for AFP, acetylcholinesterase (AChE) and karyotype as well as detailed level III ultrasonography are recommended.[18] Neural tube defects (NTD), abdominal wall defects (i.e., omphalocele or gastroschisis), sacrococcygeal teratomas, Meckel Syndrome, congenital skin defects, esophageal atresia, and fetal demise have all been reported in association with elevated AFP in amniotic fluid.[18] The combination of elevated AFP and positive AChE in amniotic fluid is by far more accurate than AFP alone in prenatal detection of NTD, and the false–positive rate is only 1:300 or less.[19,20]

Prenatal diagnosis of inborn errors of metabolism can be made by analysis of precursor levels in cell-free amniotic fluid[21] or, more commonly, by enzymatic assays of cultured amniocytes.[22] However, the diagnosis of these disorders is expensive and laborious and should be offered only when couples are at a substantial risk (25–50%) for an affected child. Hormonal changes in pregnancy may modify the expression of specific enzymes in amniotic fluid or amniocytes, causing an increase in the rate of false–negative or negative results.[23,24] Increasing use of molecular diagnoses for single-gene disorders through the use of restriction fragment length polymorphisms, gene probes, and fluorescent in situ hybridization (FISH) should reduce to a minimum the rate of false results.[25,26]

## TECHNIQUE

Amniocentesis should be preceded by genetic counseling, during which the family pedigree and genetic risk are evaluated and the advantages and risks of the procedure are explained. A detailed ultrasound examination should assess gestational age, amniotic fluid volume, fetal and placental location, and should exclude gross fetal malformations. The patient's blood type and antibody status should be known prior to amniocentesis; Rh-negative women with negative antibody screening should receive Rh immunoprophylaxis after the procedure. In Rh-negative women, the risk of Rh isosensitization is probably slightly increased by transplacental passage of the needle.[27,28]

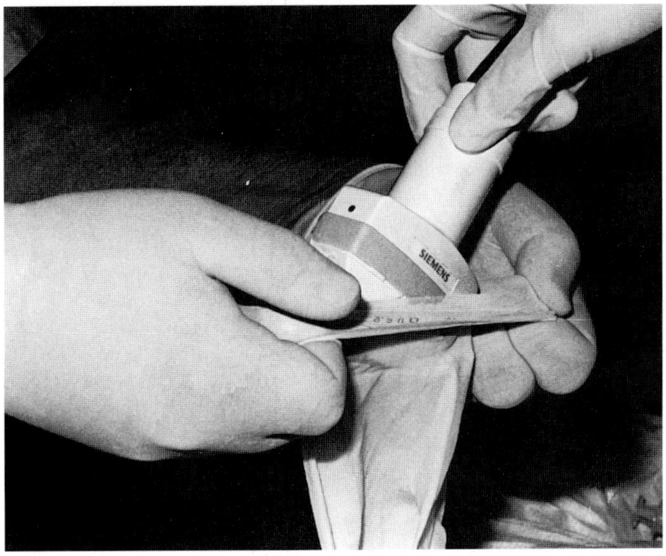

**FIG. 1–1.** Ultrasound transducer inserted into sterile glove. Gel is put into glove first to maintain solid interface between skin, glove, and transducer.

After sterile preparation of the skin, the ultrasound transducer is inserted into a sterile glove (Figs. 1–1), the physician should pick a ''spot'' on the mother's skin either by placing a finger below a linear transducer in both longitudinal and transverse planes or at least by making a mental image of the path of the ultrasound transmissions (Figs. 1–2A,B,C). The needle should not touch the skin until the insertion is begun: it hurts the patient, causing her to become tense.

The needle should be held with the index finger on top (Fig. 1–3) so that there is a direct ''feel'' of the tip of the needle and resistance can be gauged. The abdominal layers are penetrated to the amniotic cavity generally with a 20- or 22-gauge, 3.5-inch spinal needle. The experienced operator should be able to feel the needle entering the amniotic cavity by a sudden change in tissue resistance. Real-time ultrasonographic guidance during amniocentesis is, however, strongly advocated; it may reduce the frequency of multiple needle insertions, bloody taps, and failure to obtain amniotic fluid[29–32] (Fig. 1–3). The incidence of fetal trauma and fetal loss from amniocentesis[33] are apparently lowered by continuous ultrasonic visualization of the needle tip, which may also help to identify technical difficulties such as membrane tenting during the procedure.[34] In the latter situation, rotating the needle while inserting it may help.

When the needle tip, seen on ultrasound as a bright spot (Fig. 1–4), is placed satisfactorily into a pocket of amniotic fluid, the stylet is removed and a 5-mL syringe is attached. The first 2–5 mL of fluid are aspirated and discarded in order to minimize the risk of contamination from maternal cells drawn by the needle in its pathway. Twenty to 30 mL of amniotic fluid (Figs. 1–5A,B) are then gently aspirated into syringes, transferred to sterile tubes, and transported at room temperature to the laboratory for processing.

Patients are released after a brief period of observation and ultrasound documentation of fetal viability. Following amniocentesis, we recommend postponing sexual activity and strenuous exercise for 2–3 days. Patients are also instructed to report immediately signs of infection, vaginal bleeding, leakage of amniotic fluid, and regular uterine contractions.

Twinning occurs once in every 87 pregnancies of white, north-American women, and its frequency may increase with advancing parity and maternal age.[35] About 1.2–1.4% of patients presenting for prenatal diagnosis carry multiple fetuses. Separate sampling of amniotic fluid from both sacs is necessary to correctly assess the karyotype of each fetus. In general, the chance that at least one twin has an abnormal karyotype should be quoted as almost twice the age-related risk, and the danger of pregnancy loss related to amniocentesis should probably be increased accordingly.

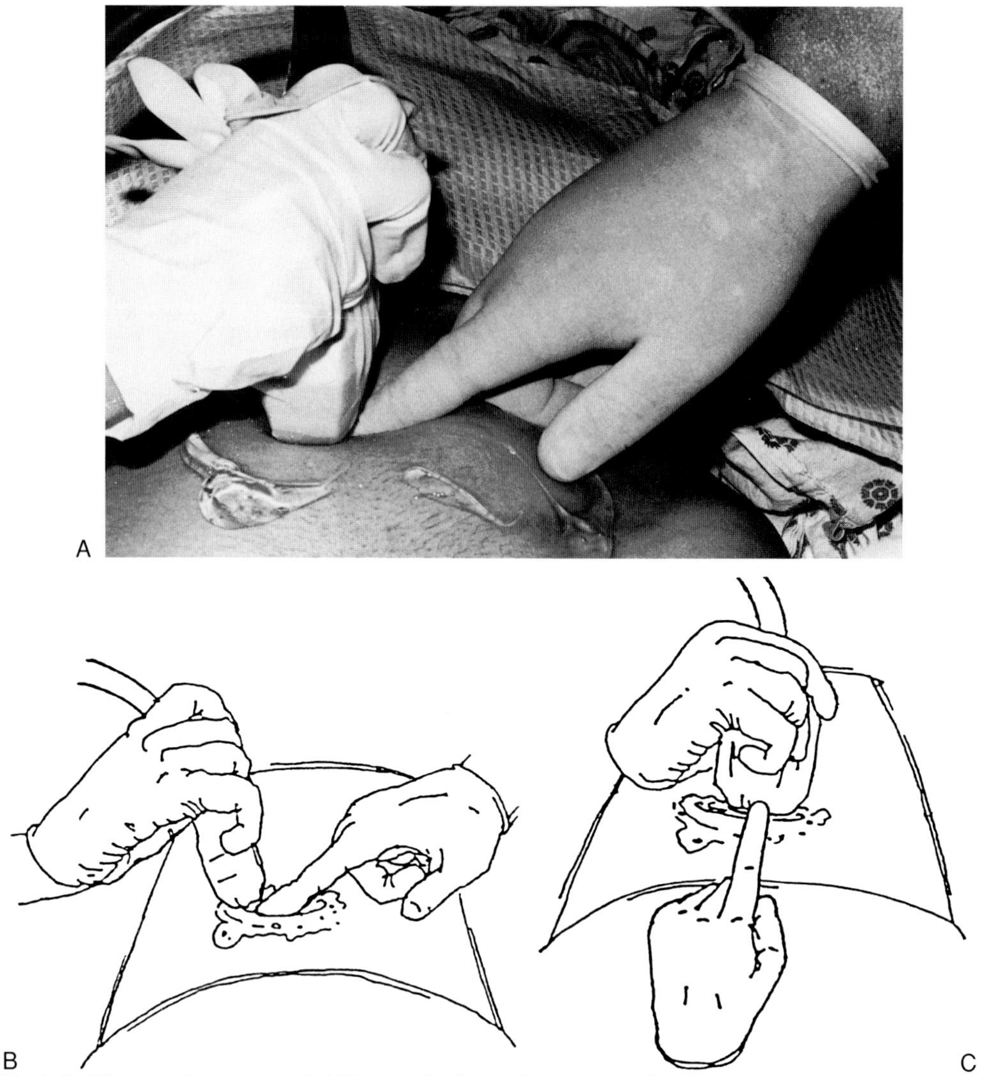

**FIG. 1–2.** Ultrasound transducer held longitudinally on abdomen (A, B) with operator's finger below linear array to see spot and path that a vertical needle would take. Transducer should then be turned 90° to make sure of accuracy of placement (C).

With continuous ultrasound guidance, it is generally easy to sample separately both sacs when the anatomic relationship of the chorioamnionic membrane between the sacs is clearly discernible (Fig. 1–6). Using a curve linear or linear array ultrasound transducer, the first needle can be left in situ while introducing another amniocentesis needle into the second sac, so that both needles are observed on ultrasound in the same plane simultaneously, with the chorioamnionic membrane between them.[36] When the relationship between the sacs is not evident, injection of dye, such as indigo carmine or Congo red, into the first sac after aspiration of amniotic fluid may be a helpful marker. After injection of dye into the first amniotic cavity, aspiration of clear fluid proves that the sample is from the second sac.[37] The use of dye in these situations should be approached cautiously, however. The use of a membrane-free maternal hemoglobin hemolysate appears to be a useful inert and safe biologic dye for this purpose.[38] In contrast, the use of methylene blue as a dye marker for genetic amniocentesis in twins has been associated with jejunal atresia in 17 of 89 twin pairs exposed.[39] Alternatively, fluid can be aspirated into the syringe and then re-expelled, thus stirring up particles and making one cavity cloudy and the other clear.

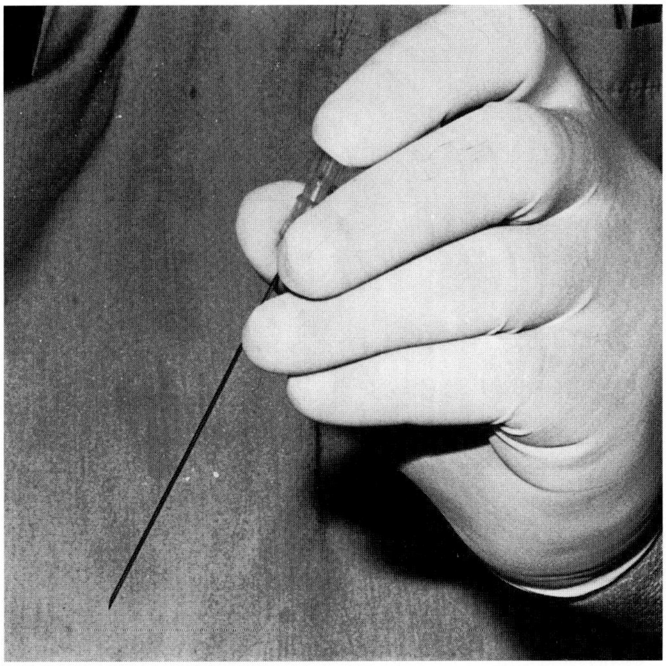

**FIG. 1–3.** Needle held such that index finger is on top of needle so that felt resistance is transmitted and accurately appreciated.

Improved ultrasound technology, increasing experience with ultrasound guided needle manipulation, and patient preference for more private earlier genetic diagnosis have motivated a shift from second trimester amniocentesis toward earlier procedures, such as chorionic villus sampling (CVS) and ''early''amniocentesis.[40] Early amniocentesis refers to procedures performed before 14 weeks gestation (most commonly at 12 or 13 weeks), with ultrasound guidance and a 22-gauge needle. We aspirate about 1 mL of amniotic fluid per every week of gestation. Increasing experience with this procedure shows it to be comparable to midtrimester amniocentesis in terms of sampling success or accurate cytogenetic diagnosis, but it can provide earlier counseling, testing, and availability of results.[41–44] Risk rates are mostly related to gestational age, not to the method of diagnosis. Our experience with over 500 such procedures also suggests that ''early'' amniocentesis is safe and reliable, with amniotic fluid samples

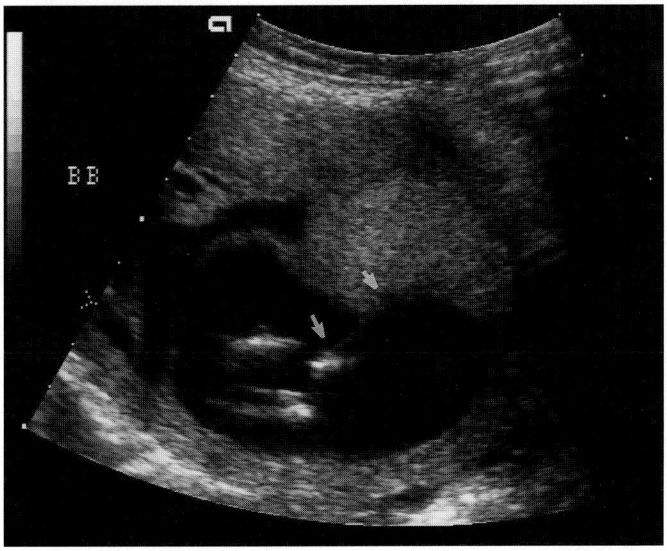


**FIG. 1–4.** Ultrasound showing tip of needle in pocket of amniotic fluid (lower arrow) and shaft of needle coursing through uterine wall and placenta (upper arrow).

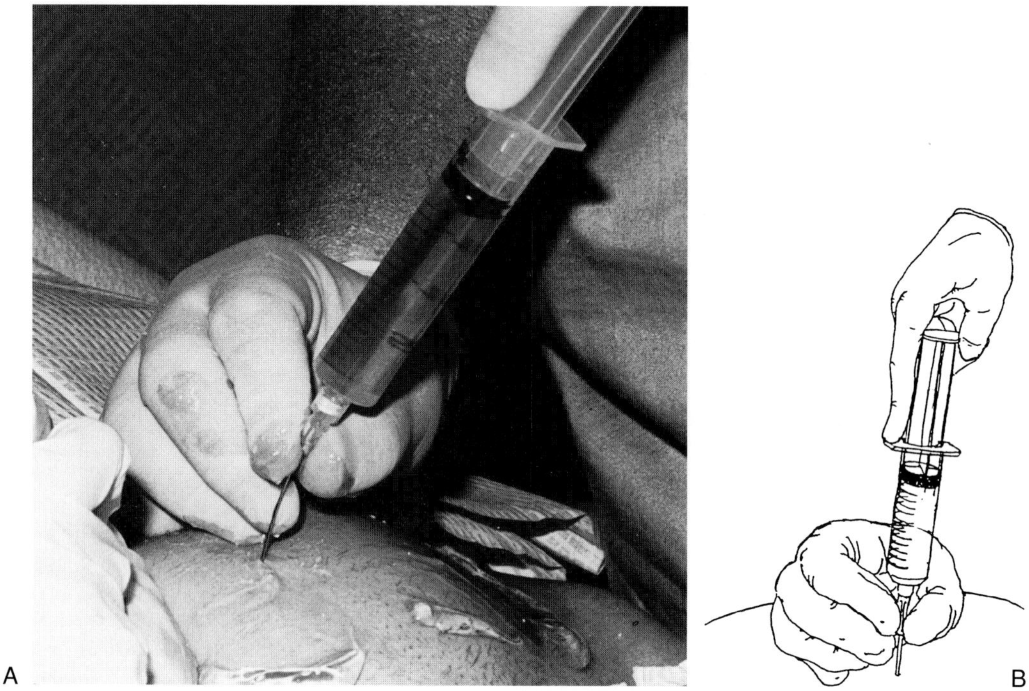


**FIG. 1–5.** 20-cc syringe attached to 20-gauge needle with aspiration of amniotic fluid (A). Using index finger abutted to syringe allows for steady withdrawal of fluid (B).

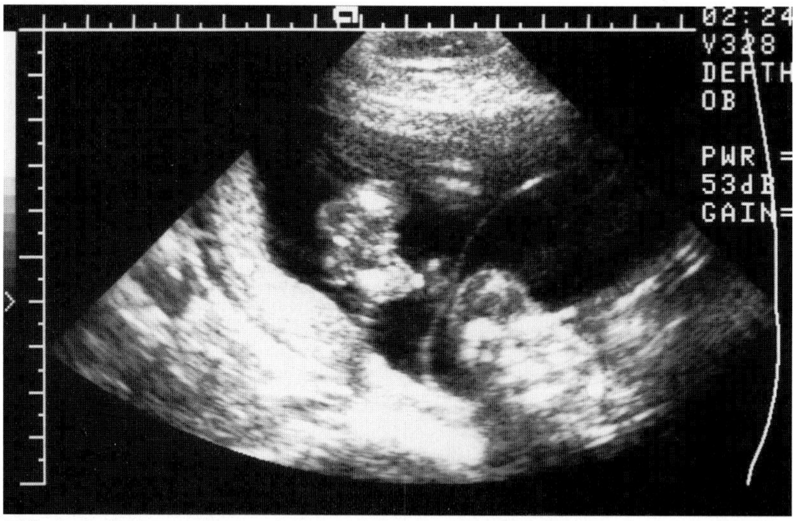


**FIG. 1–6.** Twin pregnancy ultrasound showing membrane clearly separating twins.

obtained in cases. However, because of slower growth in culture of cells obtained from early amniotic fluid, results are available 3–4 weeks after the procedure, about 1 week longer than results from midtrimester amniocentesis.[40]

## INTERPRETATION OF RESULTS

The alpha-fetoprotein (AFP) concentration and fetal karyotype are routinely evaluated on amniotic fluid specimens but the clinical interpretation of these results may not always be conclusive. The karyotype obtained in amniocytes accurately reflects fetal status in over 99% of cases.[45] One or more hypermodal cells are, however, observed in 2–3% of karyotypes analyzed.[46] Most of these cases are caused by extraembryonic nondisjunction (pseudo mosaicism) and are associated with a normal phenotype.[47] True fetal mosaicism is considered when hypermodal cells are identified in at least two colonies in the same culture flask (as encountered in 0.7% of amniotic cells cultured) or in multiple flasks (observed in 0.2% of cultures).[47,48] Even in these cases, however, mosaicism in cultured amniocytes will not always represent true fetal mosaicism. Fetal blood karyotypes evaluated after the diagnosis of chromosomal mosaicism in amniotic cell cultures were normal in 15 of 16 mosaic autosomal trisomy cases and in all 8 cases of mosaic sex chromosome trisomy diagnosed by amniocentesis.[49] Mosaicism for chromosome structural rearrangements was confirmed in fetal blood from 5 of 11 cases with mosaic translocation or inversion and in 4 of 6 cases of de novo supernumerary marker chromosome mosaicism. Although a normal blood karyotype may not exclude cases of true fetal mosaicism confined to specific fetal tissues,[47] follow-up of mosaicism in cultured amniocytes with fetal blood sampling should help to avoid termination of pregnancy of some normal fetuses.

When balanced translocations (Fig. 1–7) or inversions are diagnosed at amniocentesis, comparison with parental karyotypes is frequently needed. If the balanced structural rearrange-

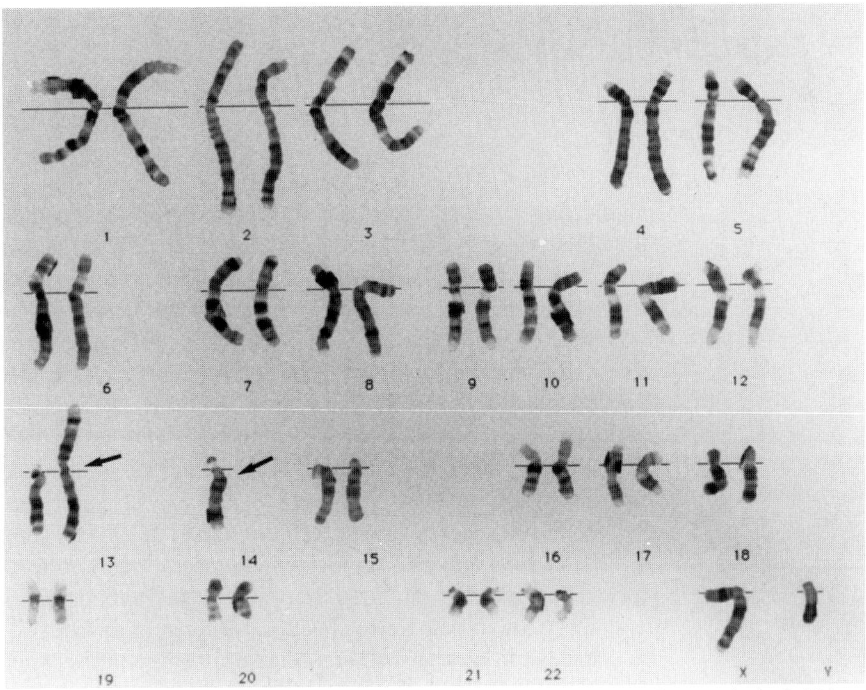


**FIG. 1–7.** Balanced translocation karyotype 45,XY(t13;14). Arrows show "missing" #14 attached to 13–14 translocation. Karyotype is from father; same finding was seen in fetus of an amniocentesis specimen.

ment is inherited from one of the parents, they may be reassured that the phenotype of the offspring will also be normal. If, however, the abnormality occurred de novo in that specific conception, the risk of major malformations and mental retardation for the fetus is probably around 8–10%.[50]

In singleton pregnancies, abnormally elevated amniotic fluid AFP indicates the need to test for AChE in amniotic fluid. An abnormally elevated amniotic fluid AFP and a positive AChE are associated in essentially all cases with fetal malformations or with fetal death. In twin pregnancies, clinical interpretation of amniotic fluid AFP and AChE results may be confused by transfer of these materials across the membranes. Discordant amniotic fluid AFP results are more common in dizygotic twins, perhaps due to the bichorionic biamniotic membrane between the sacs. AChE diffuses readily across the membranes and cannot be used to determine which twin is abnormal.[51]

An advantage of early amniocentesis is the ability to measure AFP and AChE in amniotic fluid. AFP peaks in amniotic fluid at 12–13 weeks gestation and then gradually declines, following the trend of AFP in fetal blood.[52,53] In amniotic fluid samples obtained between 10–15 weeks gestation, high amniotic fluid AFP levels have been found in association with fetal structural anomalies and low AFP values accompanied some of the pregnancies that were aneuploid, as observed in samples from pregnancies of later gestational age.[52] A faint "inconclusive" AChE band has been frequently observed on gel electrophoresis of "early" amniocentesis. This seems, however, to be less commonly associated with fetal anomalies than when this finding appears in amniotic fluid samples obtained later on in gestation.[54] Thus, until larger data bases are accumulated, results of AFP and AChE in "early" amniocentesis specimens should be interpreted with extreme caution.

Brown or green tinged amniotic fluid, aspirated in 1–6% of midtrimester amniocenteses,[5] may be associated with increased perinatal mortality and pregnancy loss (5–9%).[55,56] Analysis of discolored fluid samples indicates that in most cases the discoloring pigment is hemoglobin. Vaginal bleeding prior to amniocentesis seems to predispose for presence of discolored amniotic fluid.[57]

## SAFETY AND COMPLICATIONS

Amniocentesis is a relatively safe procedure with almost nonexistent severe sequelae. The frequency of severe chorioamnionitis following amniocentesis is about 0.1%.[5] Leakage of amniotic fluid is a relatively frequent complication, experienced by 1–2% of patients after amniocentesis, but is of minor clinical significance and usually resolves within 48–72 hours.[58] Although rare, persistent and significant amniotic fluid leakage may lead to oligohydramnios, may result in fetal pressure deformities and pulmonary hypoplasia.[59] In experienced hands, the overall procedure related pregnancy loss is 0.2–0.5% above the spontaneous pregnancy loss rate at 16 weeks gestation, the latter being estimated at 3%.[45,60] Pregnancy loss rates seem to be associated with number of failed attempts (needle insertions) at the same session and with vaginal bleeding following amniocentesis, but not with gestational age at the time of amniocentesis, the volume of fluid removed, or whether the procedure is repeated following a failed attempt at a previous date.[61] Pregnancy loss related to early amniocentesis is somewhat higher than at midtrimester, about 0.7–0.8%.[40–44] The rate of complications associated with amniocentesis is directly related to the experience of the operator.[62]

Fetal injury by the amniocentesis needle should be very rare with ultrasound-guided procedures. Traumatization of the fetus by the amniocentesis needle has, however, been reported.[63,64] Another rare complication believed to be associated with amniocentesis, the amniotic band syndrome, has been reported only a few times,[65] and other causes are suggested now as its etiology.[66]

It has been suggested that removal of amniotic fluid at amniocentesis, especially when performed early in gestation, may affect fetal lung development. Lung function tests performed after birth to babies subjected to amniocentesis apparently demonstrated lower dynamic compliance and higher resistance compared to controls.[67] Other studies could not document an effect on neonatal lung function tests, but noted a significantly higher incidence of respiratory distress and admissions to special care units for neonates subjected to chorionic villus sampling in the first trimester.[68]

## CONCLUSIONS

In summary, amniocentesis is a relatively safe, well-established, and widely utilized procedure for prenatal diagnosis, and most practicing obstetricians are familiar with it. However, failure to recognize a couple's increased genetic risk and offer prenatal diagnosis and complications arising during procedures in which a physician is not adept are areas of potential liability that bring us to question whether amniocentesis should be a routine office procedure. Thus, although amniocentesis has been labeled by Council on Research and Education in Obstetrics and Gynecology (CREOG) as a procedure that should be learned by residents, in many large cities most private practitioners do not perform it, but refer their patients to genetic centers with vast experience where many of these procedures are performed daily. Nevertheless, a practicing obstetrician who is well-experienced with amniocentesis and who has the back-up of a genetic center for counseling would certainly not be considered below the standard of care when performing amniocentesis for prenatal diagnosis.

## REFERENCES

1. Jacobson CB, Barter RH. Intrauterine diagnosis and management of genetic defects. Am J Obstet Gynecol 1967;99:795.
2. Valenti C, Schutta EJ, Kehaty T. Prenatal diagnosis of Down syndrome. Lancet 1968;2:220.
3. Nadler HL. Antenatal detection of hereditary disorders. Pediatrics 1968;42:912.
4. Nadler HL, Gerbie AB. Role of amniocentesis in the intrauterine detection of genetic disorders. N Engl J Med 1970;282:596.
5. Elias S, Simpson JL. Amniocentesis. In: Milunski A (ed). Genetic disorders and the fetus (2nd ed). New York, Plenum Press, 1986;31–52.
6. Hook EB, Cross PK, Schreimachers DM. Chromosomal abnormality rates at amniocentesis and in liveborn infants. JAMA 1983;248:2034–2038.
7. American College of Obstetrics and Gynecology Technical Bulletin. Antenatal diagnosis of genetic disorders. No. 108, September, 1987.
8. Stene J, Stene K, Mikkelsen M. Risk for chromosome abnormality at amniocentesis following a child with a noninherited chromosome aberration. Prenat Diagn (special issue) 1984;4:81.
9. Boue A, Gallano P. A collaborative study of the segregation of inherited chromosome structural rearrangements in 1356 prenatal diagnoses. Prenat Diagn (special issue) 1984;4:45.
10. Lippman A, Ayme S. Fetal death rates in mothers of children with trisomy 21. Ann Hum Genet 1984;48:303.
11. Drugan A, Koppitch FC, Williams JC, Evans MI. Prenatal diagnosis following recurrent early pregnancy loss. Obstet Gynecol 1990;75:381–384.
12. Platt LD, DeVore GP, Lopez E, Herbert W, Falk R, Alf O. Role of amniocentesis in ultrasound detected fetal malformations. Obstet Gynecol 1986;68:153.
13. Williamson RA, Weiner CP, Patil S, Benda J, Varner MW, Abu YM. Abnormal pregnancy sonogram: selective indication for fetal karyotype. Obstet Gynecol 1987;69:15.
14. Bar Hava I, Bronshtein M, Drugan A. Changing dysmorphology of trisomy 18 during midtrimester. Fetal Diagn Ther (in press).
15. Corteville JE, Dicke JM, Crane JP. Fetal pyelectasis and Down syndrome: is genetic amniocentesis warranted? Obstet Gynecol 1992;79:770–772.

16. Drugan A, O'Brien JE, Gambino RB, Evans MI. Prenatal biochemical screening. In: Evans MI, Johnson MP (eds). Prenatal diagnosis in the 90s. J Reprod Med Symp, 1992;37.
17. Kaffe S, Hsu LY. Maternal serum alpha-fetoprotein screening and fetal chromosome anomalies: is lowering maternal age for amniocentesis preferable? Am J Med Genet 1992;42: 801–806.
18. Evans MI, O'Brien JE, Dvorin E, Johnson MP. Biochemical screening, 1994. Current opinion in obstetrics and gynecology 1994;6(5):453–458.
19. Wald JN, Cuckle HS. Amniotic fluid acetylcholinesterase electrophoresis as a secondary test in the diagnosis of anencephaly and spina bifida in early pregnancy: report of the collaborative acetylcholinesterase study. Lancet 1981;2:321–324.
20. Crandall BF, Matsumoto M. Routine amniotic fluid alpha-fetoprotein assay: experience with 40,000 pregnancies. Am J Med Genet 1986;24:143.
21. Warsof SL, Larsen JW, Kent SG, et al. Prenatal diagnosis of congenital adrenal hyperplasia. Obstet Gynecol 1980;55:751.
22. Arnon J, Ornoi A, Bach G. Cultured amniotic fluid cells for prenatal diagnosis of lysosomal storage disease: a methodological study. Prenat Diagn 1986;6:351–361.
23. Wiederschain GYA, Rosenfeld EL, Brusilowski AI, et al. Alpha L fucosidase and other glycosidases in human placenta, fetus, liver and amniotic fluid at various stages of gestation. Clin Chim Acta 1971;35:99–107.
24. Hultberg B, Sjoblad S, Gustavii B. Acid hydrolases in amniotic fluid and chorionic villi at various stages of pregnancy. Clin Chim Acta 1974;53:221–227.
25. Weatherall DJ, Old JM, Their SL, Wainscoat JS, Clegg JB. Prenatal diagnosis of the common hemoglobin disorders. J Med Genet 1985;22:422–430.
26. Butler WJ, McDonough PG. The new genetics—molecular technology and reproductive biology. Fertil Steril 1989;51:375–386.
27. Golbus MS, Stephens JD, Cann HM, et al. Rh isoimmunization following genetic amniocentesis. Prenat Diagn 1982;2:149–152.
28. Murray JC, Karp LE, Williamson RA, et al. Rh isoimmunization as related to amniocentesis. Am J Hum Genet 1983;16:527.
29. Jeanty P, Rodesch F, Romero R, et al. How to improve your amniocentesis technique. Am J Obstet Gynecol 1983;146:593.
30. Benaceraff BR, Frigoletto FD. Amniocentesis under continuous ultrasound guidance: a series of 232 cases. Obstet Gynecol 1983;62:760.
31. McDicken WN, Anderson T, MacKenzie WE, et al. Ultrasonic identification of needle tips at amniocentesis. Lancet 1984;2:198.
32. Romero R, Jeanty P, Reece EA, et al. Sonographically monitored amniocentesis to decrease intraoperative complications. Obstet Gynecol 1985;64:426.
33. Williamson RA, Varner MW, Grant SS. Reduction in amniocentesis risks using real time needle guide puncture. Obstet Gynecol 1985;65:751.
34. Platt LD, DeVore GR, Gimovsky ML. Failed amniocentesis: the role of membrane tenting. Am J Obstet Gynecol 1982;144:479–480.
35. Thompson JS, Thompson MW (eds). Genetics in medicine (4th ed). Philadelphia: WB Saunders, 1986;273:281.
36. Bahado-Singh R, Schmitt R, Hobbins JC. New technique for genetic amniocentesis in twins. Obstet Gynecol 1992;79:304–307.
37. Elias S, Gerbie AB, Simpson JL. Genetic amniocentesis in twin gestations. Am J Obstet Gynecol 1980;138:169.
38. Beekhuis JR, de Bruijn HW, Van Lith JM, Mantigh A. Second trimester amniocentesis in twin pregnancies: maternal hemoglobin as a dye marker to differentiate diamniotic twins. Brit J Obstet Gynecol 1992;99:126–127.
39. Van der Pol JS, Wolf H, Boer K, et al. Jejunal atresia related to the use of methylene blue in genetic amniocentesis in twins. Brit J Obstet Gynecol 1992;99:141–143.
40. Evans MI, Koppitch FC, Nemmitz B, et al. Early genetic amniocentesis and chorionic villus sampling. J Reprod Med 1988;33:450–452.
41. Assel BG, Lewis SM, Dickerman LH, Park VM, Jassani MN. Single operator comparison of early and mid second trimester amniocentesis. Obstet Gynecol 1992;79:940–944.
42. Henry GP, Miller WA. Early amniocentesis. J Reprod Med 1992;37:305–402.

43. Bombard T, Rigdon DT. Prospective pilot evaluation of early (11–14 weeks' gestation) amniocentesis in 75 patients. Military Medicine 1992;157:339–341.
44. Hanson FW, Tennant F, Hune S, Brookhyser K. Early amniocentesis: outcome, risks and technical problems at less than 12.8 weeks. Am J Obstet Gynecol 1992;166:1707–1711.
45. Charrow J, Nadler HL, Evans MI. Prenatal diagnosis and fetal therapy. In: Emery AEH, Rimoin DL (eds). Principles and practice of medical genetics (2nd ed). London Churchill Livingstone, 1989;1959–1994.
46. Simpson JL. Amniocentesis: what it can tell you and what it can't. Contemporary Obstet Gynecol 1988;31:31–36.
47. Hsu YF, Kaffe S, Perlis ET. Trisomy 20 mosaicism in prenatal diagnosis: a review and update. Prenat Diagn 1987;7:581–596.
48. Worton RG, Stern RA. A Canadian collaborative study of mosaicism in amniotic fluid cell cultures. Prenat Diagn 1984;4:131–144.
49. Gosden C, Nicolaides KH, Rodeck CH. Fetal blood sampling in the investigation of chromosome mosaicism in amniotic fluid cell culture. Lancet 1988;1:613–616.
50. Warburton D. Outcome of cases of de novo structural rearrangements diagnosed at amniocentesis. Prenat Diagn 1984;4:69–80.
51. Drugan A, Sokol RJ, Syner FN, Ager JW, Zador IE, Evans MI. Clinical implications of amniotic fluid AFP in twin pregnancies. J Reprod Med 1989;34:977–981.
52. Drugan A, Syner FN, Greb A, Evans MI. Amniotic fluid alpha-fetoprotein and acetylcholinesterase in early genetic amniocentesis. Obstet Gynecol 1988;72:33–35.
53. Crandall BF, Hanson FW, Tennant F, Perdue ST. Alpha-fetoprotein levels in amniotic fluid between 11 and 15 weeks. Am J Obstet Gynecol 1989;160:1204–1206.
54. Drugan A, Syner FN, Belsky-Gold RL, Koppitch FC, Evans MI. Amniotic fluid acetylcholinesterase: implications of an inconclusive result. Am J Obstet Gynecol 1988;159: 469–474.
55. Allen R. The significance of meconium in midtrimester genetic amniocentesis. Am J Obstet Gynecol 1985;152:413–417.
56. Zorn EM, Hanson FW, Greve IC, et al. Analysis of the significance of discolored amniotic fluid at midtrimester amniocentesis. Am J Obstet Gynecol 1986;154:1234–1240.
57. Hankins GD, Rowe J, Quirk JG, et al. Significance of brown and/or green amniotic fluid at the time of second trimester genetic amniocentesis. Obstet Gynecol 1984;64:353.
58. Crane JP, Rohland BM. Clinical significance of persistent amniotic fluid leakage after genetic amniocentesis. Prenat Diagn 1986;6:25–31.
59. Nimrod C, Varela-Gittings F, Machin G, et al. The effect of very prolonged membrane rupture on fetal development. Am J Obstet Gynecol 1984;148:540–543.
60. Golbus MS, Loughman WD, Epstein CJ, et al. Prenatal genetic diagnosis in 3000 amniocenteses. N Engl J Med 1979;300:157–163.
61. NICHD National Registry for Amniocentesis Study Group. Midtrimester amniocentesis for prenatal diagnosis—safety and accuracy. JAMA 1976;236:1471.
62. Anandakumar C, Wong YC, Annapoorna V, Arulkumaran S, Chia D, Bongso A, Ratnam SS. Amniocentesis and its complications. Aust N Z J Obstet Gynecol 1992;32:97–99.
63. Ledbetter DJ, Hall DG. Traumatic arteriovenous fistula: a complication of amniocentesis. J Pediatric Surg 1992;27:720–721.
64. Epley SL, Hanson JW, Cruikshank DP. Fetal injury with midtrimester diagnostic amniocentesis. Obstet Gynecol 1979;53:77–80.
65. Kohn G. The amniotic band syndrome: a possible complication of amniocentesis. Prenat Diagn 1987;7:303–305.
66. Lockwood C, Ghidini A, Romero R, Hobbins JC. Amniotic band syndrome: reevaluation of its pathogenesis. Am J Obstet Gynecol 1989;160:1030–1033.
67. Milner AD, Hoskins EW, Hopkin IE. The effect of midtrimester amniocentesis on lung function in the neonatal period. Europ J Pediatr 1992;151:458–460.
68. Thompson PJ, Greenough A, Nicolaides KH. Lung volume measured by functional residual capacity in infants following first trimester amniocentesis or chorionic villus sampling. Br J Obstet Gynecol 1992;99:479–482.

*Invasive Outpatient Procedures in Reproductive Medicine,* edited by Mark I. Evans, et al. Lippincott–Raven Publishers, Philadelphia © 1997.

# 2 Chorionic Villus Sampling

Nelson B. Isada, Mark P. Johnson, Arie Drugan, Mark I. Evans

## INTRODUCTION

Since the development of amniocentesis over 25 years ago, there has been a constant desire to move prenatal diagnosis to as early in gestation as possible.[1] In the mid-1980s the combination of increasingly sophisticated ultrasound and laboratory cytogenetic advances made first-trimester sampling of chorionic villi possible. More than a decade of experience has now shown that chorionic villus sampling (CVS), in experienced hands, is both safe and effective.[3] Despite allegations of increased risk of birth defects,[2] now clearly disproven by objective data (although still disputed by some), CVS gained rapid acceptance, then declined, and now has been reaccepted in prenatal diagnosis.

In our program at Wayne State University and Hutzel Hospital in Detroit, Michigan, we have performed over 7,000 chorionic villus sampling procedures. Of these, about 85% were performed by the transcervical approach.[4] The remainder were performed transabdominally or, occasionally, by transvaginal approach.

As a result of the 1990 FDA approval of the Trophocan catheter (Concord/Portex; Keene, New Hampshire) for use in transcervical chorionic villus sampling, an increasing number of US physicians began offering the procedure. To obtain privileges to perform CVS, some states have enacted legislation requiring the performance of 50 CVS procedures in pregnancies in which the patient has already chosen first trimester abortion.[1] This practice may not be feasible because of the controversies already surrounding elective abortion or because of the increased medical costs if this experience is acquired in a hospital setting. Other states and hospitals have no guidelines at all, which may result in physicians offering and performing the procedure without the guidance and experience of practiced operators. Such inexperienced physicians can needlessly enter difficult situations and repeat known technical errors.

## INDICATIONS

The accepted reasons for genetic counseling (i.e., advanced maternal age, risk for multiple biochemical or molecularly diagnosable abnormalities) are prime indications for CVS.[1] The indications have been reviewed very extensively elsewhere and are not repeated here; they are summarized in the preceding chapter on amniocentesis.

We generally attempt to schedule patients interested in CVS to be seen at 10–12 weeks gestational age. The initial patient contact is with our genetic counselors, who discuss the risks, benefits, and alternatives to testing versus no testing. Background and procedure-related losses are reviewed. Benefits and risks of CVS versus early amniocentesis and versus routine amniocentesis are discussed.

With the exception of those patients whose primary risk is for a neural tube defect, any patient considered a candidate for amniocentesis should be offered CVS if they are seen in the first trimester. CVS has the advantage of early diagnosis, no needle (most of the time), and, most importantly, privacy. At 10–12 weeks gestation, a patient can confirm the genetic health of the gestation. If an abnormality is found they can choose to terminate by the relatively safe, easy, quick, and cheap suction method. Techniques used later in a pregnancy are more expensive, have higher complication rates, and often many of the patient's friends and relatives know of the pregnancy.

## Multiple Gestation

CVS can be performed in a multiple gestation when separate, discrete placentas are identified (Fig. 2–1). Twins remain the most common multiple gestation, even in the era of stimulated cycles and assisted reproductive technology, and comments here are confined to twins. Placental and fetal locations must be meticulously noted in order to avoid the issues of misidentification and of sampling one twin twice and the other not at all. Operators performing transcervical–transcervical CVS may run the risk of cross-contamination of samples. With twins, a transabdominal–transcervical CVS or transabdominal–transabdominal dual CVS procedure can be performed to minimize cytogenetic contamination.

In the setting of a ''vanishing twin,'' which may occur in up to 3% of pregnancies,[5] studies suggest an increased risk of aneuploidy in the remaining placental tissue of the ''vanished twin.''[6] Therefore, care must be taken during sampling when only the remaining twin is being evaluated.

## Fetal Anomalies

Another setting in which a faster diagnosis may be useful is when fetal anomalies are found. In the first trimester, we have found in the setting of a cystic hygroma or nuchal membrane the risk of aneuploidy to be as high as 60%[7] (Fig. 2–2). By use of direct analysis of villi or fluorescent in situ hybridization (FISH), one can obtain cytogenetic information (e.g., trisomies 21, 18, or 13, or monosomy X) in a matter of days when a sufficient quantity of villi is obtained at the time of CVS. However, the operator and the patient must be aware that the amount of tissue required for these studies is greater than the usual volume obtained at a ''routine'' CVS; the patient should be told that more than one sampling may be necessary.[8] The major drawback

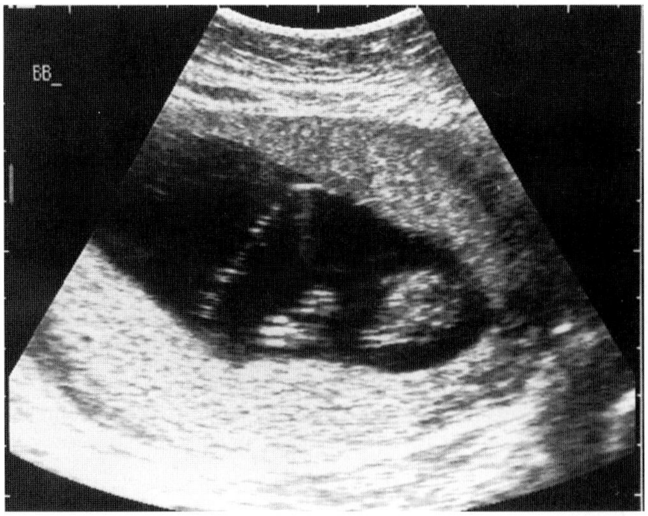


**FIG. 2–1.** First trimester ultrasound showing twin gestation, anterior placenta for twin A and posterior placenta for twin B. A membrane separating the twins, but not twin B, can be seen in the photograph.

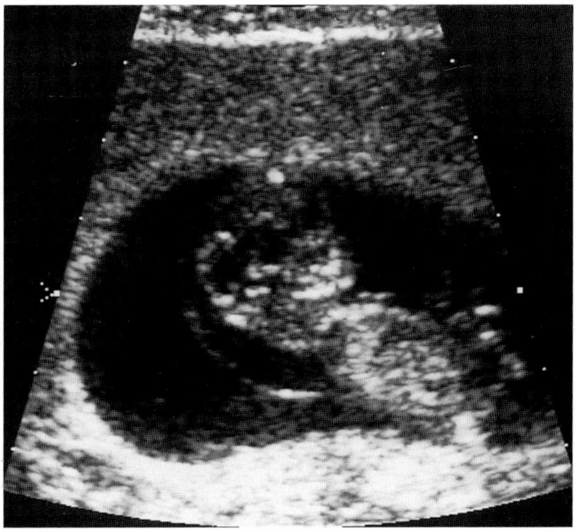

**FIG. 2–2.** Large nuchal fold extending off of back of fetal head at approximately 12 weeks gestation.

to FISH technology is that karyotypes are not generated. Thus, a banded karyotype is always required to complete the cytogenetic analysis and to rule out structural aberrations.

Alternative cytogenetic methods for rapid diagnosis include the ''direct prep.'' The direct prep specifically evaluates the rapidly dividing cytotrophoblastic component of the placenta. One must be cautious in interpreting these results and be cognizant of the recently described issues surrounding confined placental mosaicism.[9] In addition, the mitotic yield of direct preps is low and the quality of chromosome spreads and banding are often poor.

## TECHNIQUE

Thorough counseling of patients plays a crucial part in prenatal diagnosis. We believe that a full session (30–45 min.) is appropriate for patients to understand the risks and benefits of their options and the implications of their choices. If 100% of patients choose the same pathway following counseling, then the counseling is not adequate! Rational people reach different conclusions about the same data, and these differences must be respected. Approximately 85% of our patients choose to proceed with CVS testing after genetic counseling.

After (or during) counseling, patients are asked to drink 32 ounces of water. A full bladder generally optimizes the relationship between the uterus and cervix for transcervical CVS, in addition to maximizing transabdominal ultrasonic visualization.

The next step is the ultrasound evaluation. First, fetal viability is confirmed. About 7% of patients are discovered to have a blighted ovum or an embryonic or fetal demise.[10] Size and date discrepancies are also noted. Of greatest concern is the smaller than expected fetus, even in the first trimester. We have found that such fetuses are at increased risk for aneuploidy,[11] and that special studies of the chorionic villi to shorten the time to diagnosis may be appropriate.

Dating the pregnancy also has implications for special DNA studies. If the indication is prenatal testing for disorders such as sickle cell disease or cystic fibrosis, increased amounts of tissue (20–40 mg) are necessary (Fig. 2–3). If the indication is DNA analysis, we prefer to schedule the patient at 11–12 weeks gestation because the placental mass is generally larger, and multiple passes may be necessary to obtain sufficient material for DNA extraction and analysis.

Placental evaluation is of utmost importance in properly assessing patients for transcervical CVS. In general, placental location determines whether the approach will be transcervical or transabdominal. For most cases, this decision will be straightforward. If the placenta is low

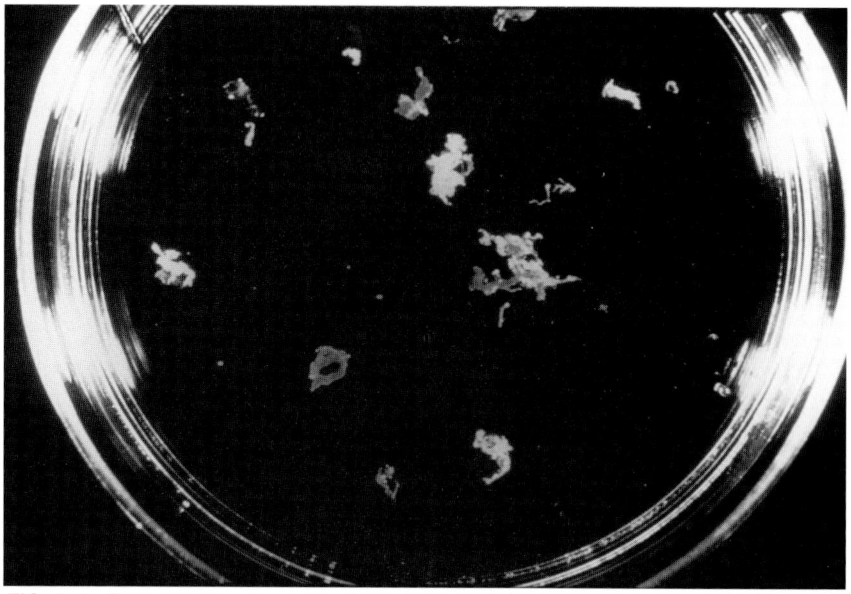

**FIG. 2–3.** Petri dish showing approximately 5 mg of chorionic villi, just aspirated by transcervical approach. Villi obtained transabdominally often are more fragmented due to damage through passage of smaller interior diameter of the needle as compared to the plastic catheter.

lying and posterior, a cervical approach is appropriate. This is the "textbook case" that should be initially attempted by novices (Fig. 2–4). If the placenta is anterior and fundal, an abdominal approach is usually indicated (Fig. 2–5). The placenta can sometimes be maneuvered into a vertical configuration by judicious manipulation of bladder volume (Fig. 2–6).

Some cases that initially appear to necessitate an abdominal approach may actually be performed transcervically. Viewed longitudinally, the placenta may appear anterior (Fig. 2–7). However, on transverse scan the placenta may lie predominantly along one uterine wall (Fig. 2–8). If the cervical canal is found to enter the uterus at a point close to the placenta, a cervical approach can be attempted. The entrance point is determined by use of a metal sound.

Potentially difficult cases arise when there is a sharp angle between the cervical canal and uterine cavity (Fig. 2–9). In this case, it is a matter of judgment and experience as to whether or not the curvature of the catheter is sufficient to negotiate the cervico-uterine junction. If the patient is nulliparous with a narrow cervical canal, a significant bend in the catheter may prevent passage through the cervical canal. However, if the patient is multiparous, sometimes the canal will more readily accommodate the curvature of the catheter. Often these cases are better performed transabdominally in order to minimize the risk of placental injury, detachment, hematoma, and subsequent pregnancy loss. When the placenta is horizontal and anterior (see Fig. 2–3) and not accessible by the transcervical route, the transabdominal method must be used.

Another placental factor that occasionally arises is when subchorionic bleeding is found, as manifested by sonolucent areas often at the placental edges (Fig. 2–10). This is usually accompanied by a history of vaginal spotting. There are no firm data on the outcome of pregnancy when CVS is performed in the presence of a subchorionic bleed, but loss rates do not appear to be significantly increased. We attempt to individualize every case and commonly, but not always, avoid the area in question. We have found that in general CVS can be safely carried out in these patients.

Other factors must be considered before attempting CVS. The patient may give a history of genital herpes simplex or recent group B streptococcus (GBS) infection. Again, all these

*Text continues on p. 21.*

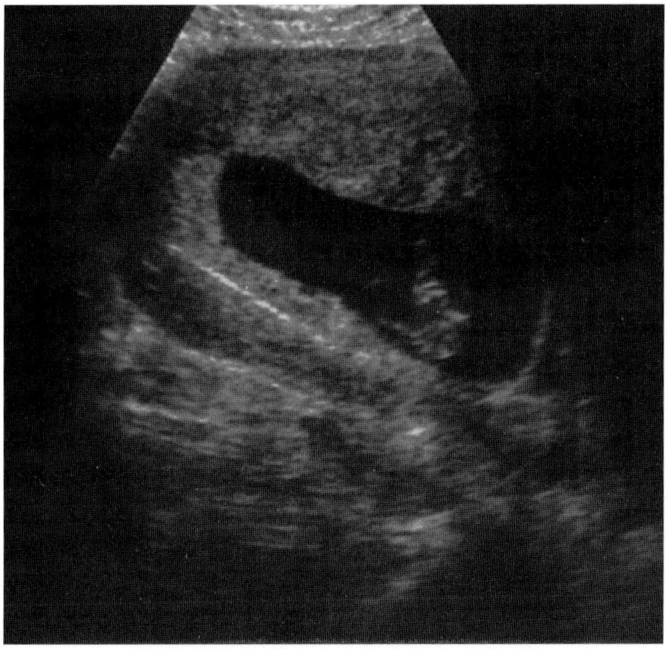

**FIG. 2–4.** Longitudinal scan of an 11-week gestation with posterior placenta. Pathway of the catheter can be seen traversing the placenta from lower right to upper left.

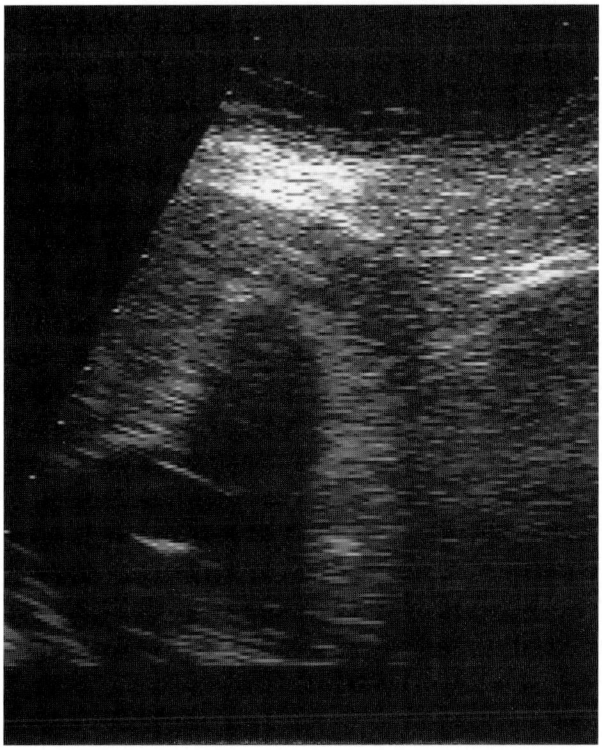

**FIG. 2–5.** Vertical placenta on transverse view, ideal for transabdominal. Tip of needle can be seen in lower portion of placenta.

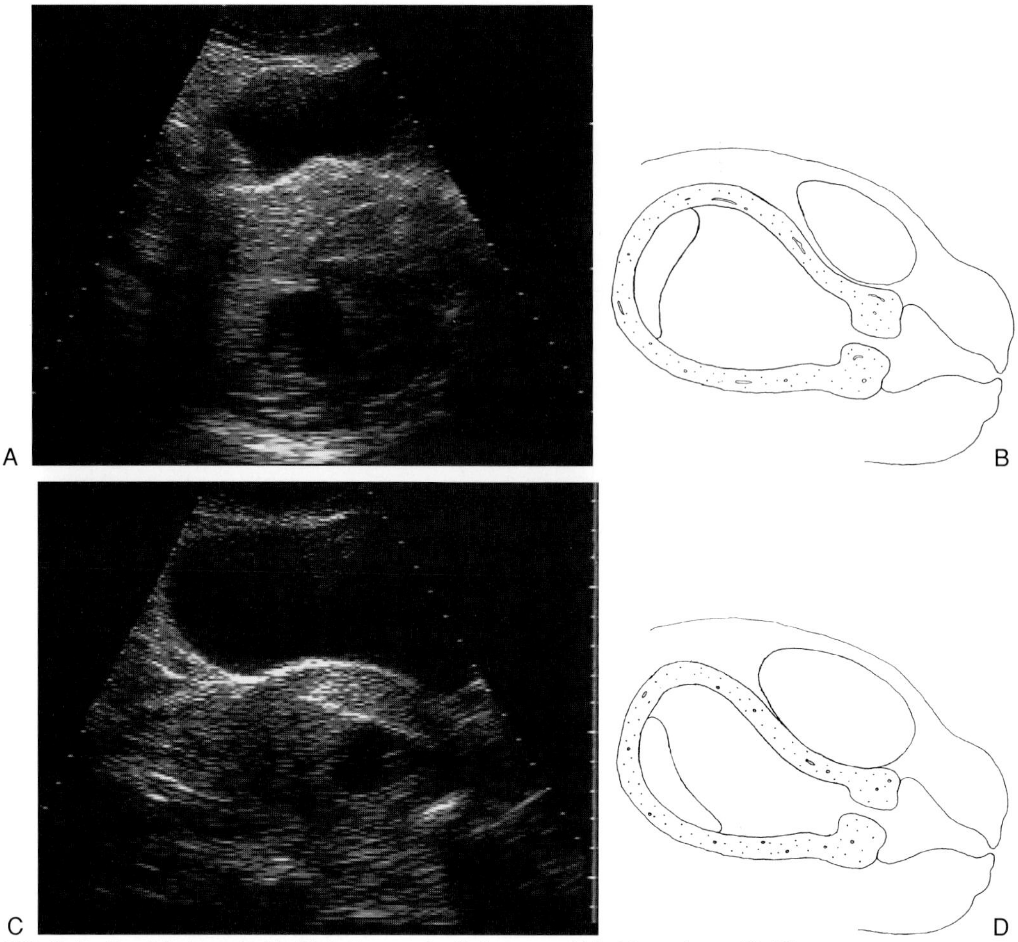


FIG. 2–6. Fundal placenta (A, B) flattens out with increased bladder volume (C, D).

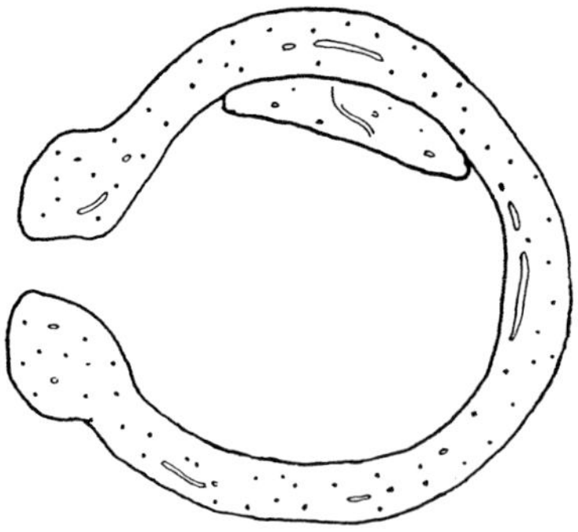

FIG. 2–7. Placenta appears predominantly anterior on longitudinal view.

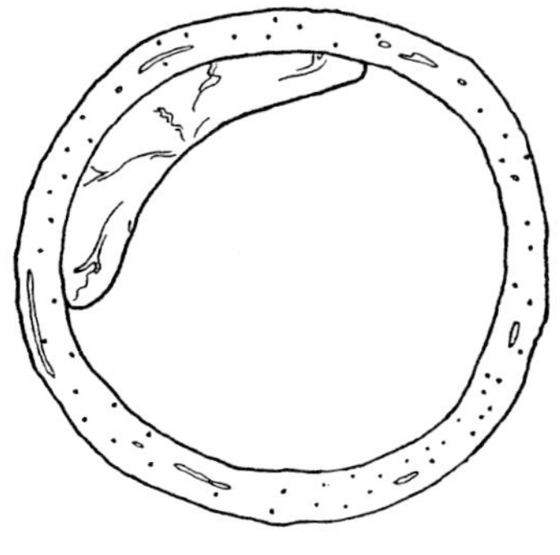

**FIG. 2–8.** On transverse view, back of placenta is actually on side-wall.

cases are individualized, and the small or theoretical risk of introduction of infection into the fetal-placental tissues is discussed. Generally we have offered transabdominal CVS or amniocentesis when a significant risk of active group B streptococcal colonization is present. When there is such a history, we prefer to initiate ampicillin therapy prior to any possible transcervical CVS procedure. We base this practice on three cases from other centers of group B streptococcal septic abortion after transcervical CVS.

## Transcervical Chorionic Villus Sampling

Once we have established that a transcervical CVS is likely to be successful, we proceed with the vaginal prep. We glove, then draw up ~2 cc of transport media into a 20-cc syringe (Fig. 2–11), and set it in a sterile field (Fig. 2–12). We use a medium Graves speculum and a povidone-iodine prep, which is also used to lubricate the speculum (Fig. 2–13). If the patient reports an iodine allergy, we use a hexachlorophene based solution. Following the prep, we change gloves and a uterine sound is guided through the cervical canal (Fig. 2–14). This metal sound, easily visualized on ultrasound exam, is used to assess the point of entry of the canal into the uterine cavity. Using the location of sound entry as the point of reference, the placental position is described as either being "toward" the ultrasonographer or "away." This is done in longitudinal and transverse planes. Both planes are important because the cervical canal often takes a variable course and may make what appears to be a straightforward CVS a most difficult one or vice-versa. For example, the placenta may wrap "toward" and the canal enter "away," increasing the difficulty of the procedure.

Specific cervical problems can also be encountered. Decreased catheter maneuverability

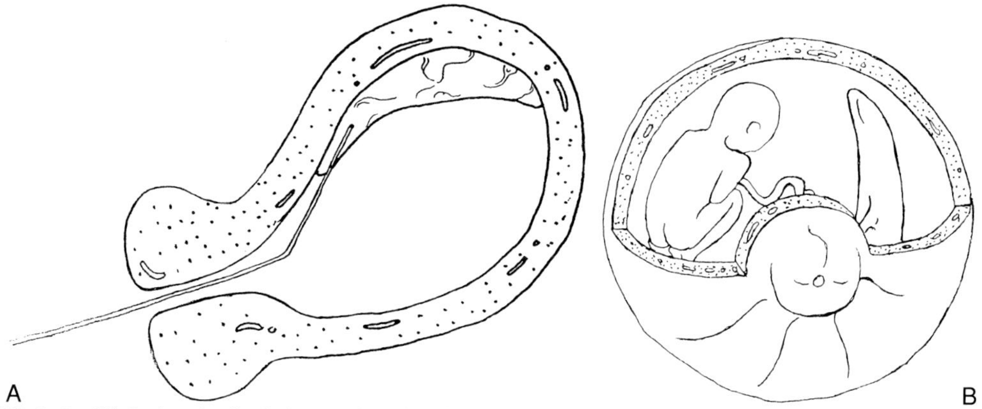

A B

**FIG. 2–9.** (A) On longitudinal view, a sharp bend in catheter is needed to go from cervical canal to placenta. (B) Head on view showing need for sharp right turn of catheter as soon as it would pass through cervix.

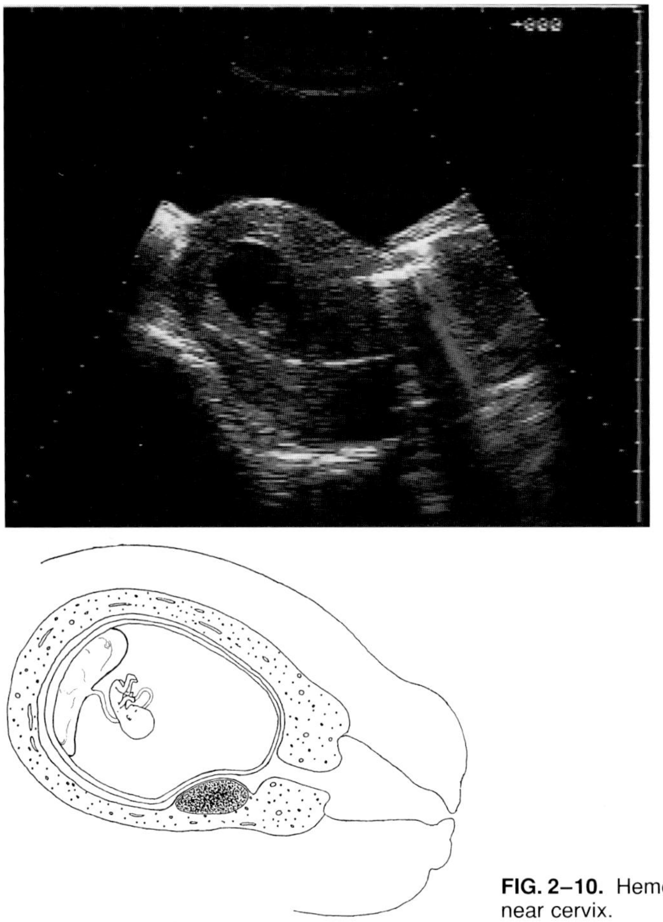

**FIG. 2–10.** Hemorrhagic area from subchorionic bleed near cervix.

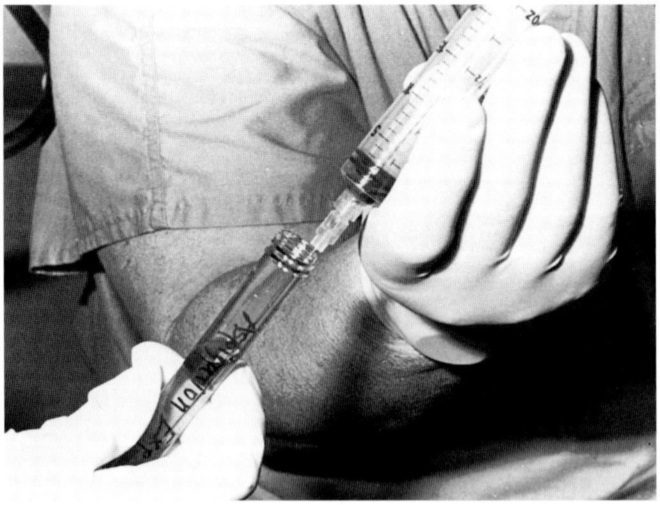

**FIG. 2–11.** Approximately 2 cc of aspiration media being aspirated from culture tube into 20-cc syringe.

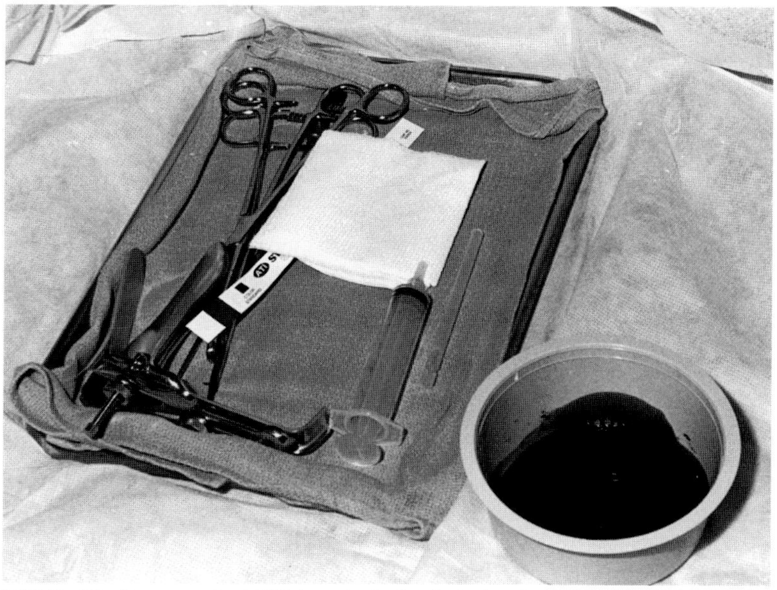

**FIG. 2–12.** Transcervical CVS tray, including betadine in prep bowl, 20-cc syringe, spinal needles for transfer of culture media into syringe, speculum, tenaculum, ring forceps, and several 4 × 4's for cleansing.

with the nulliparous cervix has been previously mentioned. Rarely, cervical fibroids may make a transcervical CVS impossible or very uncomfortable for the patient. A patient with previous cryosurgery may have a stenotic canal. Cervical polyps should be noted as specifically mentioned to the patient as they tend to bleed when touched. Care must be taken with the sound not to create a false canal. A long cervix can also pose a problem, especially when it is greater than 5 cm in length, making maneuvering of the shaped catheter more difficult. A long cervix limits catheter manipulations, and multiple passes may be required, even if the placenta covers the internal os.

We have found the uterine sound to be invaluable in evaluating the relationship of the cervix to the placenta prior to proceeding with CVS. The sound must be carefully maneuvered to the internal os sonographically and by feel to a point just short of the placenta. When the

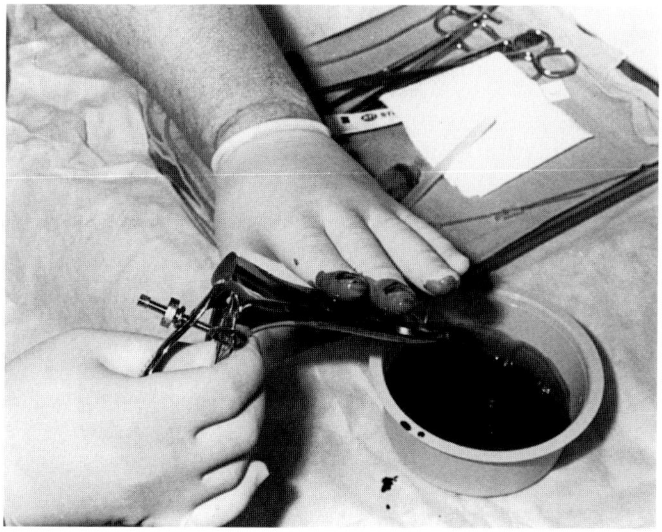

**FIG. 2–13.** Speculum being lubricated with betadine for easy entry.

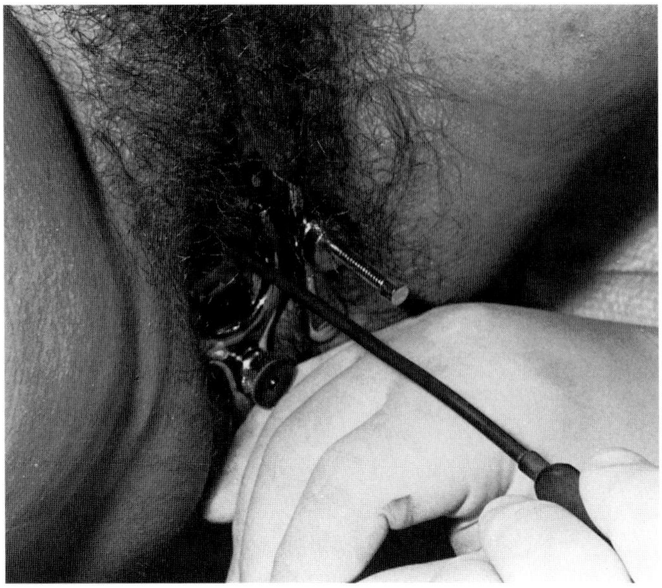

**FIG. 2–14.** Metal sound being inserted through cervix to level of internal os to help judge angle of cervical canal to placenta.

sound is in place at the internal os, the speculum can be manipulated to change cervical and uterine angles to assess the degree of subsequent mobility to facilitate manipulation of the catheter. Occasionally, pelvic relaxation or other factors such as maternal obesity can alter the relationship of the cervix to the uterus, and at times make the cervix itself difficult to visualize. In such cases, a single tooth tenaculum gently applied to the anterior lip of the cervix can greatly assist in straightening the angle between the cervix and lower uterine segment by gentle traction. In the early years of our experience it was routine to use the tenaculum. However, with experience the tenaculum is required less than 1% of the time.

Extreme uterine retroversion or retroflexion may become more obvious. If the sound enters close to the placenta, a transcervical procedure is possible. Otherwise, a transcervical procedure should be abandoned if the cervico-uterine angle appears too acute. After the angle of the uterus and cervix and the entry of the cervical canal into the uterus is established, the uterine sound is removed. The operator bends the catheter to the estimated degree necessary (Fig. 2–15), and inserts the catheter into the cervical canal. The catheter tip should be visualized

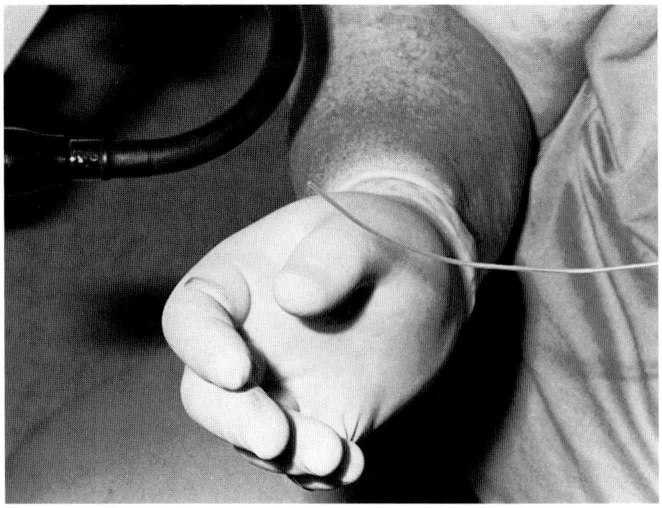

**FIG. 2–15.** Bend placed in plastic catheters held in place by metal stylet to conform to angle of cervical canal to placenta. Differing angles are needed depending upon anatomy.

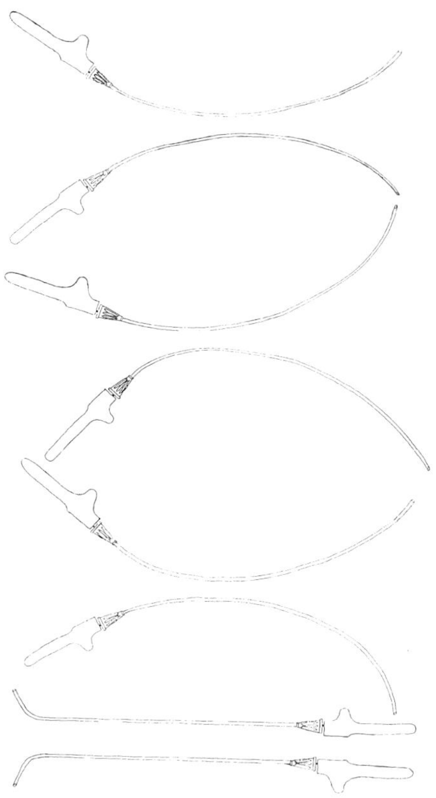

**FIG. 2–16.** Four examples of "Scanzoni" rotation of catheter that shows a minor change in the direction of the catheter at the internal os is achieved with a major rotation of the handle.

at or before the internal os. The catheter tip should be followed throughout the course of the procedure. Sometimes, because of technical reasons such as patient obesity, this is not always possible. Often tissue movement can be detected even with equivocal definition of the catheter. The operator must take care to avoid puncturing the gestational sac and make the appropriate maneuvers with the speculum and with catheter rotation to manipulate the catheter through the bulk of the placenta. If moderately acute angles are encountered, the catheter can be rotated in ''Scanzoni'' fashion, which minimizes rotational movement at the catheter tip and reduces potential placental trauma with such maneuvers (Fig. 2–16). Like mid-forceps rotations, tissue shearing can take place if a wide arc is not made at the operator's end of the instrument. In the case of transcervical CVS, failure to take a wide arc could result in placental detachment.

The operator can generally monitor the entrance of the catheter into the placenta both by ultrasound and by feel. The placenta has a definite spongy feeling and the procedure can be described as ''pushing the catheter through jello.'' If resistance is met, the catheter must be stopped. Catheter position must be reassessed and the catheter redirected. At times it is necessary to withdraw entirely and reshape the catheter.

The ultrasonographer must immediately inform the operator if the catheter appears to tent the gestational sac. The operator must pull the catheter back if this is taking place. The catheter position is then reassessed and the catheter redirected.

Ideally, the catheter should be placed through the mid-section of the placenta and the subchorionic and basal regions of the placenta avoided (Fig. 2–17). The operator must be aware that significant amounts of rotation can shear the placenta, and must be kept to a minimum. The patient should not feel any significant discomfort except possible cramping if the catheter tip touches the myometrium.

Once the catheter tip is in position, it can be gently anchored in the decidua. The stylet is then gently removed by following the course of its insertion (Fig. 2–18), and the 20-cc syringe (with ~2 cc transport media) tightly screwed to the end of the catheter (Fig. 2–19).

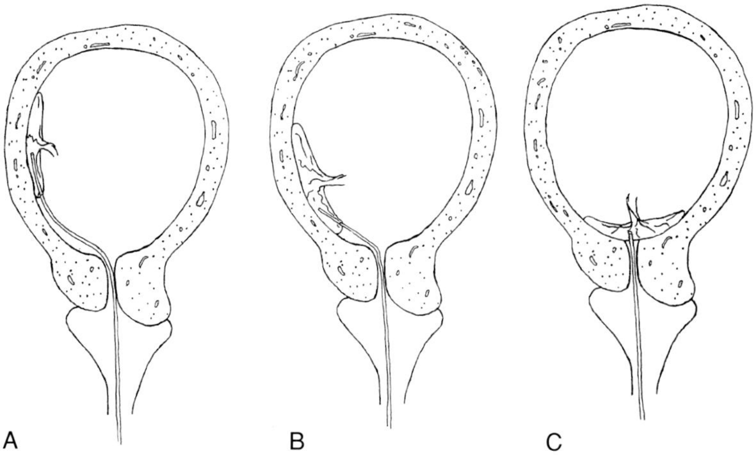

A B C

**FIG. 2–17.** Catheter can traverse placenta either transversly (A), at an oblique angle (B), or through longest approach (C). Angle depends upon relative position of cervix to placenta.

A

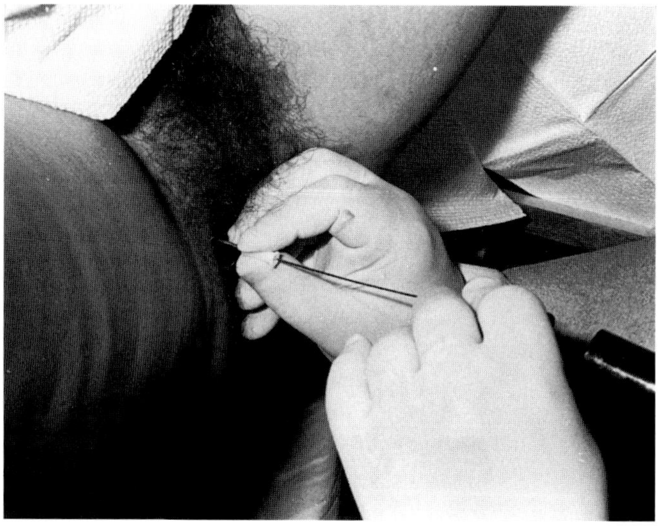

B

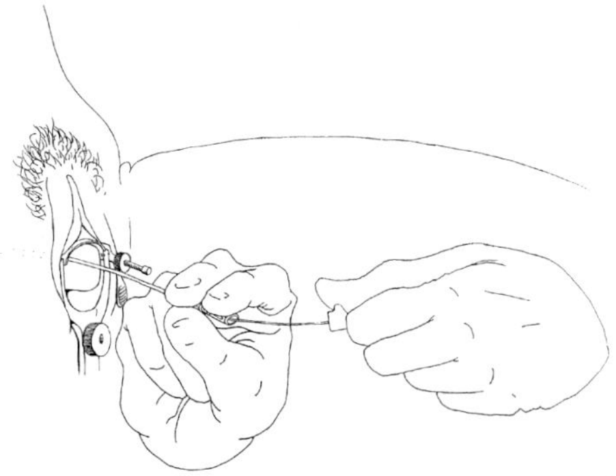

**FIG. 2–18.** Metal stylet is removed from the catheter, being careful to hold the hub of the catheter very steady, so as to ensure that the catheter position is not dislodged.

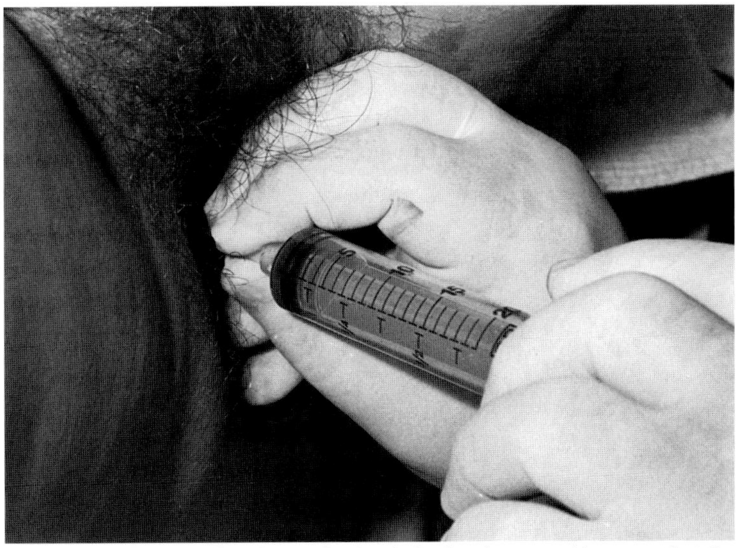

**FIG. 2–19.** 20-cc syringe is attached to hub of catheter, making sure that the fit is tight.

Care should be taken not to dislodge the catheter tip at this time. Its location must be reverified prior to application of suction. The catheter is slightly withdrawn until the tip is within the placenta. Suction should be applied by pulling the plunger out to its maximum and its position fixed with an extended index finger. A gentle rocking motion can be applied, and tissue should be seen to traverse the catheter length on ultrasound. Tissue should also be seen within the portion of the catheter in the vagina. We attempt to avoid sampling from the mid-subchorionic area beneath the cord insertion whenever reasonably possible. Gentle rocking motion and suction should be continued as the catheter is slowly withdrawn from the uterus and through the cervix and vagina. All contents of the syringe and catheter should be emptied into a tube containing transport media (Fig. 2–20). The media should then be redrawn into the syringe, swirled, and slowly re-emptied into the transport media in order to recover any tissue remaining

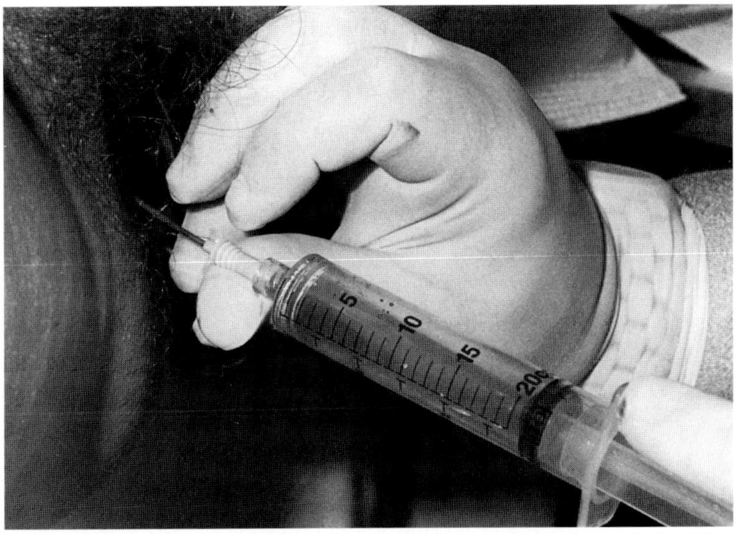

**FIG. 2–20.** Suction is created by drawing back the syringe plunger to the 20cc mark, again making sure to hold the catheter very steady. Villi can be seen within the bore of the catheter.

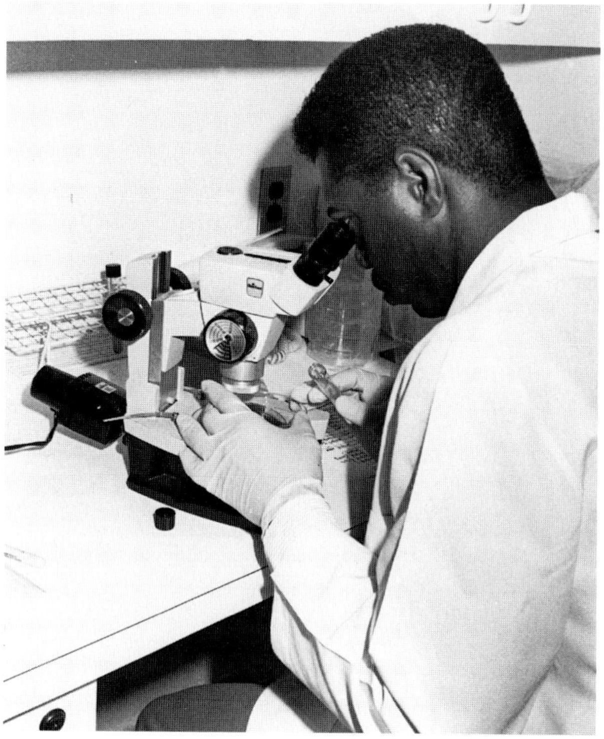

**FIG. 2–21.** Villi are immediately analyzed under a dissecting microscope in order to determine if enough villi has been obtained or if another pass is necessary.

in the syringe. The tissue is analyzed under a dissecting microscope to determine whether sufficient amounts of chorionic villi are present (Fig. 2–21). If there is an insufficient amount of tissue, the procedure must be repeated with a fresh catheter. All angles must be re-examined because the bladder continues to fill. We generally require a second pass in about 5% of cases. In DNA cases, multiple passes are usually the rule because more tissue is required. In our laboratory ~5 mg of clean tissue are sufficient for routine cytogenetic diagnosis.

Positive fetal heart rate is verified post procedure. Occasionally, a retroplacental hematoma is seen. Generally these are small and resolve spontaneously without sequelae. Post-procedure information and instructions are again reviewed, and the patient is informed that she can expect cytogenetic results in approximately two weeks.

We have found patients to have increased preference and acceptance for the transcervical approach because of the increased comfort. This has been noted by patients who have had both procedures in different pregnancies.

## Transabdominal Chorionic Villus Sampling

Our initial patient selection for transabdominal chorionic villus sampling (TA-CVS) is the same as for transcervical (TC) CVS. Because the majority of our patients (85%) are sampled transcervically, we perform TA-CVS in situations in which the placental location is fundal or anterior. Operator judgment and experience is required for selection because 60% of first-trimester placentas are in a predominantly posterior location, and 40% are in a predominantly anterior location. It is the latter group that requires a decision for TA-CVS versus TC-CVS as to whether or not the operator can ''turn the corner'' without disruption of the placenta in the lower uterine segment.

Once the appropriate approach for the patient is chosen, an angle of approach is then determined. The patient's bladder size may be manipulated by emptying or filling to improve

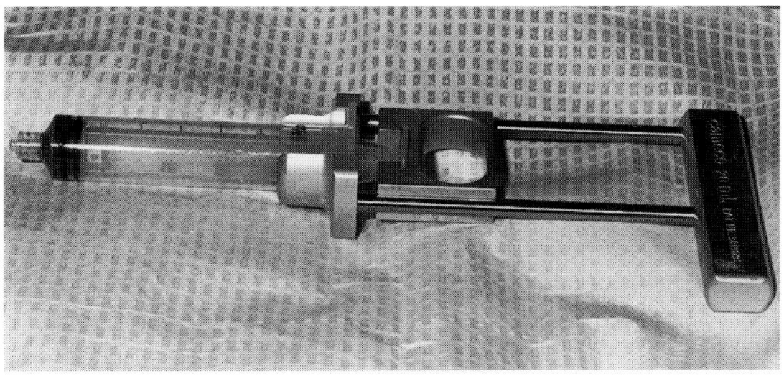

**FIG. 2–22.** 20-cc syringe in syringe gun. (Courtesy Cameco Ltd, London)

access. The angle of needle entry to the most accessible (and generally the thickest) placental site is chosen sonographically using both longitudinal and transverse views. We generally use a 18-, 19-, or 20-gauge BD spinal needle with a Quincke point (Becton Dickinson and Company, Franklin Lakes, NJ). A 20 mL syringe is loaded with 1–2 mL CVS aspiration media and placed in a syringe pistol (Fig. 2–22). The abdomen is prepped with an iodine solution (hexachlorophene if iodine-allergic), and the ultrasound transducer is covered with a sterile glove. Sterile ultrasound jelly is used, since the oxygen necessary to activate the antibacterial iodine solution results in its drying. The site is located, the needle inserted, and the tip followed and directed into the placenta sonographically, with the sonographer holding the transducer longitudinally to the patient and positioned laterally to the insertion site (Fig. 2–23). Once the needle is in the body of the placenta (and preferably not subchorionic, at the placental margin, or in maternal decidua), the stylet is removed and the syringe and syringe pistol attached (Fig. 2–24). Full suction (20 mL) is applied, and the needle is moved within the body of the placenta several millimeters with a rotating motion at the operator's wrist. The needle is steadied at the skin insertion with the opposite hand. Continuous suction is maintained. After several movements, the needle is withdrawn, and the sample is injected into the CVS transport media. Immediate microscopic examination is performed to verify the presence of an adequate amount of chorionic villi. As with the TC-CVS, the specimen is dissected prior to transport to the lab to remove decidua or clot. Blood and blood clots are more commonly found with TA-CVS specimens than with TC-CVS specimens. Up to three passes (needle insertions) may be necessary to obtain an adequate sample, especially if special genetic studies are being performed that require larger samples.

Occasionally we use an 18-gauge needle for TA-CVS. Its advantages are that a larger sample size is usually obtained per insertion and that the needle is easier to identify sonographically. Both of these advantages may be important if the operator, the sonographer, or both, are less experienced, or if a large sample is needed. Its disadvantages are that this needle size can be associated with increased patient discomfort (pain and cramping) both during and after

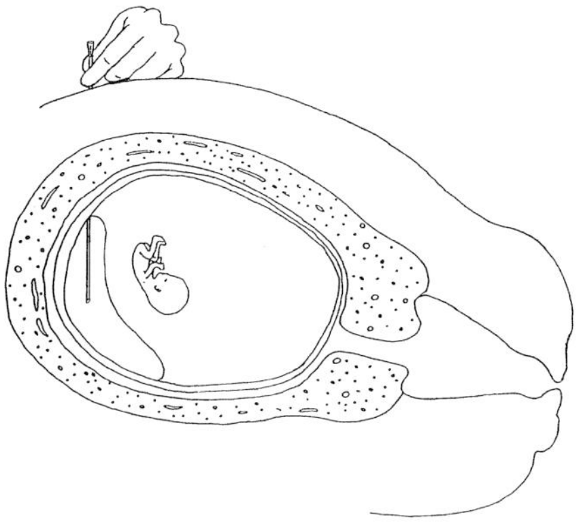

**FIG. 2–23.** Transabdominally inserted needle in placenta prior to aspiration of villi.

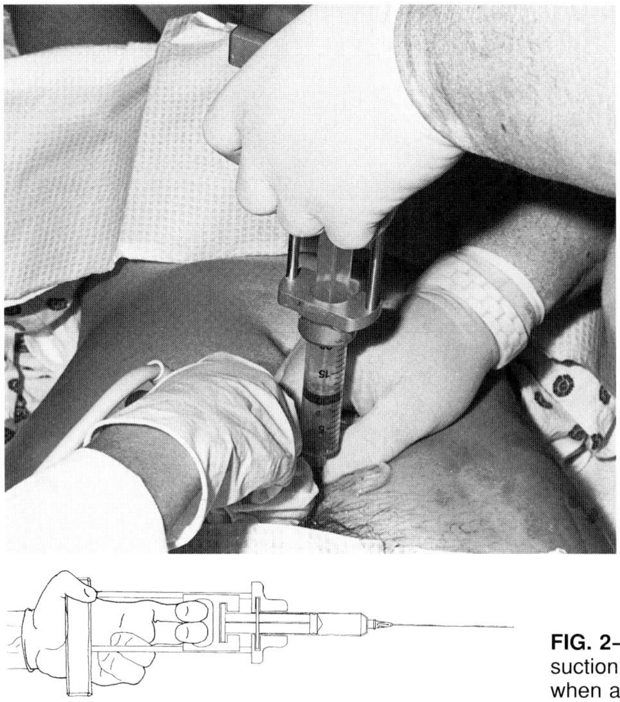

**FIG. 2–24.** Syringe gun attached to syringe with suction being created; gun is pulled back to 20 cc when aspiration of villi begins.

the procedure and that, theoretically, more placental disruption may occur because of the increased needle size.

Other approaches for TA-CVS have been utilized. The placement of the needle tip can be directed by displaying the full needle length sonographically, with the transducer placed lateral to the needle insertion site and held transversely. Some operators initially use an 18-gauge needle, leave it in the placenta, remove the stylet and then insert a smaller caliber needle for sampling.

### Transvaginal Chorionic Villus Sampling

On rare occasions, extreme uterine retroversion or retroflexion precludes TA-CVS or TC-CVS, requiring a transvaginal (TV) approach.[12] We have used a modified TA-CVS method, inserting the needle under transabdominal ultrasound guidance through the vaginal wall, and use the syringe and syringe pistol combination described above. Some authors use transvaginal ultrasound guidance (as employed in oocyte aspiration) when performing TV-CVS. In either approach, the operator must be certain that maternal bowel is not present in the cul-de-sac, and that this unusual uterine position is not a result of iatrogenic bladder overdistention.

## POST–PROCEDURE MANAGEMENT AND COMPLICATIONS

The presence of a normal fetal heart rate is verified post-procedure. Occasionally, a retroplacental hematoma is seen. Generally, these are small and resolve spontaneously without sequelae. Patients are given written and verbal instructions to call for persistent bleeding, cramping, fevers, or myalgias. Standard cytogenetic results are generally available within 10–14 days, and the patient is reminded of this. If special studies are being performed (e.g., FISH, DNA analysis, or enzymatic assays), these are also briefly reviewed. Any necessary antibiotics or Rh-immune globulin are also prescribed or administered.

A key question with any prenatal diagnostic procedure concerns its risks. Unlike many other medical procedures, the loss rates have to be factored against shifting background loss rates that are heavily dependent on both maternal and gestational age. Background loss rates (i.e., no procedure) and assuming a normal ultrasound at the time of procedure show a marked increase with maternal age from 2% at age 20 to 4% in the late 30s to over 10% in the 40s. Most authorities believe that, in experienced hands, procedure-related loss rates on top of the background vary between 0.5% to a maximum of 1%. Thus, for a 38-year-old, a background risk of about 4% would be increased to 4.5% total by the procedure. Therefore, most losses that occur after CVS would have happened anyway. Generally, we believe that a procedure-related loss will occur within several days of the procedure.

Does chorionic villus sampling cause birth defects? A few reports have proposed an increased risk of fetal abnormalities arising from chorionic villus sampling.[2,13] These are primarily limb anomalies such as abnormalities of the fingers and toes and, in more severe cases, involving the mandible (oro-facial-limb hypogenesis sequence). These abnormalities have been attributed to a disruption sequence possibly arising from CVS-related microemboli during critical periods of organogenesis. However, large studies and collaborative data from experienced centers refute these allegations and show no increased risk at the normal time of sampling.[14,15] Close review of the studies suggesting associated risk factors appear to be relative to the inexperience of the center reporting these cases (less than 500 cases), and gestational age before 9 weeks. Given these data, it seems prudent generally to perform CVS at 10 weeks gestational age or greater, to limit its use to experienced centers and operators, and to employ the techniques described above to minimize placental disruption.

## CONTRAINDICATIONS

Contraindications to CVS are few and can be divided into discrete categories. First, a transcervical or transvaginal approach is contraindicated when there is active vaginal infection such as

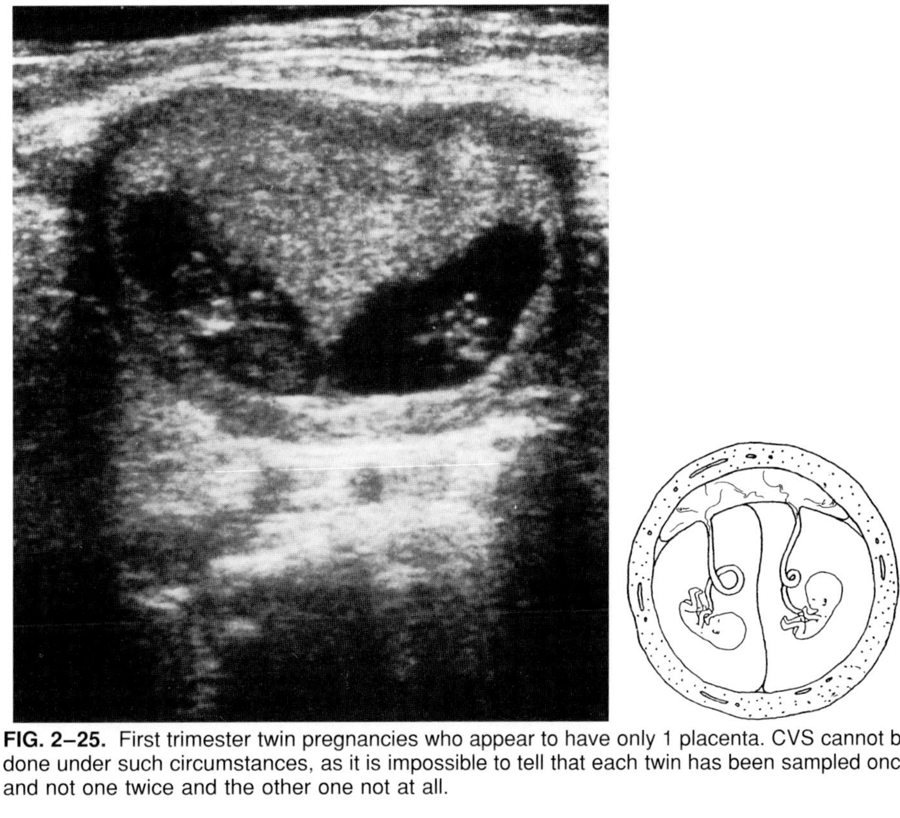

**FIG. 2–25.** First trimester twin pregnancies who appear to have only 1 placenta. CVS cannot be done under such circumstances, as it is impossible to tell that each twin has been sampled once and not one twice and the other one not at all.

a herpes or beta streptococcal outbreak. Routine culturing of the cervix, however, is not indicated and has not been shown to be useful. In most cases, transabdominal CVS or early amniocentesis can be performed for such patients.

The second category of contraindication is the multiple gestation in which no clear demarcation can be made as to which placenta belongs to which embryo (Fig. 2–25). Since such demarcation is critical for selective termination if there is an abutting, CVS should not be performed under such circumstances. Again, early amniocentesis may be appropriate then.

## CONCLUSIONS

CVS has been performed in over 200,000 cases worldwide. In experienced hands, there is an excellent record of safety and efficacy. CVS continues to be the primary invasive diagnostic method for first-trimester prenatal diagnosis.

## REFERENCES


1. Evans MI, Johnson MP. Chorionic villus sampling. In: Reproductive risks and prenatal diagnosis. Evans MI (ed.) Norwalk: Appleton & Lange, 1992;175–184.
2. Firth HV, Boyd PA, Chamberlain PF, MacKenzie IZ, Morriss-Kay GM, Huson SM. Analysis of limb reduction defects in babies exposed to chorionic villus sampling. Lancet 1994; 343:1069–1071.
3. Froster UG, Jackson L. Safety of chorionic villus sampling: results from an international registry. (Abstract) Am J Hum Genet 1994;55(3)Suppl:A3.
4. Hallak M, Johnson MP, Pryde PG, Isada NB, Zador IE, Evans MI. Chorionic villus sampling: transabdominal versus transcervical approach in more than 4000 cases. Obstet Gynecol 1992;80:349–352.
5. Landy HL, Weiner S, Carson SL. The ''vanishing twin'': ultrasonographic assessment of fetal disappearance in the first trimester. Am J Obstet Gynecol 1986;155:14.
6. Rudnicki M, Vejerslev LO, Junge J. The vanishing twin: morphologic and cytogenetic evaluation of an ultrasonographic phenomenon. Gynecol Obstet Invest 1991;31:141–145.
7. Johnson MP, Johnson A, Holzgreve W, Isada NB, Wapner R, Treadwell MC, Herger S, Evans MI. First trimester simple hygroma: cause and outcome. Am J Obstet Gynecol 1993;168:156–161.
8. Evans MI, Klinger KW, Isada NB, Shook D, Holzgreve W, McGuire N, Johnson MP. Rapid prenatal diagnosis by fluorescent in situ hybridization of chorionic villi: an adjunct to long term culture and karyotype. Am J Obstet Gynecol 1992;167:1522–1525.
9. Kalousek DK, Barrett IJ, McGillivray BC. Placental mosaicism and intrauterine survival of trisomies 13 and 18. Am J Hum Genet 1989;44:338–343.
10. Johnson MP, Drugan A, Koppitch FC, Uhlmann WR, Evans MI. Postmortem CVS is a better method for cytogenetic evaluation of early fetal loss than culture of abortus material. Am J Obstet Gynecol 1990;163:1505–1510.
11. Drugan A, Johnson MP, Isada NB, Holzgreve W, Zador IE, Dombrowski MP, Sokol RJ, Hallak M, Evans MI. The smaller than expected first trimester fetus is at increased risk for chromosome anomalies. Am J Obstet Gynecol 1992;167:1525–1528.
12. Schulman JD, Black SH, Soenksen D, Jones SL, Dorfmann AD. Transvaginal chorionic sampling during the first trimester of pregnancy [letter]. N Engl J Med 1988;319: 1612.
13. Blakemore K, Filkins K, Luthy DA, Platt LD, Medearis AL, Carlson D, Priest J, Korotkin J, Verp MS, Padilla LM, Warsof S, Weston PV. Cook obstetrics and gynecology catheter multicenter chorionic villus sampling trial: comparison of birth defects with expected rates. Am J Obstet Gynecol 1993;169:1022–1026.

14. Jackson LG, Zachary JM, Fowler SE, Desnick RJ, Golbus MS, Ledbetter DH, Mahoney MJ, Pergament E, Simpson JL, Black S, Wapner RJ, et al. A randomized comparison of transcervical and transabdominal chorionic-villus sampling. N Engl J Med 1992;327: 594–598.
15. Froster UG, Jackson L. Limb defects and chorionic villus sampling: results from an international registry, 1992–94. Lancet 1996;347:489–494.

*Invasive Outpatient Procedures in Reproductive Medicine,* edited by Mark I. Evans, et al. Lippincott–Raven Publishers, Philadelphia © 1997.

# 3 Cordocentesis

Stanley M. Berry

## INTRODUCTION

Cordocentesis is the most popular method of gaining access to the fetal circulation. The first report of ultrasound-guided cordocentesis was published by Bang et al in 1982.[1] Previous attempts to gain access to the fetal circulation included puncture of placental vessels under x-ray guidance, which was performed in the 1950s by Bevie, as well as a case from Japan in 1972, in which the uterus was surgically opened in order to gain access to the umbilical cord. Other methods of gaining access to the fetal circulation include hepatocentesis, in which a needle is guided into the hepatic vein near the anterior fetal abdominal wall, and cardiocentesis, in which the fetal heart is punctured with a needle. Gaining access to the umbilical cord with a needle under ultrasound guidance is by far the most popular method of fetal blood sampling. This procedure is known by other names, including percutaneous umbilical blood sampling (PUBS) and funipuncture.

Rh isoimmunization was the original impetus for the development of cordocentesis. In the previously mentioned article published by Bang and associates,[1] they reported their experience with the use of this technique in the management of three patients with fetal hemolytic disease secondary to maternal Rh isoimmunization. In this report, a spinal needle was inserted into the umbilical cord under direct ultrasound guidance and fetal blood was aspirated. This allowed a direct assessment of the fetal hemoglobin. They proceeded to use the needle as a port for a fetal intravascular blood transfusion. Until this time, the assessment of fetal hemoglobin level was almost always done using $\Delta OD_{450}$ measurements of amniotic fluid bilirubin content. While this continues to be an acceptable method of managing pregnancies complicated by red-cell isoimmunization, it provides only an indirect assessment of fetal hemoglobin/hematocrit levels. However, even in the most experienced centers, this method is associated with up to a 9% margin of error.[2] In addition, the accuracy of this method has been challenged when it is used prior to 27 weeks' gestation[3] or in pregnancies complicated by atypical red-cell isoimmunizations.[4] By transfusing blood directly into the umbilical cord, Bang's group was the first to report direct fetal intravascular transfusion under ultrasound guidance. Prior to this time, almost all fetal transfusions were accomplished by placing a Touhey needle into the fetal peritoneal cavity either under x-ray or ultrasound guidance and then transfusing the blood into the peritoneal cavity. This method, while effective in nonhydropic fetuses, has little efficacy once the fetus develops gross hydrops. The lack of efficacy in hydropic fetuses is thought to be due to the decreased amount of diaphragmatic movement that is characteristic of hydropic fetuses. Apparently, unhindered diaphragmatic excursion, which occurs during fetal breathing movements, is necessary for the absorption of red blood cells into the lymphatic system, which results in their eventual addition to the circulating blood volume of the fetus.

## INDICATIONS

While red-cell isoimmunization, including but not limited to Rh isoimmunization, continues to be the primary indication for cordocentesis, there are many other medical indications for

**TABLE 3–1. INDICATIONS FOR CORDOCENTESIS**

| |
|---|
| Red-cell isoimmunization |
| Platelet isoimmunization, rapid karyotype |
| Diagnosis of fetal infection |
| Determination of inherited B-cell deficiency diseases (*e.g.*, X-linked agammaglobulinemia) |
| Prediction of neonatal renal function |
| Evaluation of fetal hydrops |
| Direct injection of drugs into the fetal circulation |

which cordocentesis has been shown to be helpful in either diagnosis or treatment (Table 3–1). The list of indications for cordocentesis has grown tremendously in the fourteen years since the technique was first described. The advent of DNA probe techniques has hastened the replacement of some indications for fetal blood sampling with less invasive techniques such as amniocentesis or CVS. Given that ultrasound guided cordocentesis is almost impossible prior to 16 weeks and is not routinely performed prior to 18 weeks, DNA investigations that can be performed using amniocytes or syncytiotrophoblasts are attractive because amniocentesis or CVS can be done significantly earlier in gestation than cordocentesis. Examples of medical conditions in which a diagnosis can be made using DNA probe technology include fetal blood type determination[5] and fetal platelet antigen status in platelet alloimmunized pregnancies.[6] In addition, new technologies are now available on a research basis that may in fact replace the need for cordocentesis, amniocentesis, or CVS in some medical conditions for which they are now used. Examples include fetal blood type determination[7] and fetal karyotype determination,[8] both of which can be accomplished by fetal nucleated red cells isolated from the maternal circulation.

As some of these new genetic technologies replace some of the "traditional" indications for fetal blood sampling, other indications are being added. Examples of new indications include the prediction of neonatal renal function with the use of fetal serum $\beta_2$-microglobulin in cases of fetal urinary tract anomalies diagnosed by ultrasound.[9] It is also important to realize that for many inherited conditions that now lend themselves to prenatal diagnoses with DNA probe technology, a definitive diagnosis cannot be made without genetic material from family members. When DNA from affected family members is not available, for instance with hemophilia A, cordocentesis may still be required to make the diagnosis phenotypically. Because of the risk of spontaneous mutations and the need for DNA from an affected family member, it may be preferable to do a fetal blood sample to determine whether fetal factor VIII levels are within the normal range for a given gestational age. Table 3–1 includes a list of current indications for cordocentesis. By nature, these indications, in some cases, are dictated both by the preference of the care giver as well as the availability of alternative methods of making a diagnosis.

In combination with amniocentesis, cordocentesis continues to provide some diagnostic capabilities in the setting of possible fetal infection.[10] Although it is true that amniotic fluid culture and polymerase chain reaction (PCR) technology are now available for infections such as cytomegalovirus and toxoplasmosis, these modalities have not yet completely replaced fetal blood sampling. While the PCR technologies hold the promise of accurate and less invasive methods of diagnosis using amniocytes or syncitiotrophoblasts, cordocentesis continues to provide not only a means of diagnosing the presence of intrauterine infection, but also a means of determining how severely a fetus might be *affected* by infection. In addition, when ultrasonic signs raise the possibility of fetal infection, commonly one may not be able to determine the specific type of infection. In these cases, specific and nonspecific fetal blood parameters may be very helpful in determining first whether an infection is present and second what microbe is responsible. The nonspecific markers of fetal infection include altered liver function tests ($\gamma$-glutamyltranspeptidase [GGT], Alanine aminotransferase [ALT], Aspantate aminotransferase [AST]), anemia, thrombocytopenia, elevated nonspecific immunoglobulin-M (IgM), and alterations of fetal lymphocyte subsets.[11] Specific markers of fetal infection include IgM to specific infectious agents such as toxoplasmosis or cytomegalovirus. Fetal lymphocytes provide an excellent means of performing PCR testing if a specific infectious organism is suspected and PCR is available for the organism. It is possible that levels of the nonspecific markers outlined above can be consistent with an in utero infection, but specific markers are negative. When this situation occurs, a diagnosis of infection can be made even though the specific type of infection may remain unknown. This information may be quite helpful in counseling the parents regarding options available for the continued management of their pregnancy.

Because reference ranges now exist for levels of B-cells in the fetal circulation,[12] it is possible to diagnose several conditions, characterized by B-cell deficiencies, by performing flow cytometry on cordocentesis specimens and determining whether the percentages of B-cells are in the normal range for a given gestational age. In our institution this method allowed us to make an accurate prenatal diagnosis of Bruton's agammaglobulinemia. In this case the required DNA material from an affected family member was not available, thus making a diagnosis with DNA probe technology impossible.

Cordocentesis has rapidly increased our knowledge of fetal human physiology over the last thirteen years. Most of this information was derived from populations of fetuses who were sampled for medical indications. Because the safety record of this procedure has been excellent in centers where a large amount of experience has been gained,[13,14] recently cordocentesis has been used under Internal Review Board approved protocols for research into conditions such as preterm labor.[15] The results of further research facilitated by fetal blood sampling may truly advance our understanding of both normal fetal physiology and fetal disease states in the coming years.

In summary, the list of indications for cordocentesis is a dynamic one that will continue to change. Although there may come a time in the foreseeable future when the list of indications is greatly decreased, circumstances that limit the usefulness of DNA probe technology, the need for rapid fetal karyotype information, and the diagnosis and treatment of red cell and platelet isoimmunizations will all continue to ensure a place for cordocentesis in fetal medicine for many years to come.

## TECHNIQUE

Ultrasound-guided aspiration of fetal blood from the umbilical cord can be accomplished safely and effectively in a number of ways. The technique can be performed by having a sonographer "guide" for the operator, or the operator can hold the ultrasound transducer in one hand and direct the needle with the other. The advantage of the former technique is that the operator has a hand free to attach and detach syringes as blood is aspirated, or to connect tubing in the case of a fetal transfusion, once needle placement in the cord has been accomplished. The sonographer-guided technique has the disadvantage that needle placement is a bit more difficult for the operator. It is analogous to operating a motor vehicle with one person in control of the steering wheel while someone else is in control of the brakes and accelerator. However, like most medical procedures, this technique works well for those who have a preference for it. As one gains experience, it can be carried out both safely and very effectively.

The alternative method, as mentioned above, is the single operator free hand technique as described by Nicolaides et al,[16] in which the physician controls both the ultrasound transducer and the needle. Cordocentesis done this way is called a "6-handed procedure" because the operator finds the target and places the needle but then needs the two hands of an assistant to remove the trocar, place the syringes, aspirate blood, and connect tubing. The advantage of this technique is that the physician is able to find the target and, more easily, make any fine adjustments in needle direction that are required as the needle is inserted through the abdominal wall into the uterus and finally into the cord. This technique is easier for the operator to adapt to stereoscopically. Once mastered, it is highly effective. The disadvantage is that, with this technique, an assistant must learn to be extremely gentle with syringes and tubing that come in contact with the hub of the needle. Furthermore, the operator must be very conscious of his or her finger position on the needle hub so as not to obstruct the placement and removal of equipment. The remaining two hands are those of a second assistant (with either technique) who needs to be in the room to accept blood specimens as they are handed off, to provide any additional equipment, and to help ensure patient comfort.

## Preparation

The mother should be fully informed of the risks of this procedure, including the 1–2% risk of fetal death.[13,14]

In our institution we write a description of the procedure on the consent form using layman's terms, including a quotation of the 1–2% risk of fetal death. We have the mother sign directly across this description, as well as at the bottom of the form.

There is no specific need for maternal fasting prior to the procedure. However, if the patient is at a point in the pregnancy in which the fetus is viable and a cesarean section would be carried out for a non-reassuring fetal heart rate pattern, then it may be prudent to tell the mother not to eat several hours prior to the procedure. For all viable fetuses we perform the procedure directly adjacent to the labor and delivery unit. If an immediate cesarean section is indicated we are never more than several feet from the operating suite.

Because of the risk of inducing intra- or extrauterine infection with cordocentesis, we recommend the use of antibiotic coverage before and after the procedure for patients who have blood sampling done remote from term. We place either a heplock or an IV line. One gram of a first-generation cephalosporin with staphylococcal coverage is infused. Following the procedure, we prescribe a first-generation oral cephalosporin for 2–3 days. Since initiating this policy we have had no known procedure related infections.

## Sedation

Though sedation is not essential for this procedure, we have found that IV Diazepam and morphine are quite helpful, especially when the operator is relatively inexperienced. We use an IV dose for most women of 7 mg of Diazepam and 7 mg of IV morphine. Of over 400 cases where IV sedation was used, we have had no maternal respiratory difficulties. Using sedation in this way has two advantages; it calms the mother for what can, in some instances, be a painful procedure. It also helps to decrease fetal movement that can obstruct the intended target for needle insertion. Although at term we often dispense with the IV sedation, it is particularly helpful at early gestational ages. One of the motivations for not using sedation at term is that if an emergency cesarean section is done, there is no depressant effect on the newborn from sedative and analgesic drugs.

## Anesthesia

One percent lidocaine is used as a local anesthetic in all procedures that are carried out by our group. We use a 1 cc tuberculin syringe to anesthetize the skin and then use a 22-gauge $1\frac{1}{2}$-inch needle and 5–10 cc of 1% lidocaine to anesthetize the subcutaneous layers down the uterine wall. The lidocaine has both a local anesthetizing effect and, we believe, some psychological effect in decreasing the pain of the procedure for the mother.

## Equipment

The equipment that we prepare in a sterile fashion for this procedure is as follows: Five 1 cc tuberculin syringes, two 5 cc syringes with a 22-gauge, $1\frac{1}{2}$-inch needle for one and a 21-gauge,

$1\frac{1}{2}$-inch needle for the other. We also lay out a 20 cc syringe with an attached IV extension tubing and a 10 cc syringe. We have six gauze 4×4s on the table, as well as a 22-gauge, 5-inch spinal needle. We also have both 100% isopropyl alcohol and a Betadine surgical prep kit for the cleansing of the abdomen prior to the procedure. One pack of sterile gel is also placed on the table.

The above list is meant as a guide to the type and amount of equipment that can be used for the procedure. As one gains experience, additions and subtractions can be made to that list. The 1 cc tuberculin syringes are packaged with a 25-gauge needle attached to them. We fill one of these syringes with 1% lidocaine. Two of the other 1 cc syringes are flushed with a 1 : 10,000 solution of heparin. Care is taken not to leave a visible amount of heparin in the syringe prior to aspirating blood. The needles are removed from the two remaining 1 cc syringes. It is important to note that we leave the needles in place with covers on the two heparinized 1 cc syringes in order to make it known to the assistant that these are the heparinized syringes. The two syringes without needles are the unheparinized 1 cc syringes. This enables us to avoid confusion at the time of the actual procedure. We attach the 22-gauge, $1\frac{1}{2}$-inch needle to one of the 5 cc syringes and fill it with 1% lidocaine. This syringe is then kept in close proximity to the 1 cc syringe that was previously filled with lidocaine. We specifically use the 22-gauge needle for the 5 cc syringe that is filled with 1% lidocaine every time because, in the midst of the procedure, one can identify the syringe by the color of the hub of the needle and there is no confusion between this syringe and the second 5 cc syringe that is filled with injectable normal saline. The second 5 cc syringe is then tipped with a 21-gauge, $1\frac{1}{2}$-inch needle. The hub of this needle is green and we use the mnemonic "green for saline" to unequivocally distinguish this syringe.

It should be noted that if a transfusion is going to be performed we add the following equipment. A three-way stop cock and a 5 cc or 10 cc syringe fitted to one port of a three-way stop cock. A piece of IV extension tubing is then applied to the stop cock on one of the two remaining ports. This tubing is applied in such a way that the end with the locking sleeve is left free to later be attached to the hub of the cordocentesis needle. The remaining port on the stop cock is connected to another piece of IV extension tubing, which is then connected to the IV tubing from the bag containing the transfusate, either blood or platelets. Figure 3–1 shows a table laid out for a simple cordocentesis and Figure 3–2 shows a table laid out for an intrauterine fetal transfusion. For a transfusion we also prepare extra unheparinized 1 cc

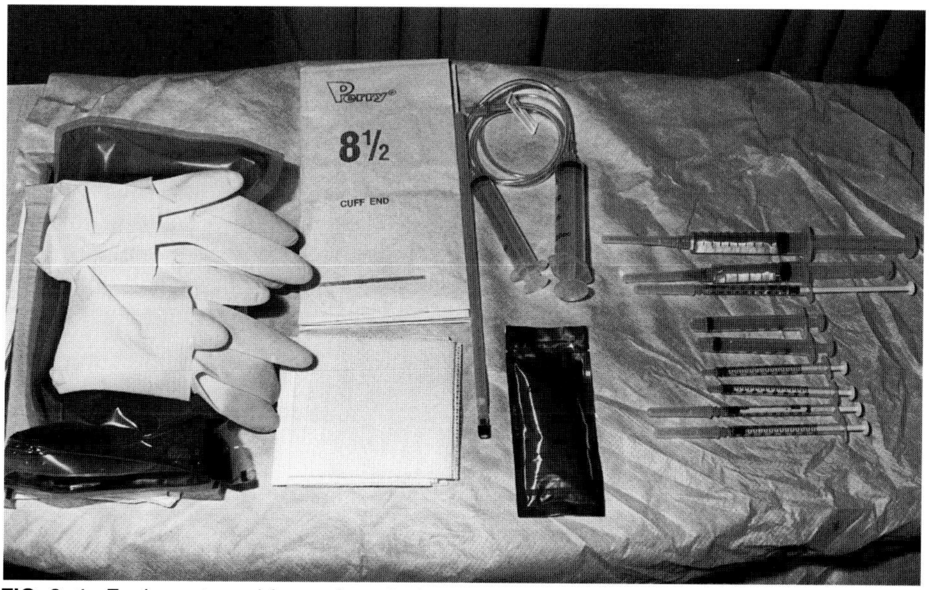


**FIG. 3–1.** Equipment used for cordocentesis.

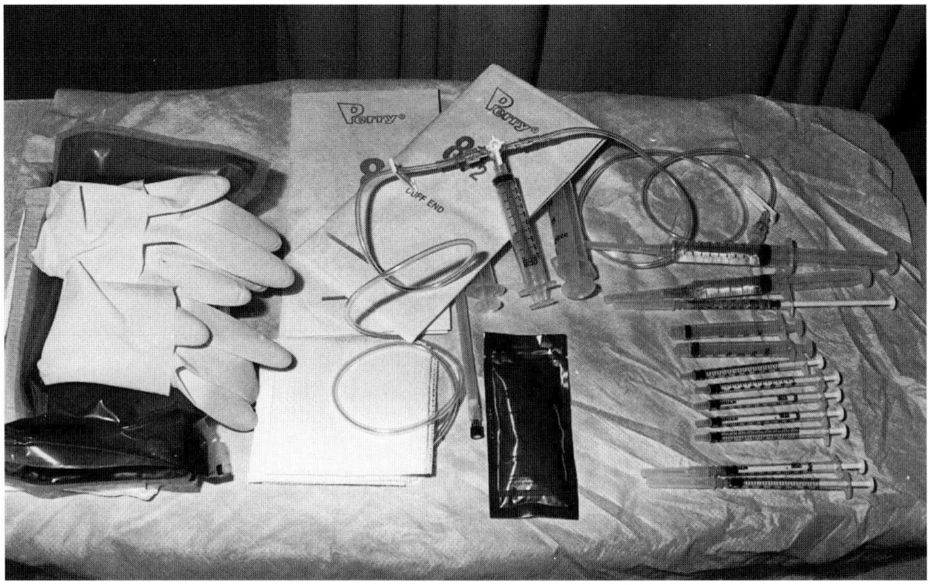

**FIG. 3–2.** Equipment used for intrauterine intravascular transfusions.

syringes without needles in order that additional samples can be taken at various points through the transfusion to determine the hemoglobin level achieved in the fetus.

## PREPARATION OF THE MATERNAL ABDOMEN

We begin by pouring warmed, 100% isopropyl alcohol over the entire abdomen. We then fan the abdomen to facilitate the evaporation of the alcohol. This leads to desiccation of bacteria on the skin. After the alcohol has dried, we use a Betadine surgical solution prep and coat the abdomen with the solution four times. We apply two coats of Betadine solution and then apply a sterile drape to absorb the excess Betadine. Two additional coats are applied and another sterile sheet is used to absorb the excess.

## ULTRASONOGRAPHY

Continuous real-time two-dimensional ultrasonography is essential to perform cordocentesis successfully. The technique can be accomplished with either a linear array, sector, or curvilinear transducer. We perform all of our procedures with a 3.5 megahertz curvilinear transducer. The field of visualization obtainable with the linear, sector, and curvilinear transducers is displayed in Figs. 3–3, 3–4, and 3–5. As depicted in Figs. 3–3 and 3–4, neither the linear nor the sector transducers allow a large visualization of the near field or the space between the maternal abdominal wall and the intended target. With experience, one can learn to perform this procedure successfully despite this lack of optimal near-field visualization. However, as depicted in Figs. 3–5 and 3–6, the curvilinear transducer allows one to get maximum near-field visualization while maintaining the intended target in view throughout most procedures. With either the linear or sector transducer, often one must move the transducer to bring the near field into view. This motion often does not allow one to keep the target in view. This advantage of the curvilinear transducer cannot be overemphasized. By having good visualization of the near field throughout as much of the needle placement portion of the procedure as possible, one can continuously make small adjustments in the angle and direction of the needle as it is

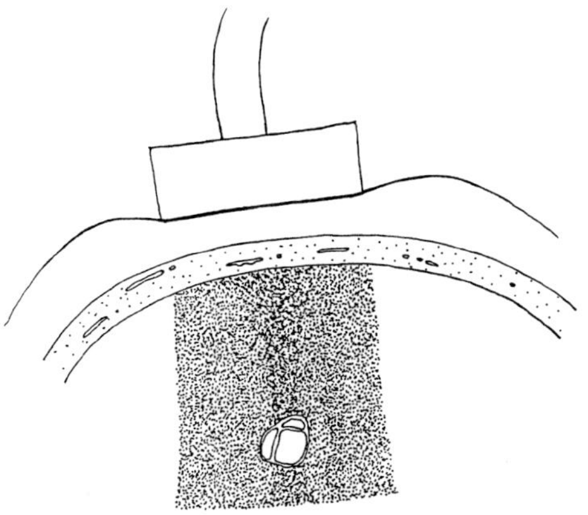

**FIG. 3–3.** Linear transducer field of visualization.

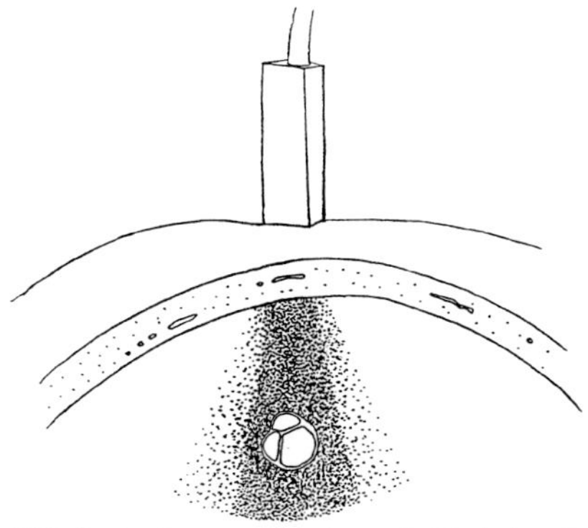

**FIG. 3–4.** Sector transducer field of visualization.

inserted closer to the target. If it is not possible to visualize the target and the needle simultaneously during insertion and, instead, the transducer must be moved to visualize the near field, the chance increases that when one goes back to bring the target into view, the placement of the needle will be off the intended path by a considerable degree. Because the curvilinear transducer, depicted in Fig. 3–6, allows for both optimal near-field and target visualization simultaneously in most cases, with a minimum amount of transducer movement, it is possible to see the tip of the needle almost immediately after it pierces the skin while keeping the target in view the entire time.

Traversing a placenta may slightly increase the complication rate and one should endeavor to avoid this whenever possible. If a transplacental approach is contemplated during the ultrasound examination, it is important to note any vessels on the chorionic plate and any placental lakes adjacent to the chorionic plate. Care must be taken to avoid puncturing these structures. They do not contain Wharton's gel and, if punctured, they can bleed profusely. It must be emphasized that it is not necessary to insert the needle at the placental umbilical cord insertion in every case. The needle can be inserted in any portion of the umbilical cord that is stable. This may be a segment of cord that is trapped between the fetal body and the uterine wall. It is possible with enough experience to gain facility with inserting the needle into a free loop or segment of floating cord. Inserting the needle successfully into a free loop of cord does take a considerable degree of experience on the part of the operator, and this technique should probably not be attempted until the operator has gained considerable experience with the procedure in general. It is possible to insert the needle at or near the fetal abdominal umbilical cord insertion also. Three potential insertion sites are shown in Figs. 3–7, 3–8, and 3–9. Fig. 3–7 shows a stable segment of cord, Fig. 3–8 shows the placental umbilical cord

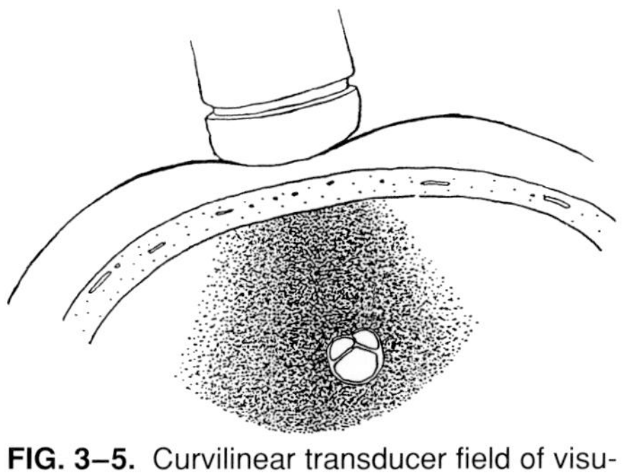

**FIG. 3–5.** Curvilinear transducer field of visualization.

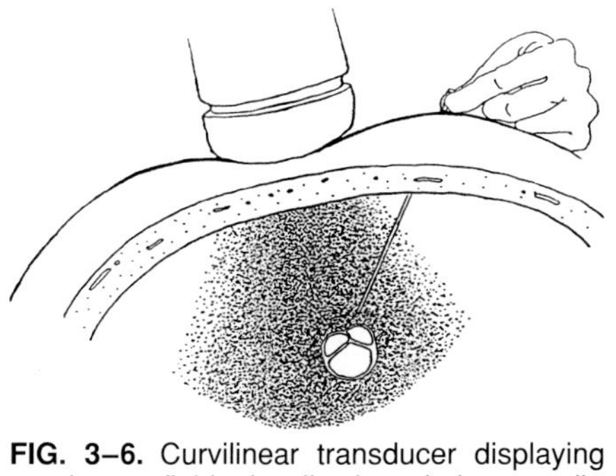

**FIG. 3–6.** Curvilinear transducer displaying good near-field visualization during needle placement.

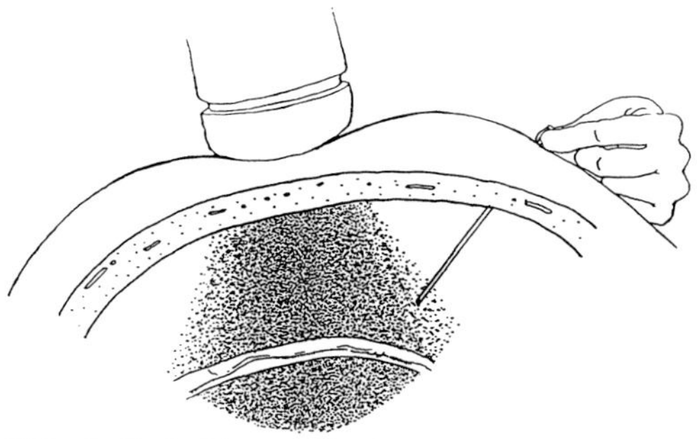

**FIG. 3–7.** Stable umbilical cord segment as intended target site with a complete transamniotic needle approach.

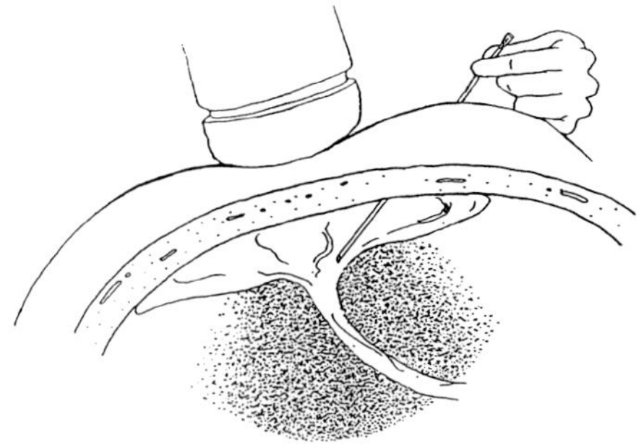

**FIG. 3–8.** Anterior placenta and umbilical cord insertion site with a complete transplacental needle approach.

insertion site with an anterior placenta and a complete transplacental approach, and Fig. 3–9 shows an anterior placenta with the umbilical cord insertion site and a transamniotic approach.

## ULTRASOUND EXAMINATION

A thorough ultrasound examination of the intrauterine contents is essential prior to beginning the procedure. This is the single most important part of this technique. As the scan is performed, the operator should become familiar with the spatial relations of potential target sites for needle insertion in the umbilical cord as well as the position of the fetus relative to possible insertion sites and the position of the placenta. This examination should be carried out prior to the sterile abdominal prep and again after the abdominal prep is finished. Once a suitable cord segment

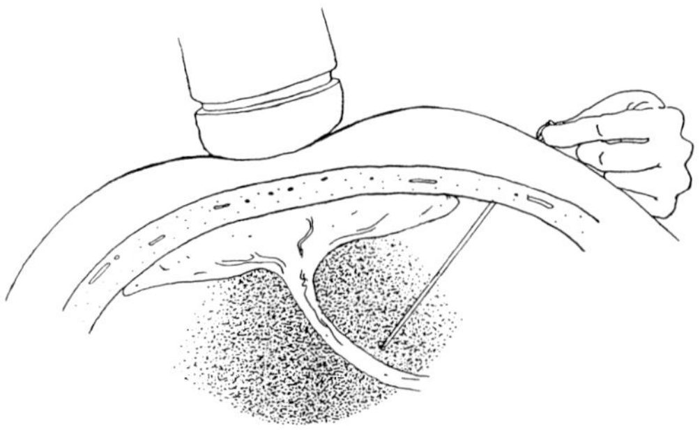

**FIG. 3–9.** Anterior placenta and umbilical cord insertion site with a complete transamniotic needle approach.

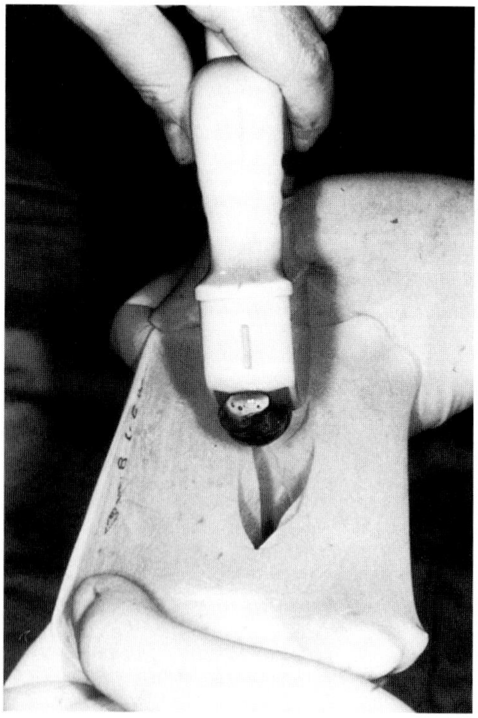

**FIG. 3–10.** Curvilinear transducer covered with non-sterile ultrasound gel being placed into a sterile glove.

has been visualized, the transducer is lined up such that the needle insertion can be done just off the end of the transducer as illustrated in Fig. 3–9.

It is most helpful to always align the image direction on the ultrasound machine in such a way that the actual direction that the needle travels during insertion is the same on the maternal abdomen as it is displayed on the ultrasound screen. To accomplish this, the image direction button on the ultrasound machine should be set such that the direction of the needle visualized on the screen is always moving away from the operator and toward the target, just as it is on the maternal abdomen. This greatly improves the spatial conception that the operator has of the needle and the intrauterine contents. To set the image in the opposite direction means that, for example, on the abdomen the needle tip is moving away from the operator while on the ultrasound image display it would be moving toward the operator. This can be very confusing and therefore should be avoided. If the ultrasound does not have an image direction button, this ''consistency of image'' can be accomplished by simply turning the transducer 180°, such that the opposite end of the transducer now visualizes the near field. One should always check for the image direction by using a finger to push in on the abdomen at the intended needle site, just off the end of the transducer, and checking the direction of the finger indentation as it shows up on the ultrasound screen.

After performing the first evaluation of the uterine contents to get a good grasp of where the optimal potential insertion sites are located, maternal sedation, if indicated, should be given. The sterile abdominal prep should then be carried out.

Although covering the transducer is not essential if a sterile ''no touch'' technique is used for the actual skin insertion site, we sterilely glove our transducers for the actual procedure in an attempt to decrease the risk of microbial contamination. There are a number of sterile transducer covers available on the market. However, we have found these to be quite expensive and no better than covering the transducer with a sterile surgical glove. This is accomplished by covering the end of the transducer with a layer of non-sterile gel and then, as depicted in Figs. 3–10, 3–11, 3–12, and 3–13, an assistant holds the transducer and places it into a sterile glove held by a gloved operator. Three of the fingers of the glove are then laid on the side of

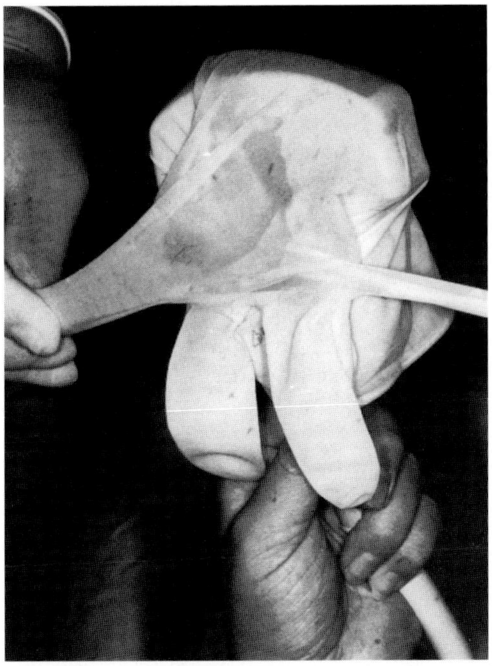

**FIG. 3–11.** Curvilinear transducer with 3 fingers of sterile glove laid against the side while the remaining fingers are stretched prior to being tied.

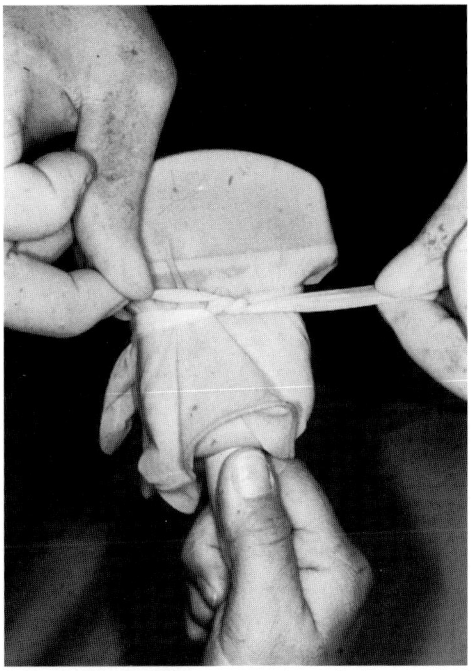

**FIG. 3–12.** Curvilinear transducer being secured inside a sterile glove.

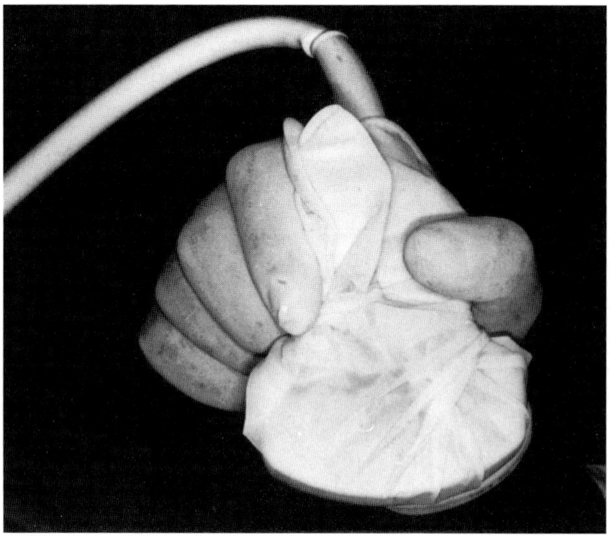

**FIG. 3–13.** Curvilinear transducer securely covered by a sterile glove and ready for use.

the transducer and the remaining two fingers are stretched and pulled around the base of the transducer and tied in such a way that the three fingers that were laid against the side of the transducer are tied down. This secures the glove to the transducer in such a way that it will not detach or loosen during the procedure. Sterile gel is then used on the maternal abdomen after the alcohol and Betadine prep has been done.

The uterine contents should be evaluated with ultrasound again using the gloved transducer with attention to which potential insertion sites are optimal. This second scan is important because usually, after maternal sedation and sterile abdominal preparation, fetal movements are at a minimum and the final intended insertion site can be chosen.

## A STEP–BY–STEP DESCRIPTION OF THE PROCEDURE

1. An explanation of the risks and benefits of cordocentesis is given to the mother and written informed consent is obtained.
2. A heplock or an IV is started and one dose of an antibiotic with staphylococcal coverage is then given.
3. A thorough ultrasound is done to evaluate the spatial relationships of the intrauterine contents and, particularly, to choose an appropriate site on the umbilical cord for needle insertion.
4. If maternal sedation is to be used, it is given.
5. The abdomen is sterilely prepped with alcohol and betadine.
6. The transducer is covered with non-sterile gel and an assistant places it in a sterile cover held by the operator wearing sterile gloves. The operator then secures the glove on the transducer.
7. Sterile gel is placed on the abdomen.
8. The final site for needle insertion is chosen.
9. Once the site is chosen the operator stabilizes the transducer position and does not move it.
10. Fingers are used to indent the abdomen and care is taken to ensure that the image direction and the actual direction of needle movement on the abdomen are consistent.
11. With the transducer hand "frozen" in position by the operator, the 1% lidocaine is then used to anesthetize the intended percutaneous and subcutaneous site of needle insertion.

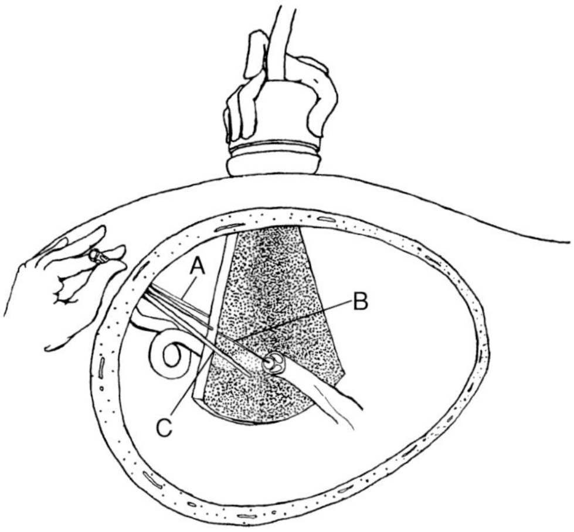


**FIG. 3–14.** Curvilinear plane of visualization with an example of proper needle position within the plane (B) and improper needle position outside the plane (A, C).

**12.** A 22-gauge, 5-inch needle is then inserted at a slight downward angle from the transducer. The needle is inserted just off the end of the transducer precisely aligned with the exact mid-point in the width of the end of the transducer. This keeps the needle in the transducer plane of visualization, as depicted in Fig. 3–14. The tip of the needle is directly visualized just after it is inserted under the maternal skin line. This is an important point. The operator must adopt a rule that the needle is not advanced more than approximately 1 inch unless the needle tip is clearly visualized on the ultrasound screen. This point can not be overemphasized. One must become brutally honest in visualizing the tip of the needle. If one advances the needle without it being under direct visualization, the chances of the tip of the needle winding up away from the target or accidently piercing a vessel on the placental surface, if the placenta is traversed, is increased. The needle can be moved back and forth laterally to bring the tip of the needle into view on the ultrasound machine. When this is done, tissue motion must not be confused for clear visualization of the needle tip. Another point to be emphasized is that one should find the transducer with the needle and not find the needle with the transducer. This means that one freezes the ultrasound transducer in position and does not move it. If one attempts to carry out the procedure by moving both the transducer and the needle in an attempt to bring the needle into view on the ultrasound screen, the target is often lost and the tip of the needle is much more difficult to visualize.

**13.** Once the needle is visualized, it is advanced down into the amniotic fluid, if a complete or partial transamniotic approach is taken.

**14.** At this point, the trocar is removed and the tip of the empty 1 cc syringe that was previously used for the first lidocaine injection can now be attached to the hub of the needle and an attempt can be made to aspirate amniotic fluid with this syringe. Once amniotic fluid is drawn back and one feels confident that it is free of blood, the 1 cc syringe is removed and the tubing that is attached to the 20 cc syringe is attached to the hub. If the end of the tubing has a sleeve lock attached to it, there is no need to screw the sleeve down to lock it onto the hub for the amniotic fluid aspiration. The tip of the tubing is inserted into the hub and gently turned approximately 30° to ensure that the seal is complete. Amniotic fluid can then be aspirated into the 20 cc syringe. Once it is full, the syringe can be detached and the 10 cc syringe can be attached to the tubing and filled with amniotic fluid. Once this is accomplished, the tubing can be removed from the needle hub and the trocar can be placed back into the needle.

**15.** The needle is then advanced down to the umbilical vein and the vein is punctured with the needle.

16. The 1 cc syringe that was used originally to aspirate amniotic fluid is emptied of its contents and reattached to the needle hub and used for a test to ensure that blood can be aspirated. Approximately 0.25 cc of blood is then aspirated into this 1 cc syringe to ensure that a pure specimen is now being obtained and also to clear the shaft and hub of the needle of any amniotic fluid that may be present.
17. At this point, we attach one of the 3 cc syringes and aspirate until the syringe is full. This is then detached and handed off. A 1 cc syringe that has been flushed with heparin is then attached to the hub of the needle and filled. This syringe is then detached and handed off. Another 3 cc syringe can be attached at this point and filled. We take between 4 cc and 8 cc of blood, depending on the gestational age. After 24 weeks it is possible to take up to 8 cc of blood. We have not had any complications from taking these amounts of blood.
18. After the final specimen is aspirated into the syringe, the syringe is detached. The syringe filled with normal saline can then be attached after a drop of saline is dripped into the chamber of the hub to clear any air that is in the chamber. A small amount of blood is first aspirated into the syringe to ensure that the needle is still seated in the umbilical vein. At this point, the normal saline can be infused into the umbilical vein for volume replacement. While volume replacement is not essential, we carry this out after the majority of procedures. If the needle should become dislodged before this is carried out, we do not replace the needle in the umbilical cord simply to replace volume.
19. The needle is now removed from the umbilical cord and the segment of the cord is visualized for several minutes to ensure that any bleeding from the cord stops in a timely fashion.

It is important to note that if a procedure extends more than approximately 5 minutes after the needle is inserted into the cord, or if multiple attempts are needed to accomplish cord puncture, the fetal heart rate must be assessed to ensure that it appears normal on the ultrasound screen. Of course, this may necessitate moving the transducer to visualize fetal cardiac motion. The transducer is then quickly moved back in the original position, and it is frozen there until needle placement in the cord is accomplished.

## Needle Guide

With most modern ultrasound transducers it is possible to obtain a device known as a needle guide. This apparatus is manufactured in such a way that it fits directly onto the ultrasound transducer. It is then possible to determine precisely the intended course of the needle from the needle guide apparatus to the point of intended insertion on the umbilical cord. This path is illustrated on the ultrasound screen. The device holds the needle and forces it to be inserted in a fixed direction. Some workers in this field feel that the needle guide is safer and more efficacious than the free-hand technique that is described in this chapter. While it is true that the needle guide may offer some advantages, particularly for less experienced operators, once the fundamentals of the free-hand technique are mastered, it holds several advantages over using a needle guide. The needle guide can be relatively difficult to position. Furthermore, if the fetus moves or changes position, the needle guide can be cumbersome to realign for proper needle placement. Those people who routinely use the needle guide and are comfortable with it believe that it is a very helpful aid. While we do not use this device in our institution, we acknowledge that for some physicians this apparatus may prove to be a useful adjunct to the performance of the procedure.

## Post-Procedure Observation

After the needle is removed, we watch the fetus with ultrasound for approximately 5 minutes to ensure that there are no bradycardias or bleeding problems. In over 1,000 procedures we have never had a cord hemorrhage complication from this procedure. However, we have had two transfusion-related fetal deaths, both of which were associated with clot formation in the umbilical cord. It is remarkable that even in fetuses with alloimmune thrombocytopenia who had platelet counts as low as 3,000 we have never had a cord hemorrhage following a cordocentesis procedure. The Wharton gel in the cord as well as factors in the amniotic fluid have been shown to have procoagulant effects. It is also theorized that the intra-amniotic pressure helps to control bleeding from the puncture site. All of these factors make the procedure potentially very safe if it can be carried out quickly with a minimum of cord trauma.

After the fetus has been observed on ultrasound for approximately 5 minutes to ensure that there are no fetal bradycardias or hemorrhages from the cord, if the fetus is pre-viable, the mother can be allowed to go home when the effects of the sedation have worn off and she is able to ambulate safely. If the fetus is at a viable gestational age, we usually observe the mothers in the labor and delivery unit on a fetal monitor for 1–2 hours. If the fetus is beyond 32 weeks, we do not discharge the patient until the fetal heart rate strip is clearly reactive. It is important to be cognizant of the fact that if the mother received IV sedation the fetal heart rate tracing may appear flat for a prolonged period of time. As long as there are no frank decelerations, this should not be a concern. Also, it is important to note that if the fetus had a bradycardia during the procedure, once the bradycardia resolves, fetuses often have a period of tachycardia in the 170–180 range that may last for an hour or more. Again, as long as there are no frank fetal heart rate decelerations and the fetal heart rate strip shows some reactivity after there has been time for the drugs to metabolize and their effects to resolve, this should not be a matter of concern.

### Procedure-Related Fetal Bradycardias

It is important to realize that if the fetus becomes bradycardic during or just after the procedure, the vast majority of these bradycardias resolve spontaneously. We routinely wait at least 5 minutes for bradycardias to resolve and have waited as long as 10 minutes. It is safe to wait for this period of time as long as the trend of the fetal heart rate is in an upward direction. A fetus can maintain cardiac output at a rate of 80 bpm. The decision to observe or proceed to cesarean section requires a lot of clinical judgment. Of course, these issues should be discussed with the mother prior to initiating the procedure, particularly if the fetus is hydropic or otherwise appears moribund and the chances for a successful outcome even with cesarean section are small.

There are several measures that one can take to help support a bradycardic fetus, which possibly help the bradycardia to resolve. The procedure should be done in an area where oxygen is available. If the fetus becomes bradycardic, the needle is removed and maternal oxygen therapy is initiated by mask at 10 L. The mother is asked to lie in the left lateral position. Some workers in this field have suggested that IV atropine in a dose of 0.4 mg should be given to the mother to help resolve a fetal bradycardia. We have used this technique but have not found it to be particularly helpful. In our experience bradycardias are frequently accompanied by uterine contractions that may be tetanic. For this reason we will often give 0.25 mg of terbutaline IV push. This helps to relax the uterus and may in fact help relieve any spasm in the umbilical cord arteries. Umbilical artery spasm is believed to be the cause of most procedure-related fetal bradycardias. This fact is the basis for avoiding puncture of the umbilical arteries whenever possible. The point to emphasize here is that the vast majority of fetal bradycardias resolve. In those fetuses for whom cesarean section would be indicated for a non-reassuring fetal heart rate pattern, one should wait at least 5 minutes before embarking on cesarean delivery. Again, clinical judgment is key in making this decision.

## CONTRAINDICATIONS

We are not aware of any absolute contraindications in performing cordocentesis as described herein. There are, however, several relative contraindications. The first of these includes a lack of operator experience with needle-guided techniques. Although anyone with a reasonable degree of hand-eye coordination can learn to perform cordocentesis, people should be comfortable with general ultrasound principles and with the performance of amniocentesis procedures before attempting cordocentesis. A fetal gestational age below 18 weeks is a relative contraindication because of the difficulties that often accompany cordocentesis procedures done prior to this period during pregnancy. Those operators who have a large experience in performing the technique are able to perform this procedure at lower gestational ages. It should be kept in mind, however, that the umbilical cord is quite fragile at early gestational ages, and there is a greater chance of tearing the cord with small amounts of lateral needle movement.

Maternal systemic infections, particularly HIV, should be viewed as a relative contraindication to fetal blood sampling. Viscerill and associates examined the risk of enhancing vertical transmission of the HIV virus after the performance of amniocentesis or cordocentesis.[17] They concluded that these invasive procedures did not appear to increase the risk of fetal HIV infection. However, it must be noted that the number of patients in their study was small and the study population did not have the statistical power to make a definitive determination that indeed the procedure does not enhance the risk of vertical transmission.

## COMPLICATIONS

There are a number of complications that can accompany the cordocentesis procedure. In our experience, by far the most common complication is fetal bradycardia. As mentioned, this appears to be related to umbilical arterial spasm. For this reason, care should always be taken to avoid puncturing the umbilical arteries during the procedure. However, as mentioned above, should the fetus become bradycardic following the procedure, the vast majority of bradycardias resolve within 5–10 minutes. Operator experience and judgment must guide one in deciding whether to perform an emergency cesarean section for a procedure-related bradycardia.

Bleeding complications can accompany cordocentesis. These have not been a problem in our series of over 1,000 cases. By performing this procedure with a minimum number of cord punctures and taking care to minimize lateral needle movement either across the surface of the cord or once the needle is inserted into the cord, one can avoid most serious cord hemorrhages. If an umbilical artery is punctured in the course of doing the procedure, once the needle is removed, often one can observe gross streaming of blood from the cord into the amniotic fluid. This usually diminishes greatly after about 30 to 90 seconds; we have not had a complication related to bleeding, even in severely thrombocytopenic fetuses. It is noteworthy that whenever fetuses with a potential for alloimmune thrombocytopenia have cordocentesis performed, we always have maternal platelets available. As soon as a cordocentesis specimen is taken, platelet transfusion is initiated while we are waiting for the platelet count results. This is done to minimize the risk of bleeding complications from the cord.

Cord thrombosis is also a risk. The occurrence of this complication can be minimized by making every effort to avoid lateral movement of the needle on the surface of the cord or lateral movement once the needle is inserted into the cord. When transfusions of either platelets or red cells are undertaken, the risk of umbilical cord thrombosis can be minimized by minimizing lateral needle movement on or in the cord and also by being very sure of needle placement within the umbilical vein prior to pushing blood into the cord. If the needle is within the substance of the cord and not seated in the vessel, blood may be transfused into the Wharton's gel and cause a thrombosis, which can result in pressure and occlusion of both umbilical arteries.

In several fetuses that we have cared for that have undergone multiple intravascular transfusions into the umbilical cord, we have noted on ultrasound examination that one umbilical artery eventually thrombosed. This has not caused any problems in the fetuses in which it has occurred, but after this condition is recognized, one must be meticulous in placing the needle into the umbilical vein without traversing the remaining umbilical artery.

Occasionally, when mothers remain in the supine position for a considerable amount of time, they may develop symptoms of the supine hypotension syndrome. This is usually accompanied by a feeling of nausea and a need to vomit. This situation occurs particularly in obese women or women with large gravid uteri near term. It also occurs more frequently in women with multiple gestations or in women with gross polyhydramnios. One of the ways to minimize the occurrence of this syndrome is to find an appropriate place for needle insertion with the mother lying in the left lateral position. If this syndrome should occur once the needle is inserted into the uterus or into the umbilical cord, one must use judgment in either rapidly finishing the procedure or terminating the procedure and allowing the mother to assume the left lateral position, if she is supine, before she begins to vomit or move on the table in response to the feeling of nausea.

## CONCLUSION

Cordocentesis is a very useful adjunct to the practice of fetal medicine. It offers the opportunity for diagnosis in a wide variety of conditions. It also offers a chance for highly effective therapy in several fetal disease states. For operators who are able to gain a reasonable amount of experience in doing this procedure there is a real chance of reducing the risks in an otherwise non-moribund fetus to less than 0.5%. While several methods can be used to accomplish cordocentesis, the free-hand technique wherein the operator controls both the transducer and the needle, offers many advantages in terms of flexibility in finding a proper insertion site and the opportunity it provides for puncturing the cord in a very short time. It is our hope that this chapter offers some helpful guidance for the performance of this procedure; however, it must be emphasized that this chapter cannot be a substitute for training from an experienced operator for anybody who wishes to develop an expertise in performing cordocentesis.

## REFERENCES


1. Bang J, Bock JE, Trolle D. Ultrasound-guided fetal intravenous transfusion for severe rhesus haemolytic disease. BMJ 1982;284:373–374.
2. Bowman JM. Hemolytic disease (erythroblastosis fetalis). In: Creasy RK, Resnik R (eds). Maternal–fetal medicine (3rd ed). Philadelphia: WB Saunders, 1994:711–743.
3. Nicolaides KH, Rodeck CH, Mibashan RS, Kemp JR. Have Liley charts outlived their usefulness? Am J Obstet Gynecol 1986;155:90–94.
4. Berkowitz RL, Beyth Y, Sadovsky E. Death in utero due to Kell sensitization without excessive elevation of the $\Delta OD_{450}$ value in amniotic fluid. Obstet Gynecol 1982;60: 746–749.
5. Bennett PR, Le Van Kim C, Colin Y, Warwick RM, Cherif-Zahar B, Fisk NM, Cartron JP. Prenatal determination of fetal RhD type by DNA amplification. N Engl J Med 1993; 329:607–610.
6. Bennett PR, Warwick R, Vaughan J, Chana H, Lubenko A, Fisk NM. Prenatal determination of human platelet antigen type using DNA amplification following amniocentesis. Br J Obstet Gynaecol 1994;101:246–249.
7. Geifman-Holtzman O, Berstein IM, Berry SM, Holtzman EJ, Vadnais TJ, DeMaria MA, Bianchi DW. Fetal RhD genotyping in fetal cells flow sorted from maternal blood. Am J Obstet Gynecol 1996;174:818–822.
8. Bianchi DW, Mahr A, Zickwolf GK, Houseal TW, Flint AF, Klinger KW. Detection of fetal cells with 47,XX, +21 karyotype in maternal peripheral blood. Hum Genet 1992; 90:368–370.
9. Berry SM, Lecolier B, Smith RS, Bercau G, Dombrowski MP, Puder KS, Kithier K, Bidat L, Johnson MP, Cotton DB. Predictive value of fetal serum $\beta_2$-microglobulin for neonatal renal function. Lancet 1995;345:1277–1278.

10. Isada NB, Berry SM. In utero diagnosis of congenital infection. In: Gonik B (ed). Viral diseases in pregnancy (1st ed). New York: Springer-Verlag, 1994:24–49.
11. Thilaganathan B, Carroll SG, Plachouras N, Makrydimas G, Nicolaides KH. Fetal immunological and haematological changes in intrauterine infection. Br J Obstet Gynaecol 1994; 101:418–421.
12. Berry SM, Fine N, Bichalski JA, Cotton DB, Dombrowski MP, Kaplan J. Circulating lymphocyte subsets in second and third-trimester fetuses: comparison with newborns and adults. Am J Obstet Gynecol 1992;167:895–900.
13. Daffos F, Capella-Pavlovsky M, Forestier F. Fetal blood sampling during pregnancy with use of a needle guided by ultrasound: a study of 606 consecutive cases. Am J Obstet Gynecol 1985;153:655–660.
14. Ghidini A, Sepulveda W, Lockwood CJ, Romero R. Complications of fetal blood sampling. Am J Obstet Gynecol 1993;168:1339–1344.
15. Berry SM, Romero R, Gomez R, Puder KS, Ghezzi F, Cotton DB, Bianchi DW. Premature parturition is characterized by in utero activation of the fetal immune system. Am J Obstet Gynecol 1995;173:315–320.
16. Nicolaides KH, Soothill PW, Rodeck CH, Campbell S. Ultrasound-guided sampling of umbilical cord and placental blood to assess fetal wellbeing. Lancet 1986;1:1065–1067.
17. Viscarello RR, DeGennaro NJ, Griffith SM, Andiman W, Hobbins JC. Does an antepartum invasive procedure increase the risk of perinatal transmission of HIV-1? Am J Obstet Gynecol 1992;166:394.

*Invasive Outpatient Procedures in Reproductive Medicine,* edited by Mark I. Evans, et al. Lippincott–Raven Publishers, Philadelphia © 1997.

# 4 Embryoscopy

Yves Dumez, Jean-Francois Oury, Marc Dommergues

## INTRODUCTION

Of all the newly developed prenatal diagnostic techniques, none has had more emotional impact than visualization of actual fetal form fetoscopically in utero.[1–4] The original development of fetoscopy in the 1970s was particularly dramatic because ultrasound images were very poor, and, by comparison, the fetoscopic images were very clear.[5] Unfortunately, the quality of the optics was overall very poor, and the technique was largely abandoned in the early 1980s in favor of the steadily improving images seen on ultrasound.[6]

In the early 1990s, technological leaps in fiberoptics have again made fetoscopy or embryoscopy (depending on gestational age) feasible with the potential for extremely clear images.[1–4] Exactly what role direct visualization of the fetus will have in the overall armamentarium of prenatal diagnosis remains to be seen. Important factors will include its accuracy, costs, and risks.

## INDICATIONS

In our opinion, prenatal diagnosis by embryoscopy should generally only be offered to patients with a high genetic risk, particularly for limb or face malformation, or in cases in which fetal laparoscopy or cytoscopy would significantly add to the diagnosis. Genetic counseling is crucial to identify accurately the index case and to assess the risk of recurrence in the couple. Four types of indications should be considered:

1. Isolated abnormalities of the extremities whose inheritance is likely to be dominant (*e.g.*, ectrodactily, syndactily, adactily, acromesomelia).
2. Isolated cleft lip with suspected dominant inheritance.
3. Polymalformation syndromes, which include anomalies of the face, with probable hereditary transmission. This includes autosomal recessive diseases such as Carpenter or Mohr syndromes, or syndromes with syndactyly and cleft lip. Autosomal dominant disorders include Nager syndrome (radial ray agenesis and cleft lip) or EEC syndromes (ectodermic dysplasia and cleft lip).
4. Polymalformative syndromes, which include anomalies of the extremities, with probable hereditary transmission. These include recessive autosomal syndromes (*e.g.*, Baller-Gerold, Saldino-Noonan, Barbet-Biedl, Rothmund-Thomson, Mekel, Quazi, Ellis van Creveld, Smith-Lemli-Opitz), and X-linked disorders with polydactily, such as Golaby-Rosen syndrome.

## TECHNIQUE

***Principles.*** Embryoscopy consists of observing the embryo through the intact amniotic membrane via an endoscope introduced across the chorion into the extraembryonic coelom.

While the chorion is opaque and flimsy, the amniotic membrane is transparent and strong. These anatomical features permit introduction of the endoscopic device across the chorion without damaging the amnion. Because of the relatively large size of the extraembryonic coelom, it is also possible to freely move the tip of the endoscope without tearing the amnion.

Embryoscopy should be performed after the major external features of the embryo's body have been established (*i.e.,* after 8 menstrual weeks) but before the extraembryonic coelom is obliterated by the growth of the amniotic cavity (*i.e.,* before 11 menstrual weeks). Moreover, in order to prevent potential eye damage from excessive light exposure, we believe that endoscopic lighting of the amniotic cavity should be avoided until the development of the embryo's eyelids has been completed (9 menstrual weeks). Because at 9 weeks the maximal size of the extraembryonic coelom is achieved, this is the ideal gestational age for performing embryoscopy.

***Material.*** We use a rigid fiberoptic endoscope with a zero-degree wide-angle lens (Needlescope, Olympus, France), measuring 17 cm in length and 1.7 in diameter, which is introduced through a cannula (2 mm outer diameter). The cannula is equipped with a side channel, allowing for the injection of normal saline while the endoscope is in place. Our group uses a Combison 320, with a 5 MHz sector probe (Kretz, Vienna, Austria) for ultrasound guidance.

***Methods.*** Embryoscopy is an outpatient procedure performed either transcervically or transabdominally. Preoperative ultrasonic evaluation is required to rule out a multiple pregnancy, check the size of the embryo and extraembryonic coelom, and confirm fetal vitality. Intraoperative ultrasound is also needed to guide the endoscope directly into the coelom, to avoid the trophoblast, and to orient the tip of the device towards the part of the embryo to be viewed.

### TRANSCERVICAL EMBRYOSCOPY

The originally described technique was transcervical, which is appropriately used unless the thickest part of the trophoblast is located in direct contact with the internal cervical os. No anesthesia or sedation is required. The cervix is exposed by a single valve weighted speculum and carefully cleaned. The endoscope, within the cannula, is then gently introduced under ultrasound guidance through the cervix, and directed towards the lowest part of the ovum in contact with the chorion (Fig. 4–1). The entire device is then briskly pushed forward in order to cross the chorion and to enter the coelom. The smooth and relatively large tip of the endoscope may reach the amnion but will not damage it. Direct visual inspection of the extraembryonic coelom confirms the proper placement of the endoscope. If needed, the cannula can be flushed with 1–2 mL of normal saline to remove blood and particles. The tip of the endoscope is then brought in direct contact with the amniotic sac, through which the embryo can be observed. The initial inspection is made directly through the endoscope. A video camera is

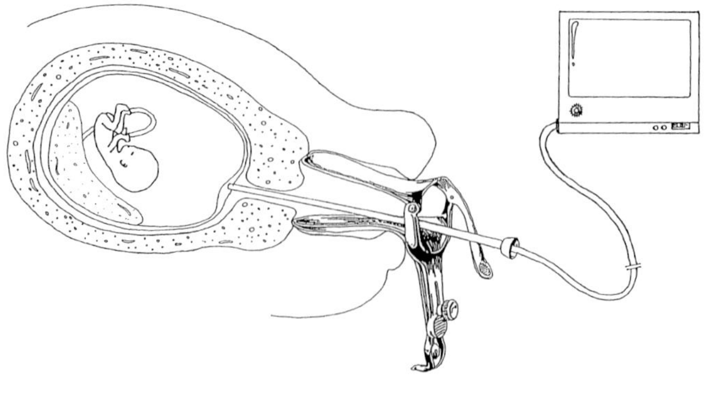

**FIG. 4–1.** Schematic of embryoscope inserted transcervically through chorion but stopping short of amnion.

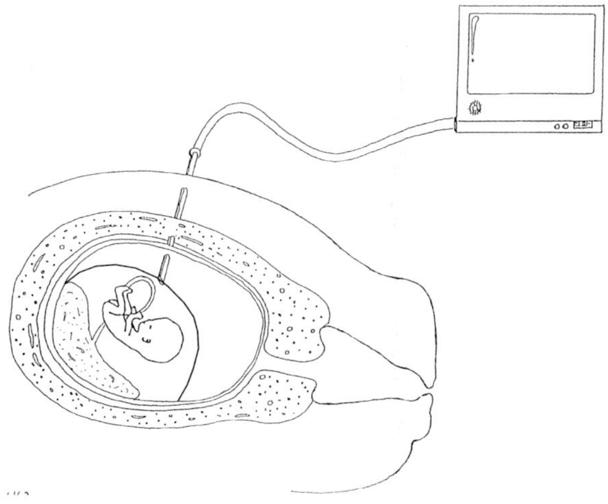

**FIG. 4–2.** Transabdominal needle insertion into the chorionic space. Later in gestation the needle is inserted transamnionicly.

then attached to the endoscope, allowing the mother to view the embryo on a television monitor and to obtain a video tape recording when a malformation has been discovered. If the fetus is found to be normal, the duration of the procedure should be kept as short as possible in order to minimize the risk of miscarriage.

### *TRANSABDOMINAL EMBRYOSCOPY*

A transabdominal approach can also be used whenever the thickest trophoblastic area is not located on the anterior aspect of the uterus. After administering local anesthesia with 1% lidocaine solution, the cannula, containing a sharp trocar, is introduced into the coelom. The trocar is then removed and replaced by the endoscope. After confirming the integrity of the amniotic sac, the endoscopic tip is placed in contact with the transparent amniotic membrane and the remainder of the procedure is the same as described above (Fig. 4–2). Later in gestation the procedure is performed transamnioticly.

Whichever route is used, the patient is discharged after a follow-up ultrasound scan. Antibiotics are given following transcervical procedures.

## INTERPRETATION OF RESULTS

### *NORMAL PREGNANCY*

***Extraembryonic Coelom and Yolk Sac.*** Through the embryoscope, the extraembryonic coelom appears to be a clear space in which thin trabeculae may sometimes be observed. Numerous vessels run on the inner aspect of the chorion, which are easily identified by their red color. The embryo can be seen through the whitish amniotic sac that limits the coelom opposite the chorionic plate. The two vessels of the vitelline duct can be identified at the insertion of the amnion around the umbilical cord. The vitelline duct runs freely in the coelom and connects the yolk sac to the fetal circulation. The yolk sac looks like a yellowish sphere, with a rich vascular network connected to the vascular pedicle of the vitelline duct (Fig. 4–3, Color Fig. 1). Later in gestation, the vascular network of the yolk sac diminishes. By following the vitelline duct from the yolk sac, the cord insertion on the chorionic plate will be reached. At 9 menstrual weeks, the umbilical cord adjacent to the chorionic plate is located within the coelom, and outside the amniotic cavity. The umbilical vein appears deep blue while the umbilical arteries are bright red.

***Embryo.*** After observing the coelom, the tip of the endoscope is moved in contact with the amnion. A nearly complete wide-angle view of the embryo can be obtained, when crown-

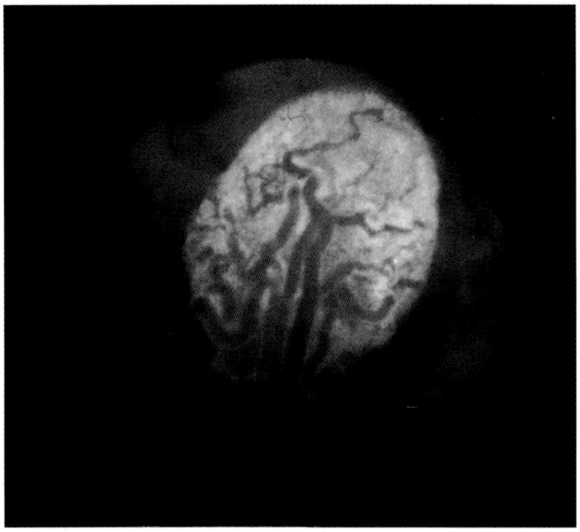

**FIG. 4–3.** Yolk sac with vascular network. See Color Fig. 1.

rump length does not exceed 35 mm. A detailed examination of the four extremities and the face can be performed within a few seconds of direct observation.

### *EMBRYONIC EXTREMITIES*

When the endoscope approaches an embryonic hand or foot, the region studied occupies the whole visual field, and morphologic details can be studied with great accuracy. At 9 weeks, the hands are found in a symmetrical position in front of the embryonic face, with the radial borders being directed cranially. Small spontaneous movements of the fingers, forearm, and arm are often observed. The fingers can be visualized and easily counted, and the phalangae can also be clearly identified (Fig. 4–4, Color Fig. 2). The thumb has a typical 2 phalangeal appearance and is opposed to the other digits. The size of the entire limb as well as the relative dimensions of each portion can be assessed. Both pre- and post-axial aspects of the hands and forearms can be observed in detail. Earlier, at 7 weeks, the fingers are normally fused at the distal end of the upper limb bud, but the outlines of all 5 future digits are already clearly visible. Later in gestation, at 10 weeks, the primary nail fields can also be identified.

The feet have a different appearance. At 9 weeks their plantar surfaces face each other,

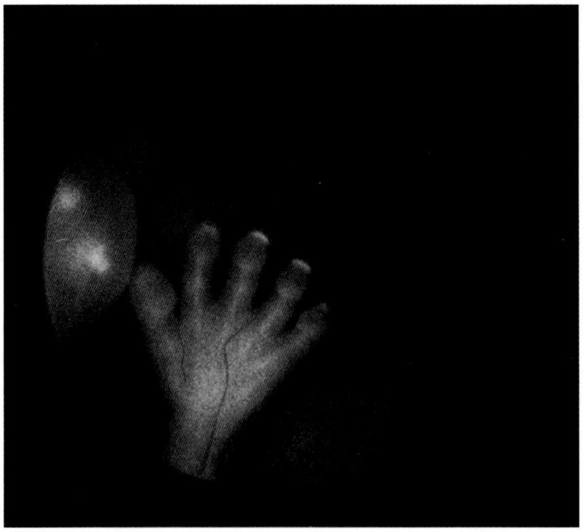

**FIG. 4–4.** Direct visualization of fetal hand at 9 weeks. See Color Fig. 2.

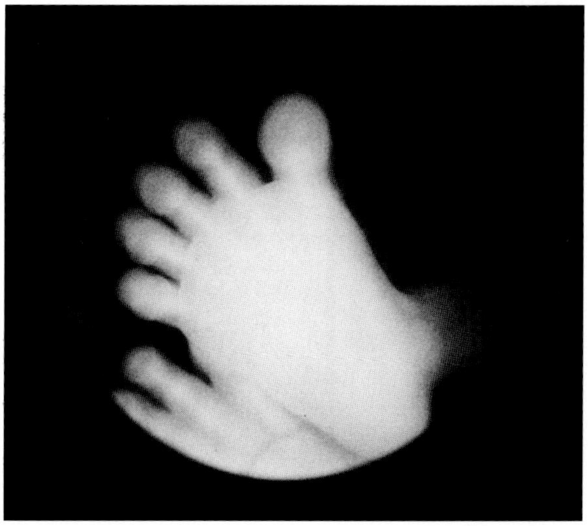

**FIG. 4–5.** Fetal toes at 9 weeks. See Color Fig. 3.

and the tibial border of the leg is directed cranially. After visualizing the heel, however, it can be seen that the foot is oriented perpendicularly to the leg, forming a right angle in the region of the ankle. The toes can be clearly identified (Fig. 4–5, Color Fig. 3), and both their size and shape can be assessed. The pre- and post-axial borders of the leg can also be observed. Earlier in gestation, at 7 weeks, the distal end of the hind limb bud has a grossly triangular shape with the future toes still appearing as united rays.

## *EMBRYONIC FACE*

The face can be thoroughly analyzed (Fig. 4–6, Color Fig. 4). At 9 weeks the eyes are located in the anterior aspect of the face, and the eyelids are fused, completely covering the eyes. The nose, nostrils, mouth, and ears are well established, and the upper lip is fused. The chin looks prominent. Earlier, at 8 weeks, the eyelids have not been formed, and deep blue eyes can be observed on the lateral aspect of the face. The eyes look like convex discs covered by a thin transparent membrane, which is the corneal ectoderm.

## *EMBRYONIC ABDOMEN AND EXTERNAL GENITALIA*

At 9 weeks, the midgut is normally herniated into the embryonic insertion of the umbilical cord, and the small intestine can be observed through the transparent wall of this physiologic,

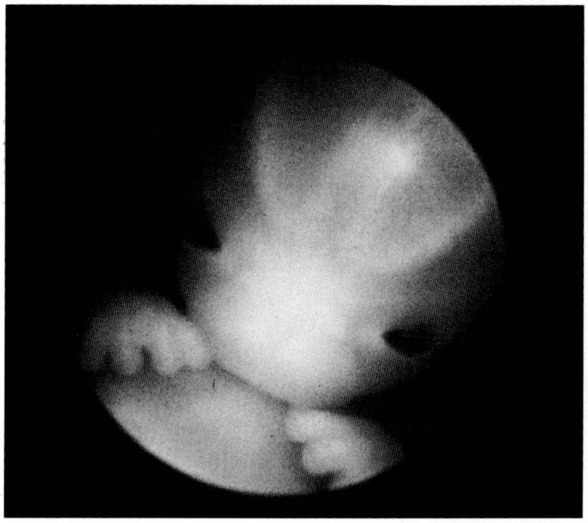

**FIG. 4–6.** Frontal view of face. See Color Fig. 4.

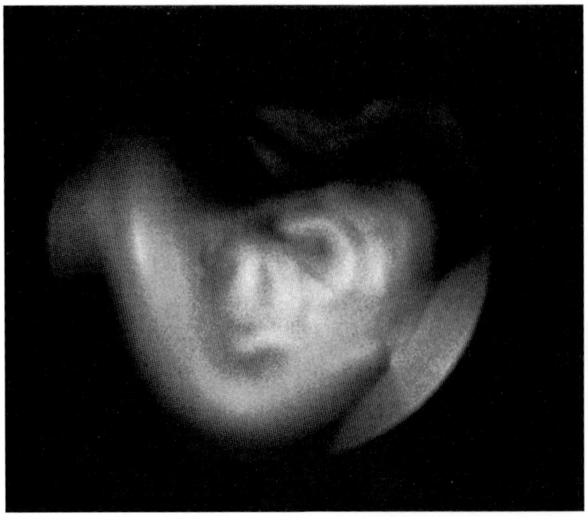

**FIG. 4–7.** Physiologic umbilical hernia at 9 weeks. See Color Fig. 5.

umbilical hernia (Fig. 4–7, Color Fig. 5). At 11 weeks the hernia has usually, but not always, completely disappeared. When this has occurred, the abdominal wall is completely closed. At 10 weeks, during the process of reduction of the physiological hernia, a vestigial sac may persist adjacent to the umbilical cord.

At 9–10 weeks the external genitalia are not yet differentiated and consist of a genital tubercle with 2 labioscrotal swellings (Fig. 4–8, Color Fig. 6). At this age, the embryonic sex cannot be phenotypically diagnosed.

## SKULL AND BACK

The shape of the skull is round; it is covered by thin skin through which subcutaneous blood vessels as well as the large sagittal suture can be seen. The neural tube is closed at 9 weeks, which can be observed through the skin. Earlier in gestation, the neural tube is still open in its cranial and caudal regions.

## MALFORMED EMBRYOS

**Extremities.** The quality of embryoscopic imaging allows prenatal diagnosis of any foot or hand congenital defect at 9 weeks.[8–12]

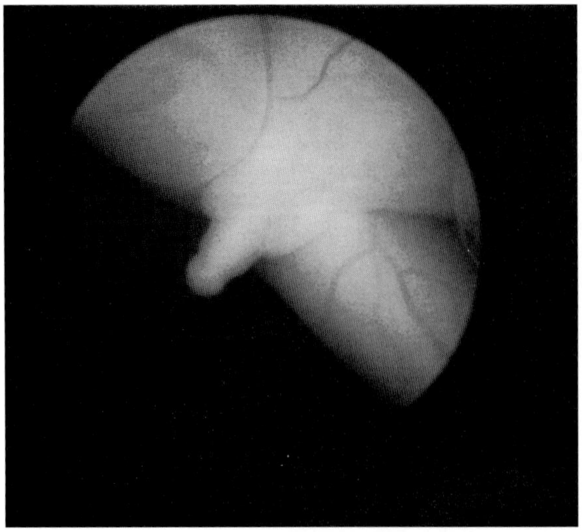

**FIG. 4–8.** External genitalia at 9 weeks. Ultimate phenotype is not certain at this gestational age. See Color Fig. 6.

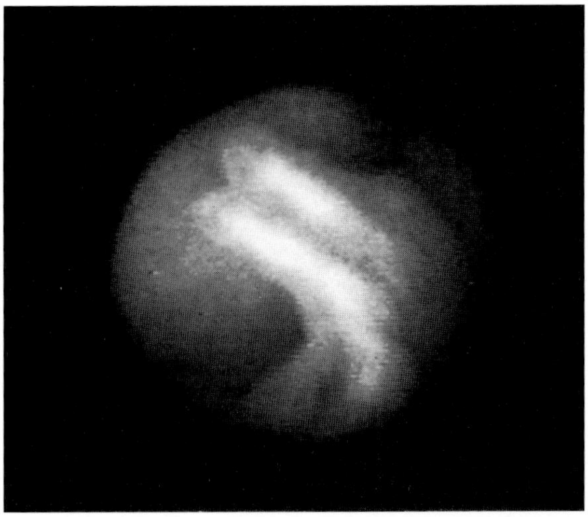

FIG. 4–9. Digital anomalies—syndactyly. See Color Fig. 7.

Gross anomalies such as ectrodactily, monodactily, adactily (Fig. 4–9, Color Fig. 7) are obvious at the first glance. However, because the expression of the disease may differ from one extremity to the other, the four extremities must always be studied. Hexadactily is also easy to diagnose. The sixth digit is usually found on the ulnarian border of the hand (Fig. 4–10, Color Fig. 8), but can also be located on the radial border.

Syndactily is slightly more difficult to diagnose. However, the appearance of the hand is globally abnormal. Part of the digits or all the digits are fused. The hand appears wide but does not look flat like the distal end of the limb bud earlier in pregnancy.

More subtle anomalies can be diagnosed by embryoscopy such as hypoplasia of one digit, nail hypoplasia, or a short phalanx.

***Face.*** The face may be slightly more difficult to observe than the extremities. A cleft lip can be unequivocally diagnosed based on a divided upper lip at 9 weeks. Anophtalmy has not yet been diagnosed by embryoscopy, and the fusion of the eyelids is a potential limitation for such a diagnosis. Ear hypoplasia or aplasia can be diagnosed. However, in the absence of a well defined malformation, facial dysmorphy cannot be demonstrated by embryoscopy.

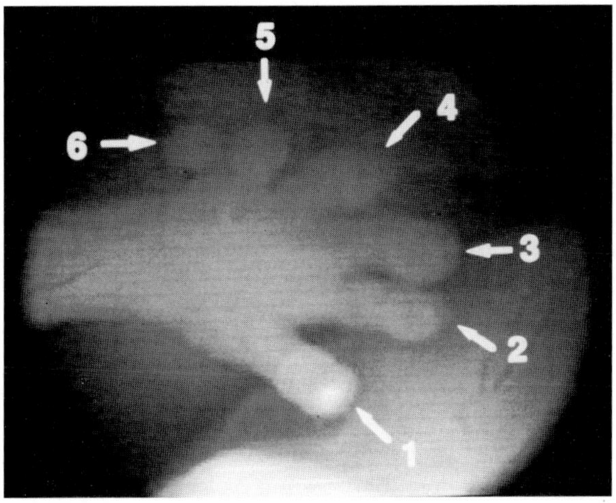


FIG. 4–10. Polydactyly showing 6th digit. See Color Fig. 8.

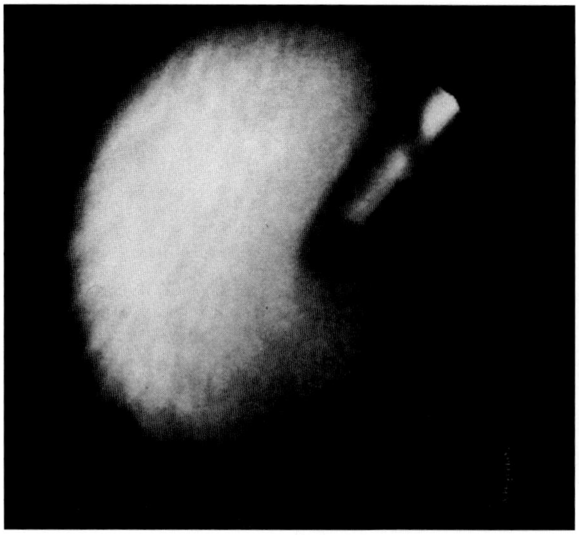

**FIG. 4–11.** Fetal muscle biopsy gun about to enter fetal skin at 19 weeks gestation. See Color Fig. 9. (Photograph courtesy of Dr. Ruben Quintero).

## DIAGNOSTIC VALUE AND COMPLICATIONS

Because of the small number of indicated cases, our experience with ongoing pregnancies is limited to 57 cases over a period of 10 years. The diagnostic value of this technique, however, seems to be excellent. In our series, all positive diagnoses were confirmed by postmortem examination, and no morphologic abnormality was missed. Six miscarriages occurred, all in procedures performed after 10 menstrual weeks. Postnatal follow-up did not reveal any pediatric morbidity associated with the procedures.

## CONTRAINDICATIONS

Patients who are actively bleeding, have leaked fluid, or are infected would appear to be poor candidates for embryoscopy. Because there is still such little experience with the procedure, there are no good statistics to quantitate such risks.

## CONCLUSIONS

Embryoscopy permits prenatal diagnosis of facial and limb defects to be made as early as 9 weeks. Although invasive, this approach has clinical utility in couples with a high risk of having infants affected with severe disorders that cannot be diagnosed by any other means in the first trimester.

Embryoscopy may have considerable importance for future developments in fetal diagnosis and therapy. In the future, thanks to the use of new, very small optical fibers, the procedure will become easier and safer and this will allow for new developments. This procedure may permit sampling of fetal blood or the yolk sac during the first trimester, as well as injection of cells into the embryo. This latter approach has potential applications for early therapy of a variety of genetic disorders, including those involving the hematologic, metabolic, or immune systems.

Later in gestation operative fetoscopy has begun to be utilized, and has been reported in the treatment of acardiac twins, endoscopic fulguration of posterior urethral valves from inside the fetus, and for direct observation of in utero fetal muscle biopsies for the diagnosis of muscular dystrophies (Fig. 4–11, Color Fig. 9).[13–15]

## REFERENCES


1. Dumez Y, Oury JF, Dommergues M. Diagnostic embryoscopy: 50 cases of early diagnosis. International Symposium: From Gametes to Embryo, May 18–20, 1992, Milan.
2. Dumez Y, Dommergues M, Beuzard Y. Study of a method for early first trimester fetal blood sampling and intravascular injection. Symposium on Fetal Therapy and Development: Outlook for the 21st Century, November 27–30, 1988, Chicago.
3. Reece A, Tormensch S, Whethman J, Cullen M, Hobbins J. Embryoscopy: a closer look at first-trimester diagnosis and treatment. Am J Obstet Gynecol 1992;166:775–780.
4. Cullen M, Reece A, Whetham J, Hobbins J. Embryoscopy: description and utility of a new technique. Am J Obstet Gynecol 1990;162:82–86.
5. Rodeck CH, Campbell S. Sampling pure fetal blood by fetoscopy in second trimester of pregnancy. BMJ 1978;2:722–730.
6. Chervenak FA, Isaacson GA, Streltzoff J. Second trimester ultrasound. In: MI Evans (ed). Reproductive risks and prenatal diagnosis. Norwalk; Appleton & Lange, 1992;151–174.
7. Cullen M, Whetham J, Viscarello R, Reece A, Sanchez-Ramos L, Hobbins J. Transcervical endoscopic verification of congenital anomalies in the second trimester of pregnancy. Am J Obstet Gynecol 1991;165:85–87.
8. Cullen M, Green J, Whetham J, Salafia C, Gabrielli S, Hobbins J. Transvaginal ultrasonographic detection of congenital malformations in the first trimester. Am J Obstet Gynecol 1991;163(2):446–447.
9. Timor-Tritsch I, Monteagudo A, Peisner D. High frequency transvaginal sonographic examination for the potential malformation assessment of the 9 week to 14 week fetus. J Clin Ultrasound 1992;20:231–238.
10. Gorlin R, Cohen M, Lewine S. Syndromes of the head and neck (3rd ed.). Oxford University Press, 1990.
11. Smith DW. Recognizable patterns of human malformation: genetic, embryologic, and clinical aspects. Philadelphia: WB Saunders, 1982.
12. Dumez Y, Dommergues M, Gubler MC, Bunduki V, Narcy F, Lemerrer M, Mandelbrot L, Berkowitz R. Meckel Gruber syndrome: prenatal diagnosis at 10 menstrual weeks using embryoscopy. Prenat Diagn 1994;14:141–144.
13. Quintero RA, Reich H, Puder KS, Bardicef M, Evans MI, Cotton DB, Romero R. Brief report: umbilical cord ligation of an acardiac twin by fetoscopy at 19 weeks of gestation. N Engl J Med 1994;83:134–137.
14. Quintero RA, Hume R, Johnson MP, Smith C, Bardicef M, Cotton DB, Romero R, Evans MI. Percutaneous fetal cystoscopy, and endoscopic fulguration of posterior urethral valves. Am J Obstet Gynecol 1995;172:206–209.
15. Evans MI, Hoffman EP, Cadrin C, Johnson MP, Quintero RA, Golbus MS. Fetal muscle biopsy: collaborative experience with varied indications. Obstet Gynecol 1994;84: 913–917.

*Invasive Outpatient Procedures in Reproductive Medicine,* edited by Mark I. Evans, et al. Lippincott–Raven Publishers, Philadelphia © 1997.

# 5 Fetal Shunt Procedures

Mark P. Johnson, Alan W. Flake, Ruben A. Quintero, Mark I. Evans

## INTRODUCTION

The field of fetal medicine has changed rapidly over the past two decades. The late 1970s saw the introduction of midgestational prenatal diagnosis, which marched into the late first trimester during the 1980s. The decade of the 90s has seen not only continued improvement in our prenatal diagnostic capabilities, but has witnessed the next stage of development in which prenatally diagnosed disorders have been treated in utero. Thus, the fetus has now achieved the status of ''potential patient,'' and numerous congenital conditions, previously associated with little hope of survival, are being re-evaluated for possible in utero treatment.

Most congenital malformations do not lend themselves to definitive in utero surgical correction, but the destructive impact of several conditions may be significantly reduced by simple interventions resulting in dramatically improved outcomes in fetuses whose prognosis was otherwise quite dismal. One such intervention involves the use of diverting shunts whose sole purpose is to chronically drain fluid-filled spaces. Such diverting shunts, which can be placed percutaneously with a minimum of uterine invasion, have been shown to be safe and reliable, and have resulted in the births of numerous infants who otherwise had little chance of survival. While the actual placement of the shunt is undoubtedly the most challenging aspect of these cases, considerable experience has shown that one must understand the underlying pathologic processes at work, and that careful diagnostic evaluation and patient selection are the most important aspects of this type of in utero therapy. In this chapter we discuss the mechanisms of damage, the prenatal evaluation, criteria for selecting those fetuses who may benefit from intervention, the invasive technique, potential complications, and recommended follow-up after shunt placement for pregnancies complicated by idiopathic pleural effusion, congenital cystic adenomatous malformation (CCAM), and obstructive uropathy.

## IDIOPATHIC PLEURAL EFFUSION

### *MECHANISMS*

Pleural effusion(s) can present as isolated sonographic findings or as part of a more generalized picture of non-immune fetal hydrops (Fig. 5–1). The etiologies of pleural effusions (Table 5–1) are those of non-immune hydrops and include association with underlying fetal aneuploidy, in utero infections, cardiovascular malformations, lymphatic anomalies, and hematologic perturbations resulting in fetal anemia. Isolated pleural effusions that do not progress to fatal fetal hydrops pose a threat to the developing fetus by intrathoracic compression of the developing lungs, interference with fetal swallowing resulting in polyhydramnios, and potential disturbances in blood flow secondary to increased intrathoracic pressure or mediastinal shift of the heart and great vessels.

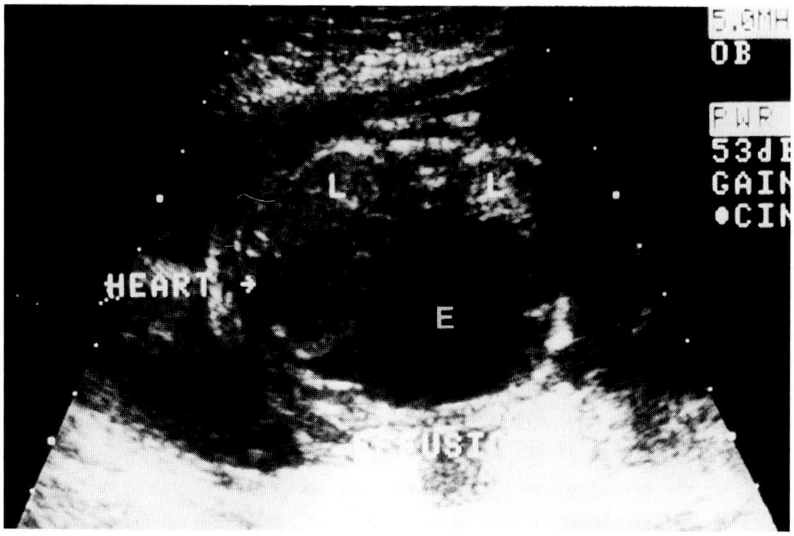


**FIG. 5–1.** Fetal pleural effusion (E = left effusion, L = lungs, the oblong compressed heart is shown by arrow).

## *PRENATAL EVALUATION*

Prenatal evaluation focuses on identifying cases of isolated, idiopathic pleural effusion(s) by searching for the other etiologies mentioned previously. Detailed, high-resolution study of the fetus is essential to rule out other associated anomalies that may contribute to the effusions or identify the fetus as at risk for a more complex underlying genetic syndrome. A fetal echocardiogram will allow detailed evaluation of the heart and associated major vessels to identify those effusions that may be secondary to cardiovascular malformations. Cordocentesis is a particularly important component of the work-up because it allows for rapid evaluation of fetal karyotype, hematologic abnormalities by hematocrit and reticulocyte count, and fetal infection by IgG/IgM titers for specific pathogens as well as liver enzymes, albumin, and total protein values.

Weiner[1] has suggested measurement of umbilical venous pressure (UVP) before and after thoracocentesis drainage of the pleural effusion(s) as a diagnostic or prognostic tool when selecting patients for in utero intervention. He suggests that fetuses with normal UVP prior to thoracocentesis drainage or those in which the UVP remains elevated following thoracocentesis do not represent good candidates for intervention as the underlying mechanism for the effusion(s) may not be correctable or will not benefit by simple chronic drainage. In contrast, they found that fetuses in which the UVP was elevated prior to and decreased following thoracocentesis drainage of the effusion had much better outcomes after thoracoamniotic shunt placements, suggesting this criteria can be used in patient selection prior to in utero treatment. This, however, would require two cordocentesis procedures and an increased risk of complications from a second procedure.

The interventive goal for unilateral or bilateral placement of thoracoamniotic shunts

**TABLE 5–1. POTENTIAL ETIOLOGIES OF ISOLATED PLEURAL EFFUSIONS**

| |
|---|
| Infectious |
| Hematologic |
| Chromosomal |
| Cardiac anomalies |
| Metabolic disorders |
| Lymphatic anomalies |

**TABLE 5–2. SELECTION CRITERIA FOR PLEURAL EFFUSIONS**

| |
|---|
| Normal karyotype |
| Negative viral cultures |
| Normal echocardiogram |
| Normal laboratory evaluation |
| Effusion(s) recur following drainage |
| Normal phenotype on ultrasound exam |

would be continuous chronic drainage of idiopathic pleural effusion(s), allowing reexpansion and normal development of compressed pulmonary tissues in fetuses during the critical transition phase from canalicular to alveolar lung development occuring between 18–24 weeks' gestation, the reduction in intrathorasic pressures that may inhibit fetal swallowing leading to polyhydramnios and increased risk for preterm delivery, or the resolution of mediastinal shift and improved hemodynamic status, which may otherwise result in lethal fetal hydrops. Selection criteria for identifying fetuses who may benefit from such intervention are listed in Table 5–2.

An important component of the evaluation involves the performance of a fine-needle thoracocentesis (Fig. 5–2). Under continuous ultrasound guidance, a 22-gauge needle is passed into the lower, lateral aspect of the hemithorax between the midclavicular and midaxillary lines. This entrance point is important in that this is the most dependent portion of the thorax into which the effusion will collect as you aspirate, allowing the maximum amount of fluid to be removed while avoiding intrathoracic structures that may begin to return to their normal anatomic positions during the aspiration. Sonographic reevaluation is then done 48–72 hours later to evaluate for recurrence of the effusion. In some cases, the effusion(s) will not recur and the single thoracocentesis is curative. In others, the effusion(s) will not recur for several weeks. In these cases, therapeutic thoracocentesis may be performed every few weeks as clinically indicated by the volume of effusion present and the development of secondary complications such as polyhydramnios or those suggestive of fetal hydrops. When multiple interventions are necessary during the course of the pregnancy, antibiotic prophylaxis is recommended utilizing an agent known to achieve therapeutic levels in the amniotic fluid. Cases in which the effusion(s) rapidly reaccumulate following thoracocentesis represent those in which the fetus will most likely benefit from chronic drainage through thoracoamniotic shunt placement.

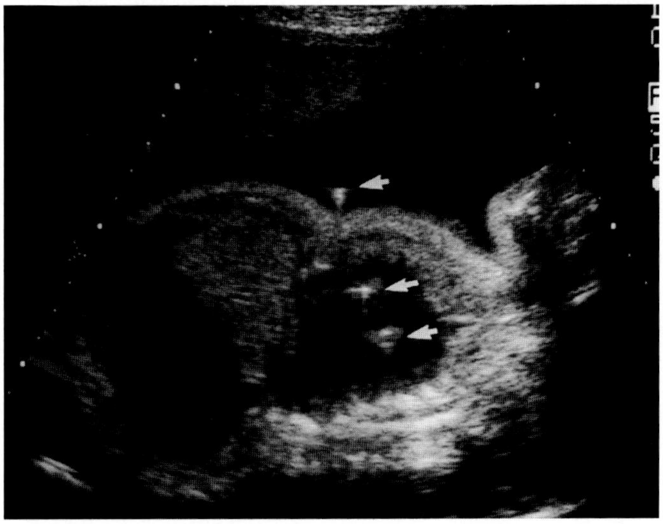

**FIG. 5–2.** Fetal thoracocentesis. Needle can easily be identified (arrows) within the effusion fluid during drainage.

### *TECHNIQUE*

We are currently using the Rodeck catheter (KCH fetal bladder drainage catheter, Rocket of London Ltd., Watford, England) and trocar apparatus for our shunting procedures. The advantages of this catheter are its high-density plastic composition with open, metal-tipped proximal and distal ends, which assist in sonographic identification. The ''memory'' of the plastic allows the catheter to return to original shape after exposure to the warm environment of intrauterine fluids following the straightening of the catheter, which is required for trocar passage. Also, the orientation of proximal and distal pigtail segments are at right angles such that the internal segment prevents complete collapse of the fluid cavity to promote drainage and prevent occlusion of the tip, while the distal segment lies somewhat flattened against the outer chest or abdominal wall. This orientation significantly improves function and reduces the risk of displacement when compared to other simple double pigtail catheters.

Using continuous ultrasound guidance, a spot is chosen on the maternal abdomen that will allow the linear passage of the shunt trocar into the amniotic space immediately adjacent to the hemithorax, into which the shunt catheter is to be placed. If the fetus is very active, it may be necessary to use pancuronium to temporarily paralyze the fetus prior to attempting shunt placement. Once a spot is identified that allows straight access to the fetal thorax, the maternal skin is anesthetized using 1% Xylocaine, and a small 3 mm incision through the skin is made to allow easy passage of the trocar apparatus. Using continuous ultrasound guidance, the shunt trocar is slowly advanced into the appropriate position in the amniotic space just lateral to the fetal hemithorax. An appropriate position is then chosen in the lower mid-axillary line and the sharp tip of the shunt trocar is anchored between the two chosen ribs at the entrance site. If the catheter is to be placed into the left hemithorax, a position at or just slightly posterior to the mid-axillary line should be chosen as placement anteriorly may interfere with return of mediastinal structures to their normal anatomical positions.

Again, using a gentle twisting action, the trocar is carefully advanced above the inferior rib through the chest wall such that the tip lies about 5 mm within the chest cavity. The stylet is then removed and the Rodeck shunt inserted into the trocar sheath. At this point it is quite common for effusion fluid to flow quite briskly out the end of the catheter and it is important to proceed quickly so that the effusion pocket does not drain, which would make catheter placement more difficult and the proximal catheter end within the chest cavity would not be able to resume its original coiled shape. Prior to inserting the catheter into the trocar sheath, it must first be straightened to allow passage through the sheath. We leave the wire stylet within the catheter until the proximal tip is well into the trocar sheath (approximately 2 cm) before removing the stylet wire. Removal of the stylet wire prior to this point may result in difficulty inserting the catheter into the trocar sheath, while failure to remove it as suggested may result in kinking of the wire and distortion of the catheter tip, which will prevent further passage down the sheath.

Once the catheter has been fed into the trocar (Fig. 5–3), a short push rod is introduced into and slowly advanced down the trocar sheath, which displaces the proximal segment of the catheter into the intended cavity. The metal tip and high-density composition of the Rodeck catheter make visualization of its entrance into the fluid cavity quite straightforward. The catheter will begin to resume its original coiled configuration on exposure to the warm environment of the effusion cavity (Fig. 5–4). The short push rod is then removed and a long push rod inserted and advanced until the distal tip of the catheter is encountered within the trocar sheath. At this point the catheter needs to be stabilized with the push rod while the trocar sheath is backed out through the chest wall a distance of approximately 1–1.5 cm, which represents the straight portion of the Rodeck catheter. Once outside within the amniotic cavity, the tip of the trocar sheath is deviated slightly away from the entrance site and the remainder of the catheter passed from the trocar using the long push rod. If the tip of the trocar sheath is not deviated slightly away from the entrance site, the catheter may be further advanced into the chest cavity instead of being dropped into the amniotic space. Once placed, the effusion can generally be noted to begin drainage, a process that begins rapidly because of the initial

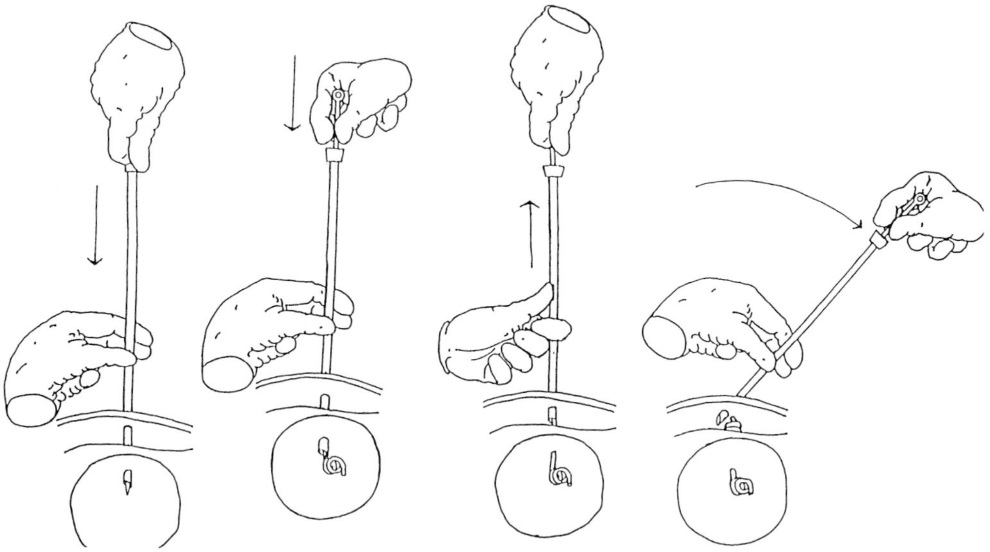

**FIG. 5–3.** Four-step shunt trocar technique (see text for detailed description).

increased intrathorasic pressure, but may take 12–24 hours to complete (Fig. 5–5). Again, prophylactic oral antibiotic therapy is recommended for these invasive fetal procedures.

## COMPLICATIONS

Occasionally the catheter will become displaced into the amniotic cavity and need to be replaced if the effusion(s) recur. If the catheter has been in place for a period of time, it may not need replacement as occasionally an epithelialized tract remains, which serves as a fistulous drainage tract. Less commonly, if the catheter was improperly placed initially, it may migrate into the thoracic cavity becoming an indwelling foreign body with recurrence of the effusions

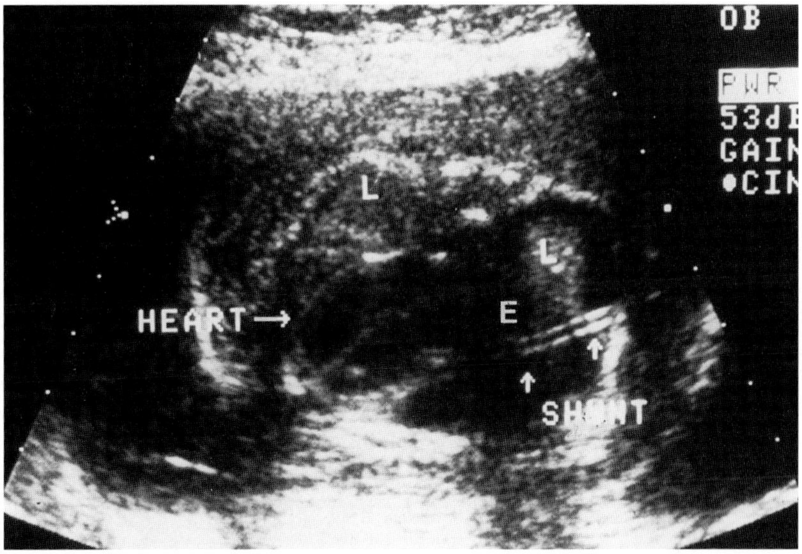


**FIG. 5–4.** Thoracoamniotic shunt. Shunt has been introduced into the left fetal chest and the proximal end can be seen (arrows) beginning to resume its coiled shape within the effusion space. Note the change in shape of the heart compared to Figure 5–1, as intrathorasic pressure is relieved and the effusion fluid drains (L = lungs, E = effusion).

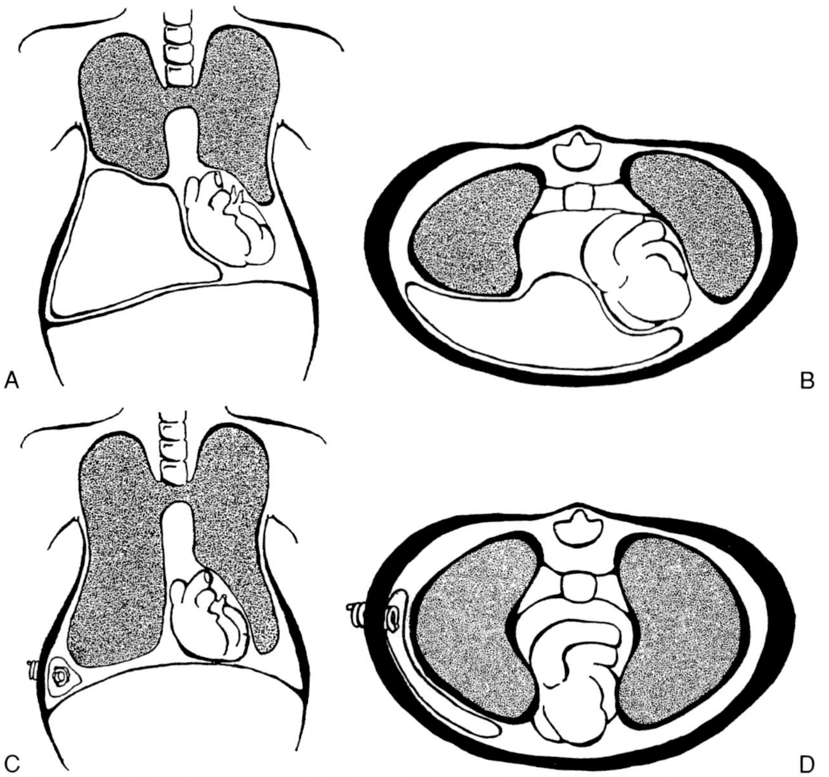


**FIG. 5–5.** Thoracoamniotic shunting of a right pleural effusion. (A,B) Frontal and transverse views showing space occupied by effusion with displacement of the lungs and heart. (C,D) Frontal and transverse view showing thoracoamniotic shunt properly placed into the lower lateral aspect of the effusion, allowing maximal drainage of effusion. Note return of lungs and heart to their appropriate positions.

necessitating a second shunt placement. Care must be taken to stay lateral during catheter insertion as medial insertions may result in placement within the mediastinum, thus isolating the shunt from the pleural space requiring drainage. Also, placement too high or posteriorly in the chest cavity may result in incomplete drainage as the catheter tip may become occluded by the fetal lung as it expands to fill the space made by the draining effusion. Certainly one must stay well away from the paraspinal regions because of the possibility of vascular and nerve-root damage. Lastly, it is possible that the catheter may become occluded by proteinacious material within the effusion or by thrombus if bleeding occurred during shunt placement, resulting in loss of function, although sonographically the catheter appears to be optimally placed.

### *FOLLOW–UP*

Follow-up sonographic evaluation is initially done 48–72 hours later to confirm successful catheter placement and function as evidenced by the resolving effusion, re-expansion of the fetal lungs, and restoration of normal mediastinal relationships. After, the patient is generally rescanned at weekly intervals to confirm catheter placement and function.

Route of delivery of the infant is dictated by obstetrical factors. If the catheter is not pulled out during the delivery process, it may be temporarily left in place and treated as an indwelling chest tube during the immediate postpartum neonatal evaluation, or simply removed with wound management similar to that of a removed neonatal chest tube.

## CONGENITAL CYSTIC ADENOMATOUS MALFORMATION (CCAM)

### *MECHANISMS*

Congenital cystic adenomatous malformations are benign, space-occupying tumors of bronchial origin. They are generally classified into microcystic, macrocystic, and mixed types, depending on the size of the cysts they contain. CCAMs can occasionally contain a single or several macrocysts, which fill with fluid, progressively enlarging until they form very large space-occupying lesions within the fetal chest. Such large lesions, particularly within the lower-left lobe, can cause rapid mediastinal shift and compromise the hemodynamic state of the fetus, resulting in the development of non-immune hydrops. Once the fetus has developed hydropic changes, the prognosis becomes quite poor and the risk for intrauterine demise high. Early development and enlargement of lesions can result in significant compression of fetal lung tissues, which, if present during the critical transition from canalicular to alveolar stage between 18–24 weeks gestation, may result in lethal pulmonary hypoplasia. In addition, large macrocysts can lead to compression of the fetal esophagus, resulting in decreased fetal swallowing and the development of polyhydramnios and risk of preterm delivery of a compromised infant.

The goal of shunt therapy in such cases focuses on chronic drainage of large macrocysts. Early therapy would be directed at preventing pulmonary hypoplasia, while later interventions would be done for hemodynamic disturbances resulting in evolving hydrops or progressive polyhydramnios due to esophageal compression.

## PRENATAL EVALUATION

The differential diagnosis for echogenic, cystic intrathoracic masses includes cystic ademomatous malformation, teratoma, bronchogenic cyst, diaphragmatic hernia, and bronchopulmonary sequestration (Table 5–3). Prenatal evaluation of such cases includes a complete high-resolution sonographic fetal survey to rule out additional fetal anomalies that may indicate the presence of a more complex genetic syndrome. Detailed fetal echocardiography is necessary because cardiac anomalies may be associated with such lesions; it is also an important component of the evaluation in the presence of fetal hydrops. Detailed Doppler flow studies of the lesions may help differentiate nonvascular CCAMs from other masses, such as lung sequestrations, which are usually associated with an anomalous artery originating off the fetal aorta. Lastly, rapid fetal karyotyping is recommended to rule out aneuploidy, and is generally accomplished by transabdominal chorionic villus sampling in early cases or by cordocentesis in later cases, when such is part of the evaluation of associated hydropic changes.

## PATIENT SELECTION CRITERIA

In utero surgical interventions should be reserved only for those fetuses who have developed secondary complications that worsen the pregnancy prognosis, such as early onset pulmonary compression, evolving hydrops, or progressive polyhydramnios, and in whom simple chronic drainage of a dominant macrocyst would potentially correct the underlying physical disturbances that lead to the secondary complications. It must be stressed that such intervention is only temporizing and not corrective in nature, and that the fetus continues to be at risk for subsequent complications and poor outcome due to the primary underlying lesion. The fetus must have the diagnosis of macrocytic CCAM confirmed by high-resolution ultrasound; fetuses afflicted with the other potential lesions will not benefit and could be harmed by attempted intervention using transthoracic shunts. The fetus must have a normal karyotype and an otherwise negative workup for fetal hydrops, including hematologic, infectious, and cardiovascular etiologies.

**TABLE 5–3. DIFFERENTIAL DIAGNOSIS IN CONGENITAL CYSTIC ADENOMATOUS MALFORMATION**

| |
|---|
| Teratoma |
| Bronchogenic cyst |
| Diaphragmatic hernia |
| Bronchopulmonary sequestration |
| Congenital cystic adenomatous malformation |

### *TECHNIQUE*

Once a fetus is identified who meets the above criteria and intervention holds the potential for benefit, the first step in therapy involves the initial drainage of the macrocyst. The initial step is very important because the cyst may not reaccumulate fluid and this minimally invasive drainage may be the only intervention needed; or the cyst may rapidly reaccumulate fluid demonstrating the need for chronic drainage. The initial cyst drainage is done under continuous high-resolution ultrasound guidance in which a 22-gauge spinal needle is carefully introduced into the amniotic cavity at the appropriate angle to allow a single linear entrance into the fetal thorax between the mid-axillary and mid-clavicular lines. Once positioned at the fetal chest, the appropriate space between adjacent ribs should be selected and the needle passed through the fetal chest wall just above the inferior rib, avoiding the nerve and vessels that lie along the inferior margin of the superior rib. The point of entrance through the fetal chest and into the macrocyst should be chosen with careful consideration given to how the cyst will predictively shrink (Fig. 5–6) during the drainage process such that the cyst can be completely drained of essentially all its fluid while retaining the original position of the needle insertion and eliminating the need for needle repositioning and multiple transthoracic passages, which would significantly raise the risk of fetal trauma and potential complications. In addition, prior to entering the fetal chest, color-flow Doppler should be utilized to assure the operator that no large vessel or vascular formation lies between the chest wall and intended target. We have not found that having the aspirated fluid analyzed for biochemical markers or cytologic components is useful in confirming or changing our diagnosis and treatment plan, and therefore do not advocate such studies on the aspirated specimen.

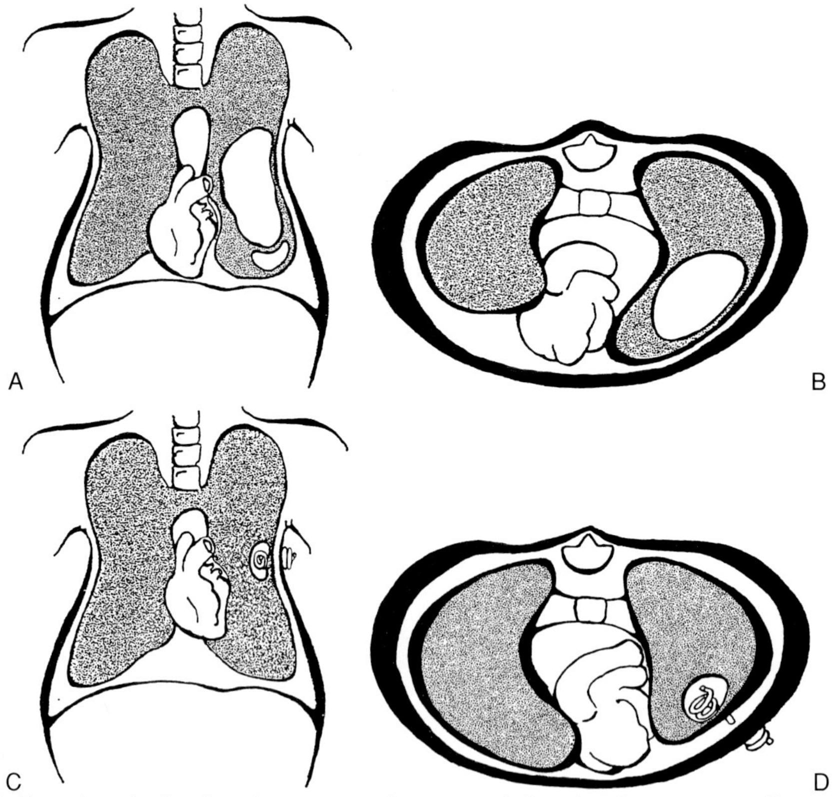


**FIG. 5–6.** Transthoracic shunting of a macrocyst in a congenital cystic adenomatous malformation. (A,B) Frontal and transverse views showing large macrocyst in left lung, which displaces mediastinal structures and compresses developing tissues within the left lung. (C,D) Frontal and transverse views following shunt placement, showing maximal drainage of the macrocyst with reexpansion of the left lung and reestablishment of normal mediastinal anatomic relationships.

Following fine-needle aspiration, we generally reevaluate the fetus 3–5 days later to determine whether fluid has reaccumulated within the macrocyst or whether there has been a change in secondary complications following the decompression of the macrocyst. If the fluid has not reaccumulated and secondary complications are resolving, then no further intervention is necessary and weekly sonographic surveillance is suggested to follow the growth of the underlying CCAM and to monitor for additional complications. If the fluid does not return but fetal hydrops or polyhydramnios does not resolve, then the prognosis is guarded and alternative etiologies for these problems should be pursued. If the fluid reaccumulates over the course of several days and secondary findings persist, then the fetus should be considered a candidate for chronic shunt drainage.

Prior to attempting shunt placement, the patient should be carefully and thoroughly counseled about the purpose and potential benefits of such surgery, as well as the potential risks and complications of the procedure to both the mother and fetus. These include technical failure in placement or function of the shunt, possible infection, preterm labor, traumatic injury, and possible fetal death. In addition, the patient should be aware that the shunt may become displaced into the fetal chest or out into the amniotic cavity, which may necessitate the placement of an additional shunt if the macrocyst and associated secondary complications recur.

Prior to placement, the fetus is reevaluated sonographically to determine position and the best single linear approach for trocar insertion, which will result in the most optimal placement with the least amount of trocar manipulation and potential trauma to the fetus. If the fetus is extremely active, it may be necessary to temporarily paralyze the fetus using pancuronium (single intramuscular injection into the fetal thigh or deltoid muscle at a dose of 1mg/Kg estimated fetal weight), although we have rarely found this to be necessary. Careful consideration needs to be given to the predicted pattern of cyst involution during drainage based on the previous fine-needle cyst aspiration procedure such that the shunt can be placed at the macrocyst's predicted position on achieving minimum size following successful shunt placement. If this is not done, the macrocyst can potentially move away from the catheter where it enters the fetal chest as the cyst drains, resulting in less of the proximal pigtail within the cyst and a much higher risk of shunt displacement out of the cyst cavity. In addition, when draining a macrocyst within the left thorax, one must position the catheter to enter the fetal chest at the superior and lateral left aspect of the macrocyst to encourage the expected upward and lateral involution of the cyst, thus allowing resolution of mediastinal structures to their normal position within the left chest (see Fig. 5–6). Placement of the catheter in the mid-clavicular line low within the fetal chest could potentially interfere with restoration of normal mediastinal positions and put the catheter at increased risk for displacement. The actual mechanical technique for catheter placement is the same as that described for thoracoamniotic shunts as described for pleural effusions except that the proximal end of the Rocket catheter is placed into the macrocyst at the position that will allow optimal involution of the cyst and continued drainage.

### COMPLICATIONS

If the catheter is not optimally placed initially, it is possible that it will be displaced and drawn into the chest cavity as the macrocyst involutes with drainage. This could result in a potential pleural effusion with its associated complications and may necessitate the placement of a thoracoamniotic shunt. Also, the fetus may actively or passively participate in the displacement of the catheter out of the chest such that it is free within the amniotic space necessitating the placement of an additional shunt if the macrocyst and associated secondary complications recur. In our experience, such displaced catheters do not pose a risk to the fetus. Other potential complications include vascular trauma if one is not careful when choosing a site to place the catheter, and it is recommended that color-flow Doppler be used prior to insertion of the catheter into the chest to identify any large vessels along the chosen route of shunt placement. Although not directly contraindicated, all efforts should be made to avoid trocar passage through the placenta; this may result in hematoma formation or vascular damage to the placenta, resulting in fetal death. If no other access to the fetus is available, then the placenta should be traversed in a single pass as far away from cord insertion as possible, using color-flow Doppler to identify and avoid large vessels coursing through the placenta at the chorionic plate. In addition, all insertions should be done as high in the fundal region of the uterus as possible; this will reduce the risk of amniotic fluid leakage and associated risks of oligohydramnios and chorioamnionitis.

As with all major in utero interventions, good sterile operative technique and oral antibiotic prophylaxis is recommended to reduce the risk of infection. Lastly, if intervention occurs in the later second or third trimester, uterine irritability may occur, which could progress to preterm labor and delivery. We therefore moniter our patients for 1–2 hours and utilize aggressive tocolytic therapy as indicated.

### *FOLLOW–UP*

After shunt placement, we routinely have the patient return for follow-up evaluation in 2–3 days to document catheter placement and function. Following this postoperative exam, we recommend weekly sonographic evaluations to document continued shunt function, resolution of associated problems (polyhydramnios/hydrops), and to continue close monitoring of the underlying CCAM lesion and potential additional complications that might arise due to these lesions. Mode of delivery for an infant with an indwelling catheter should be determined by obstetrical indications only, and most would be expected to deliver vaginally. It is highly recommended that the neonatal team be notified well in advance of the delivery as many infants with CCAM have special pulmonary needs in the immediate postnatal period. In most cases, the catheter can simply be removed postnatally and the entrance site treated similarly to a pediatric chest-tube removal.

## OBSTRUCTIVE UROPATHY

### *MECHANISM*

Fetal obstructive uropathies are a diverse and heterogeneous group of developmental abnormalities that generally involve obstruction of the proximal urethra in the male fetus. The more common etiologies involve urethral atresia, posterior urethral valves, or prune-belly syndrome. Cloacal anomalies may be part of the underlying disorder, reflect the presence of a more complex underlying genetic syndrome, and must be ruled out during prenatal evaluation because such cases have not been found to benefit from shunt therapy. Other etiologies can include anterior urethral valves, chromosomal abnormalities, complex genetic causes such as megacystis/microcolon syndrome, or partial obstructions or strictures that restrict flow through the urethra as may rarely occur in abnormalities of the urethral meatus such as hypo- or epispadius.

Complete urethral obstruction or significant restriction of urethral flow results in accumulation of urine within the fetal bladder, leading to megacystis. Prolonged obstruction results in smooth-muscle hypertrophy and hyperplasia within the bladder wall, and eventual impairment of contractile capacity as well as compliance and elasticity. Bladder distention results in elevated intravesicular pressures, which may overcome the delicate physiologic valve mechanism at the ureterovesical junctions. Bladder wall distortion-associated hypertrophy and hyperplasia may contribute to the loss of these physiologic valves. Reflux eventually results, contributing to the development of hydroureters and hydronephrosis.

Ureteral distention due to reflux also elicits smooth-muscle hypertrophy and hyperplasia, particularly in the distal ureter where smooth muscle is more prevalent. This appears to result in further distortion of the delicate ureterovesical angles as well as diminished elasticity of the ureters.

Ongoing studies at our center indicate that there is a subset of male fetuses in which no anatomical obstruction can be demonstrated on fetal autopsy, although these fetuses appear sonographically identical to those in which complete obstruction is confirmed postnatally. Histologically, these fetuses appear to have a basic underlying defect in the development and response of smooth muscle throughout the upper and lower urinary tract, resulting in dilation of the bladder and subsequent reflux hydronephrosis. In cases of true anatomical obstruction, there is a marked hypertrophic and hyperplastic response of the smooth muscle component in the walls of the bladder and distal ureters to obstruction, which is progressive and reflective of the duration of the obstructive process (Fig. 5–7). In fetuses without anatomical obstructions, which we refer to as "true prune-belly syndrome" fetuses to differentiate them from those with anatomical obstructions, we have found no change in the smooth muscle component when compared to age-matched non-obstructed controls.[2]

Long-term prognosis in cases of true prune-belly syndrome following shunt intervention

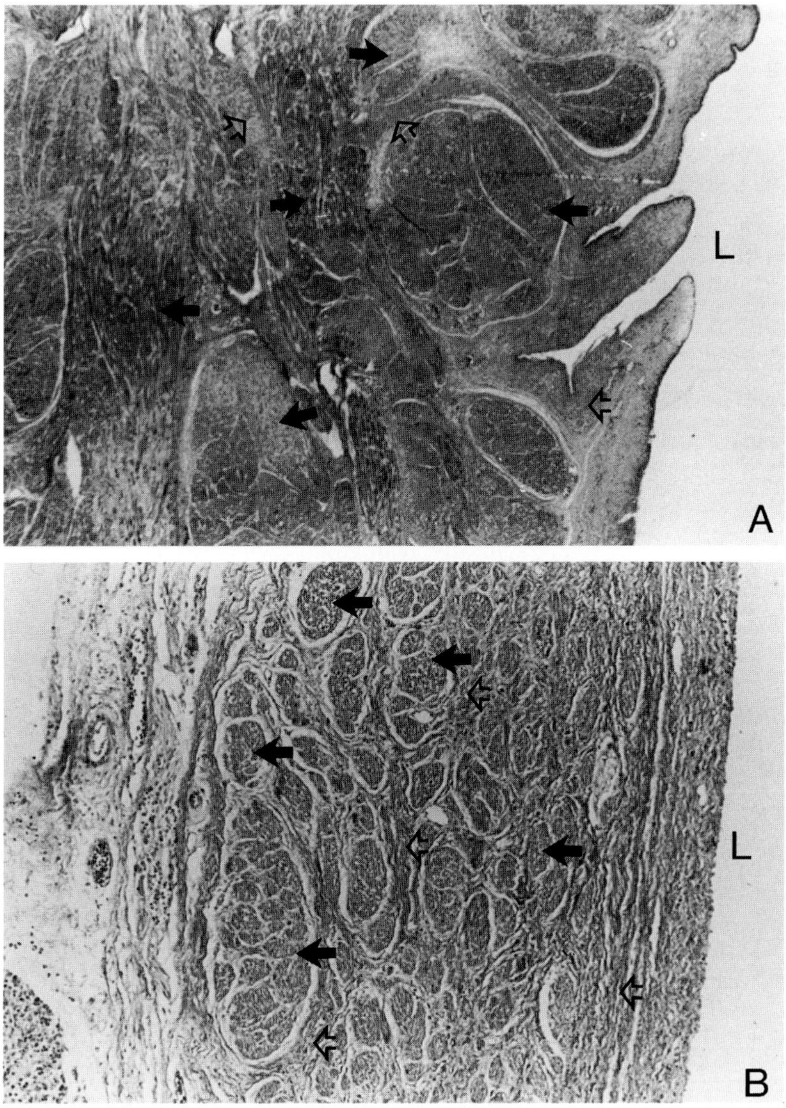


**FIG. 5–7.** Histologic changes in the bladder wall observed in fetal obstructive uropathies. (A) Marked thickening of the bladder wall seen due to hyperplasia and hypertrophy of the smooth muscle component in cases of complete urethral obstruction (magnified ×20). (B) Mild increase in wall thickness due to a balanced smooth-muscle and connective-tissue response to bladder enlargement observed in cases of prune-belly syndrome with urethral patency (incomplete to minimal obstruction [magnified ×100]).

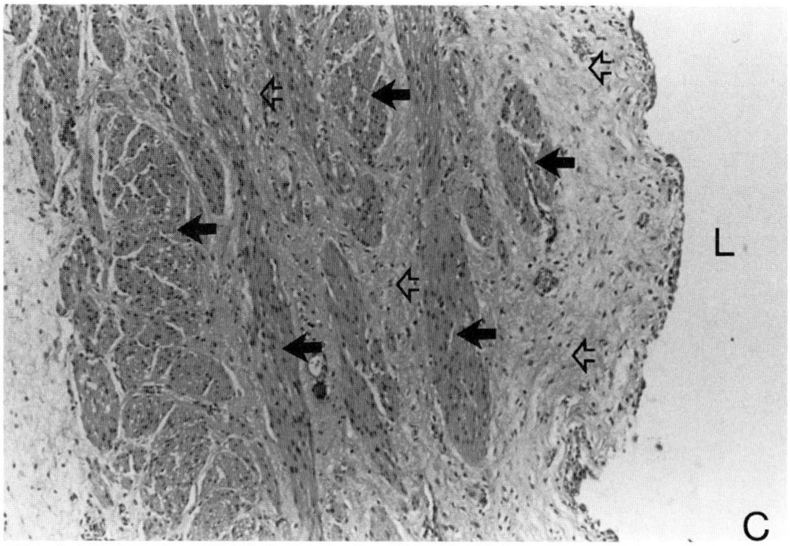


**FIG. 5–7.** *(continued)* (C) Age-matched bladder from a normal fetus (magnified ×100). L = bladder lumen, open arrows = connective tissue component, filled arrows = examples of smooth-muscle bundles.

appears to be better than outcomes in cases of anatomical obstruction, and it would therefore be helpful to be able to identify reliably these two groups prenatally.[3] We have recently introduced the use of fine-needle fetoscopy to perform in utero fetal cystoscopy during the prenatal evaluation to directly examine the bladder mucosa, ureteral orifaces, and proximal urethra.[4] In cases of true urethral obstruction, the proximal urethra has been markedly dilated with trabeculations noted in the trigone of the bladder (Fig. 5–8, Color Fig. 10). In cases subsequently confirmed to be urethra-patent true prune-belly syndromes, the proximal urethra and bladder neck was much less distended and the trigone was without trebeculations (Fig. 5–9), although sonographically, both groups demonstrated the characteristic ''keyhole'' sign associated with proximal urethral distention (Fig. 5–10). The capability of differentiating these two major groups of fetuses prenatally may allow future changes and refinements in our interventive approaches so as to optimize long-term outcomes.

Hydronephrosis develops from continued urine production in the face of obstructed drain-

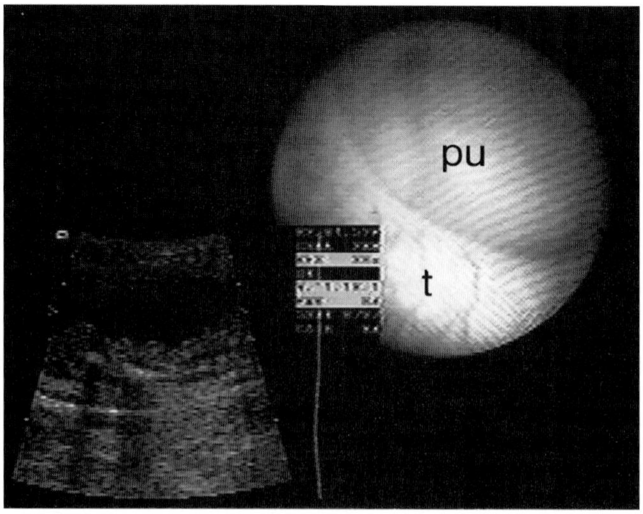


**FIG. 5–8.** Fetal cystoscopy in a 23-week pregnancy complicated by posterior urethral valves. Note tense dilation of proximal urethra and marked trabeculations of the trigone due to long-standing urethral obstruction. pu = proximal urethra, T = trigone region of posterior bladder. See Color Fig. 10.

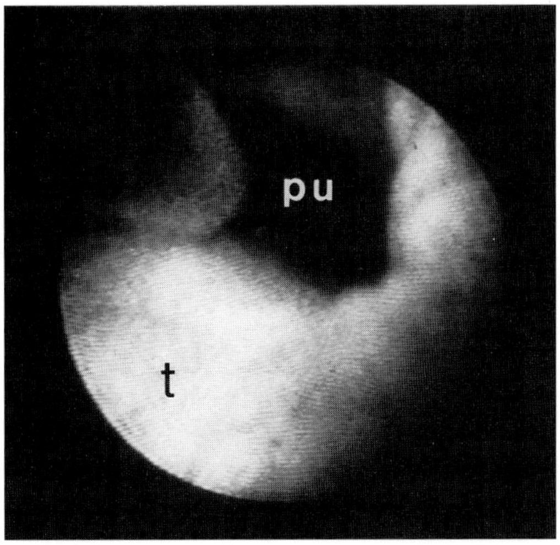


**FIG. 5–9.** Fetal cystoscopy in a 22-week pregnancy complicated by prune-belly syndrome (enlarged bladder, bilateral hydroureters, and hydronephrosis) and a narrow but patent urethra and low-normal amniotic fluid volume. Note the "puckered" appearance of the moderately dilated proximal urethra (pu) and smooth appearance of the trigone (t) region of the posterior bladder.

age as well as reflux from the distended bladder. The renal pelvises and calyceal systems become progressively distended and compress the renal parenchyma against the distended renal capsule. Histologic studies indicate a progressive dilation of the distal to proximal renal tubules associated with the development of peritubular and interstitial fibrosis (Fig. 5–11). Sonographically, the degree of compression and associated fibrosis is reflected by the echogenic appearance of the parenchyma. Eventually, these processes lead to type IV cystic degeneration of the kidneys and renal insufficiency at birth.

After 14 weeks' gestation, amniotic fluid volume is principally from fetal urine production. In cases of obstruction, fetal urine cannot replenish amniotic fluid volume lost by membrane reabsorption, fetal swallowing and fetal breathing, and amniotic fluid volume progressively falls. Subsequent severe oligo- or anhydramnios and massive megacystis leads to physical deformations and physiologic changes characteristic of the prune-belly sequence, which include a markedly protuberant abdomen with apparent decrease in skeletal muscle present within the rectus sheath, joint contractures, compressive facial abnormalities, and pulmonary hypoplasia from intrathoracic pressure alterations and inability to take in amniotic fluid during fetal breathing, which appears to play an important role in lung development and maturation. The presence of severe oligohydramnios during the transition from canalicular to alveolar phase of development, which occurs between 18 and 24 weeks' gestation, results in severely underdeveloped lungs and respiratory insufficiency at birth.[5]

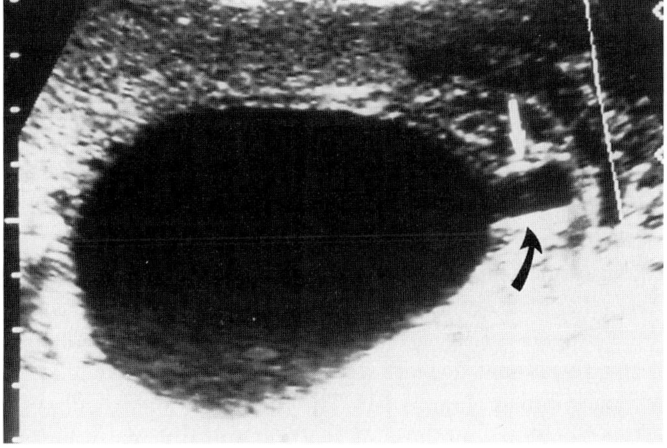

**FIG. 5–10.** Sonographic image of a dilated fetal bladder and the characteristic "keyhole" (arrow) appearance of the dilated proximal urethra in a case of posterior urethral valves.

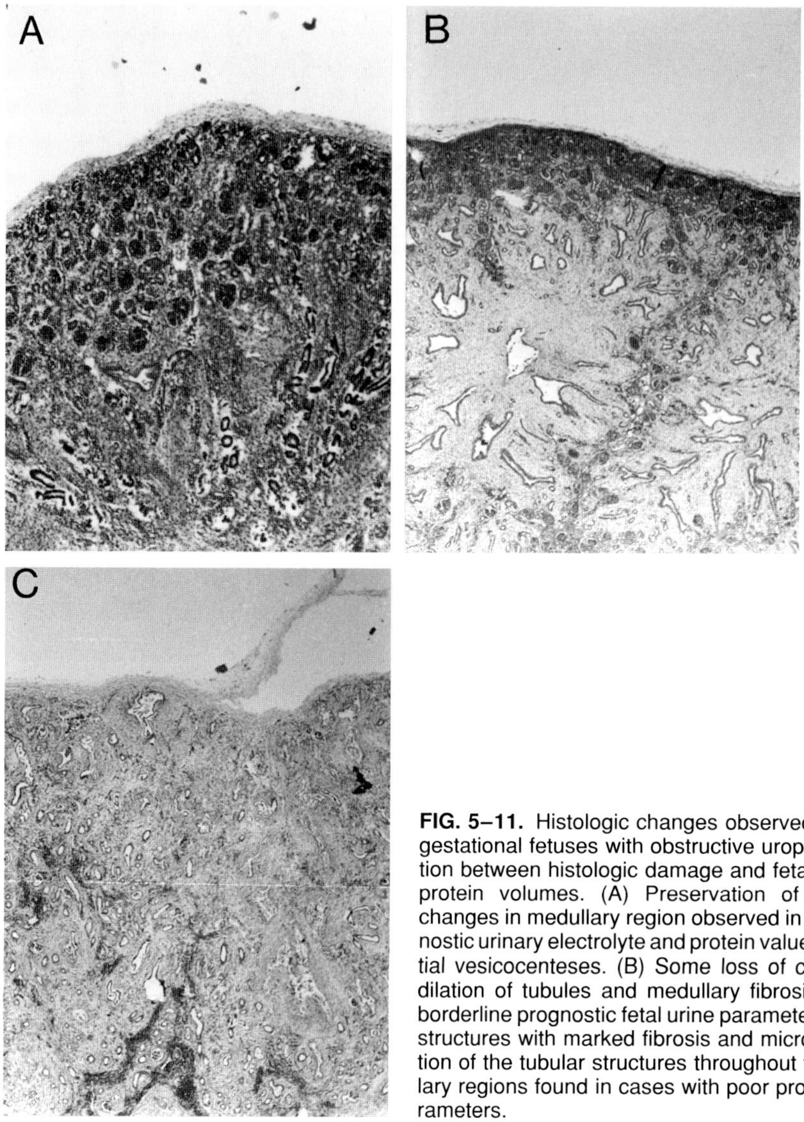


**FIG. 5–11.** Histologic changes observed in kidneys from midgestational fetuses with obstructive uropathy, showing correlation between histologic damage and fetal urine electrolyte and protein volumes. (A) Preservation of cortex with minimal changes in medullary region observed in cases with good prognostic urinary electrolyte and protein values obtained by sequential vesicocenteses. (B) Some loss of cortical structures with dilation of tubules and medullary fibrosis seen in cases with borderline prognostic fetal urine parameters. (C) Loss of cortical structures with marked fibrosis and micro- or macrocystic dilation of the tubular structures throughout the cortex and medullary regions found in cases with poor prognostic fetal urine parameters.

## *PRENATAL EVALUATION*

The antenatal evaluation consists of three basic steps: high-resolution sonographic survey to rule out additional congenital anomalies, fetal karyotyping, and renal function analysis. Detailed fetal sonographic survey is necessary to rule out the presence of other anomalies, such as neural-tube or cardiac defects, which would dramatically impact on the long-term prognosis for that fetus. Certainly, in utero intervention would not be warranted when the fetus is afflicted with another life-threatening anomaly. One must also look carefully for other, more subtle phenotypic signs, such as limb shortening or facial abnormalities that may indicate the presence of an underlying genetic syndrome, which might adversely affect the clinical prognosis. The urinary tract is then carefully evaluated from the kidneys to the distal urethra. Long axis measurement of the kidney is useful in evaluating the underlying hydronephrosis and, in general, kidneys that measure large for gestational age and are less hyperechogenic are associated with a better prognosis (Fig. 5–12). Kidneys that are hyperechogenic and measure appropriate or small for gestational age are generally found to have poor underlying function due to advanced renal fibrosis (Fig. 5–13). The finding of small kidneys in such cases likely reflects the underlying contraction phase of scarring and fibrosis in these severely damaged tissues.

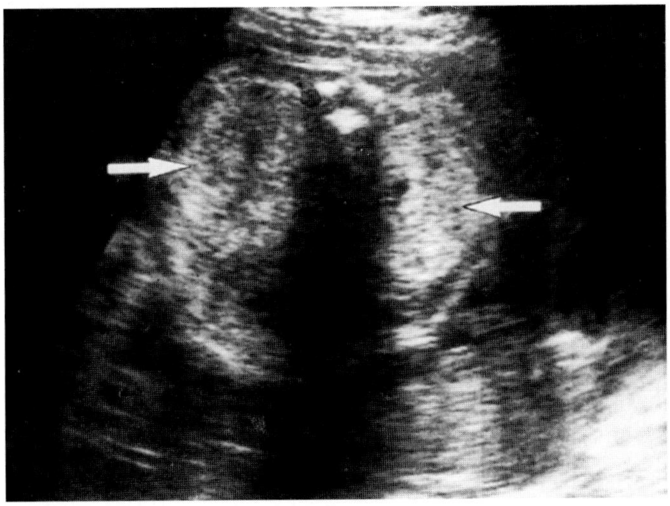

**FIG. 5–12.** Sonographic cross section of fetus with early obstructive bilateral hydronephrosis. Kidneys (arrows) are large for gestational age and have a "fluffy" echodensity without significant dilation of the renal pelvis or major and minor calyces.

The renal parenchyma is then examined for the degree of echogenicity, compression, and the absence of discrete cortical cysts. Care must be taken when possible microcystic changes are noted to ensure that what the sonographer is seeing is not dilated minor calyces. The presence of cortical cysts is associated with irreversible, advanced renal damage, which renders the fetus not amenable to interventive therapy (Fig. 5–14). Occasionally, a large, unilocular cystic structure can be found adjacent to the renal capsule. In many cases, this represents a subcapsular urinoma and must be differentiated from a large pyelectasis or cortical macrocyst (Fig. 5–15). Such urinomas may result from increased intrarenal pressures from obstructive hydronephrosis and may transiently decrease intrarenal pressure and associated damage, serving a temporary protective function for the kidney. We routinely drain urinomas to allow evaluation of the underlying renal parenchyma and have consistently found much better than expected renal function in these kidneys. Also, following placement of a vesicoamniotic shunt and diminished hydronephrosis, we have not found the urinomas to recur, supporting the probable role of increased renal pressures in their etiology.

Next, the ureters are carefully examined for abnormalities. The presence of massive pyelectasis in the absence of minimal hydroureters may indicate the presence of an obstructive

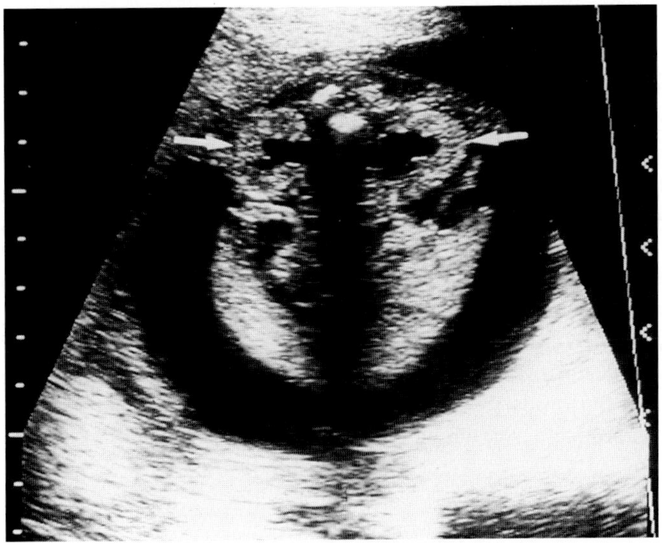

**FIG. 5–13.** Sonographic cross section of fetus with late obstructive bilateral hydronephrosis. Kidneys (arrows) are normal to small for gestational age, with very echodense parenchyma and dilated renal pelvises, major and minor calyces.

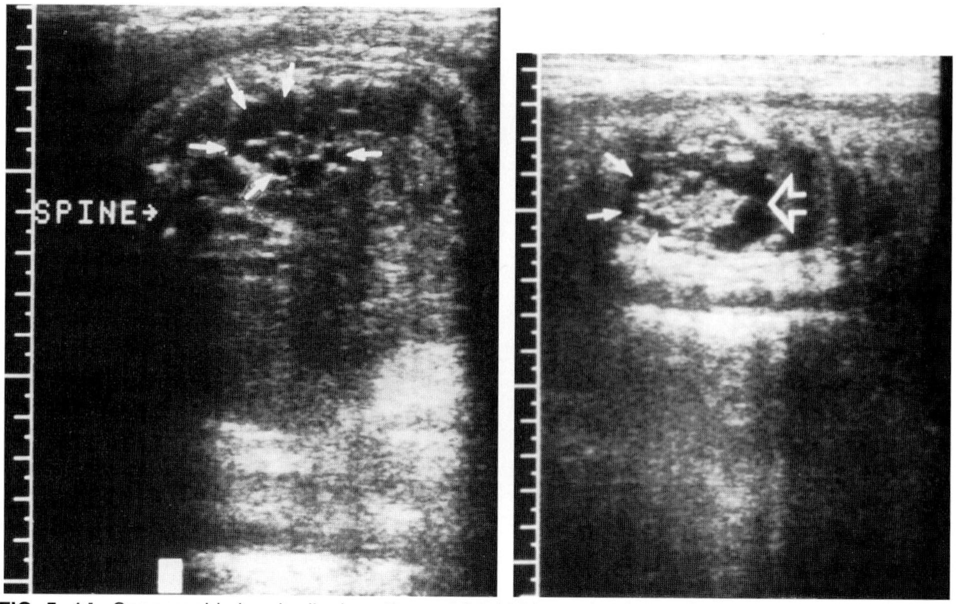


**FIG. 5–14.** Sonographic longitudinal sections of fetal kidneys in obstructive uropathy, showing cystic changes. (A) Arrows show cystic degeneration in the renal cortex in kidneys later shown histologically to have severe fibrosis and macro- or microcystic degeneration throughout. (B) Small arrows indicate renal cortical cysts; large arrow shows dilated major and minor calyces within the renal medulla, which are sometimes misinterpreted as representing renal cystic change.

component at the level of the ureteropelvic junction (UPJ). Successful vesicoamniotic shunting in the presence of a complete or high-grade UPJ obstruction would not allow renal drainage, and bladder shunting would therefore fail to prevent further damage to that kidney. Megaureters and obvious distortion of the ureterovesical junctions (Fig. 5–16) indicate severe reflux, which is generally associated with more advanced renal damage and a poorer prognosis.

The bladder is carefully evaluated prior to and following complete drainage by fine-needle vesicocentesis. Prior to drainage, overall size is assessed as well as degree of apparent proximal urethral dilation (*i.e.*, keyhole sign) as an indication of level and etiology of apparent obstruction. In addition, the presence of abnormal bladder shape (Fig. 5–17) or urachal abnormalities (Fig. 5–18) may indicate the presence of an underlying developmental abnormality of cloachal differentiation, which represent more complex anomalies that have not benefited from simple diverting procedures, such as vesicoamniotic shunting. The penile urethra is also evaluated for dilation or abnormalities indicating a distal etiology, such as stenosis of the urethral meatus or anterior urethral valves (Fig. 5–19). Following vesicocentesis, the extent and uniformity of bladder wall thickening can be assessed.

The second major component of the prenatal evaluation is the fetal karyotype. Female fetuses are rarely found to have simple urethral obstructions and usually have complex developmental abnormalities of the cloaca. Past attempts at in utero shunt therapy have proven unsuccessful in improving the prognosis for these fetuses, and therefore are not indicated. We have also encountered fetuses with trisomy 21, trisomy 18, and Klinefelter syndrome with apparent isolated megacystis, hydronephrosis, and decreased amniotic fluid volume in the absence of other major sonographic markers. As most cases of early onset obstructive uropathy have severe oligohydramnios by the time they are identified, amniocentesis is not an option. We routinely perform chorionic villus sampling via the transabdominal approach, which provides us with a preliminary result in 2–3 days and a final karyotype in 7–10 days. Other options include cordocentesis, which can prove difficult given the typical situation of severe oligohydramnios, as well as vesicocentesis with culturing of the cells from the fetal urine. Although successful in most cases, fetal urine specimens are more difficult to grow and results are therefore delayed.

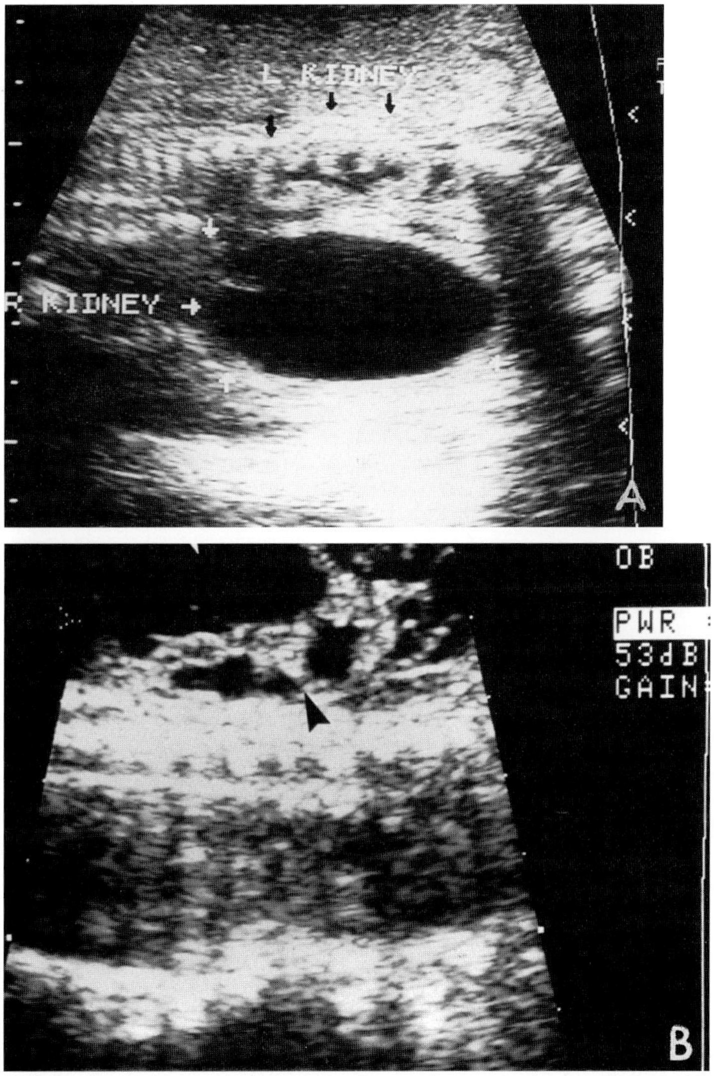


**FIG. 5–15.** Sonographic image of subcapsular renal urinoma. (A) Left kidney is very echodense with dilated calyces and right kidney appears to be replaced by a large cystic structure. (B) Following fine-needle drainage of the right renal cyst, the remaining fluid-filled region (white arrow) can be differentiated from the underlying renal parenchyma (highly echogenic with dilated calyces, black arrow) as a subcapsular urinoma. Note absence of amniotic fluid in this case of complete urethral atresia.

The last step in the work-up is the evaluation of underlying renal function. We do this utilizing sequential vesicocenteses in which the fetal bladder is completely drained at 48–72-hour intervals on a minimum of three occassions.[6] The urine is then analyzed for electrolyte and protein values as a reflection of the level and severity of damage in the fetal kidneys (Table 5–4). Fetuses who demonstrate progressive hypotonicity on sequential urine samples and have final values that fall below recommended thresholds (Fig. 5–20) have been shown to benefit from in utero intervention.[7] Occasionally, especially later in midgestation, it is necessary to perform four or five bladder drainages in order to establish a clear pattern of improving hypotonicity or increasing hypertonicity prior to final counseling of the patient as to underlying renal status and prognosis. We have been able to demonstrate histologically that there is strong correlation between progressive hypo- or hypertonicity and final urine values in predicting the presence or absence of significant, advanced renal damage.[8] We have found

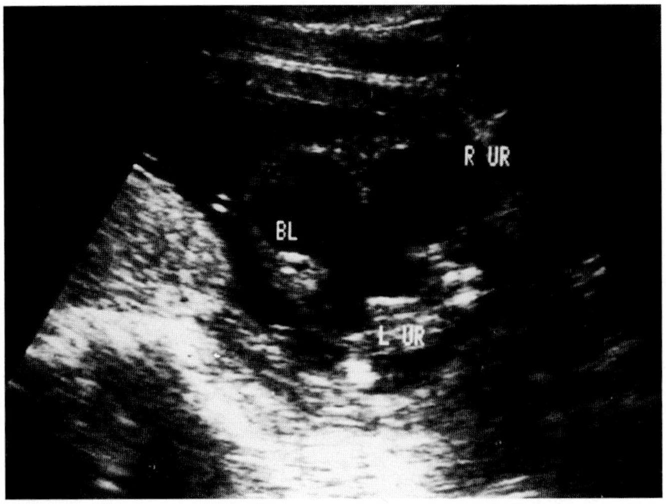


**FIG. 5–16.** Sonographic cross section of a fetal bladder (BL) showing grossly dilated ureterovesical junctions and reflux in both the right (R UR) and left ureters (L UR).

that once electrolyte levels approach threshold values (*i.e.* sodium > 85 mg/dl, osmolality > 170 mOsm/L), urinary proteins (total protein, albumin, microglobulins) may provide a better reflection of the degree of underlying damage, and may reflect impairment that has extended past the level of the proximal tubule to involve the glomerulus.[9] With such information, one can reliably counsel the patient about the futility or potential benefits of vesicoamniotic shunt placement.

## PATIENT SELECTION

Fetuses with isolated megacystis, bilateral hydronephrosis, decreased amniotic fluid volume, absent associated congenital anomalies, a 46, XY (male) karyotype, and serially improving hypotonicity with values below recommended thresholds would be considered potential candidates for vesicoamniotic shunt placement. Fetuses who meet all other criteria but have urine values demonstrating minimal improvement and cluster about the threshold cutoffs (see Fig. 5–20), can be counseled that placement of a vesicoamniotic shunt may help ensure a live birth with a decreased chance of pulmonary insufficiency, but that the infant would be expected to

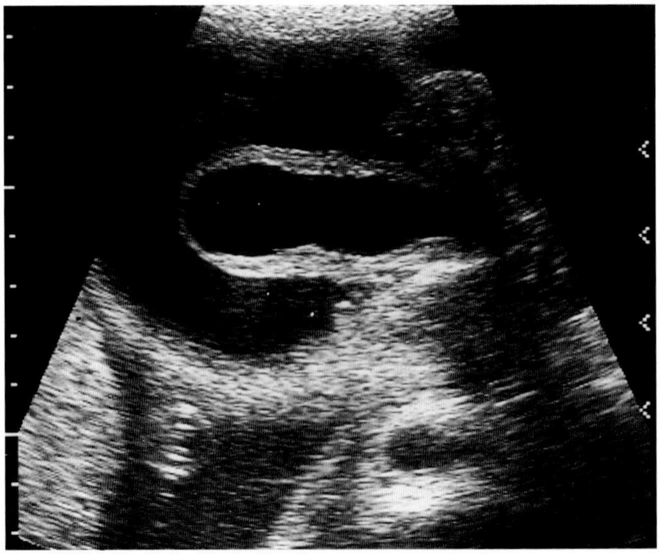

**FIG. 5–17.** Sonographic image of a bladder in a fetus with prune-belly syndrome and urethral hypoplasia. Note unusual elongated, tubular appearance and "snowman" shape of inner bladder cavity. Also present is urinary ascites due to a transient leak in the bladder dome at the site of fine-needle vesicocentesis performed 2 days earlier. Such leaks close in 48–72 hours and progressive bladder enlargement recurs secondary to urethral obstruction or restricted urethral flow as shown in this case. Urinary ascites generally resolves in 10–14 days.

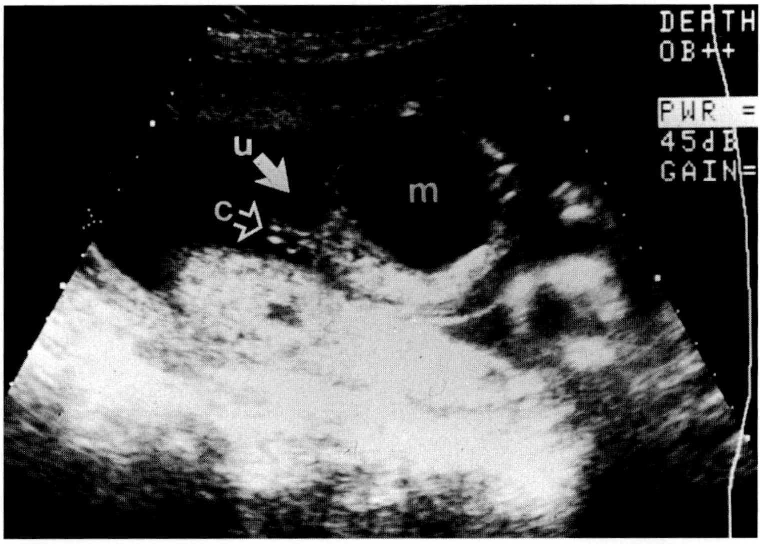


**FIG. 5–18.** Sonographic cross section of fetal abdomen showing markedly distended fetal bladder (m) and large urachal cyst (u) adjacent to the umbilical-cord (c) insertion site. Note presence of fluid in amniotic cavity following amnioinfusion, which significantly improved anatomic visualization in this pregnancy with anhydramnios and obstructive uropathy.

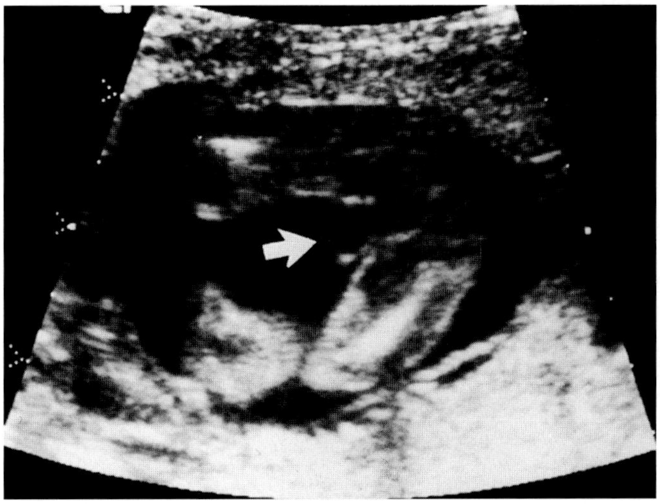

**FIG. 5–19.** Sonographic image of fetal penis showing megalourethra (arrow) due to anterior urethral valves. Again, note improved imaging due to presence of fluid in amniotic space following amnioinfusion.

**TABLE 5–4. FETAL URINE PARAMETERS**

| | |
|---|---|
| Sodium | ≤100 mg/dl |
| Osmolality | ≤200 mOsm/L |
| Chloride | ≤90 mg/dl |
| Calcium | ≤8 mg/dl |
| Total protein | ≤20 mg/dl |
| B-2 microglobulin | ≤6 mg/L |

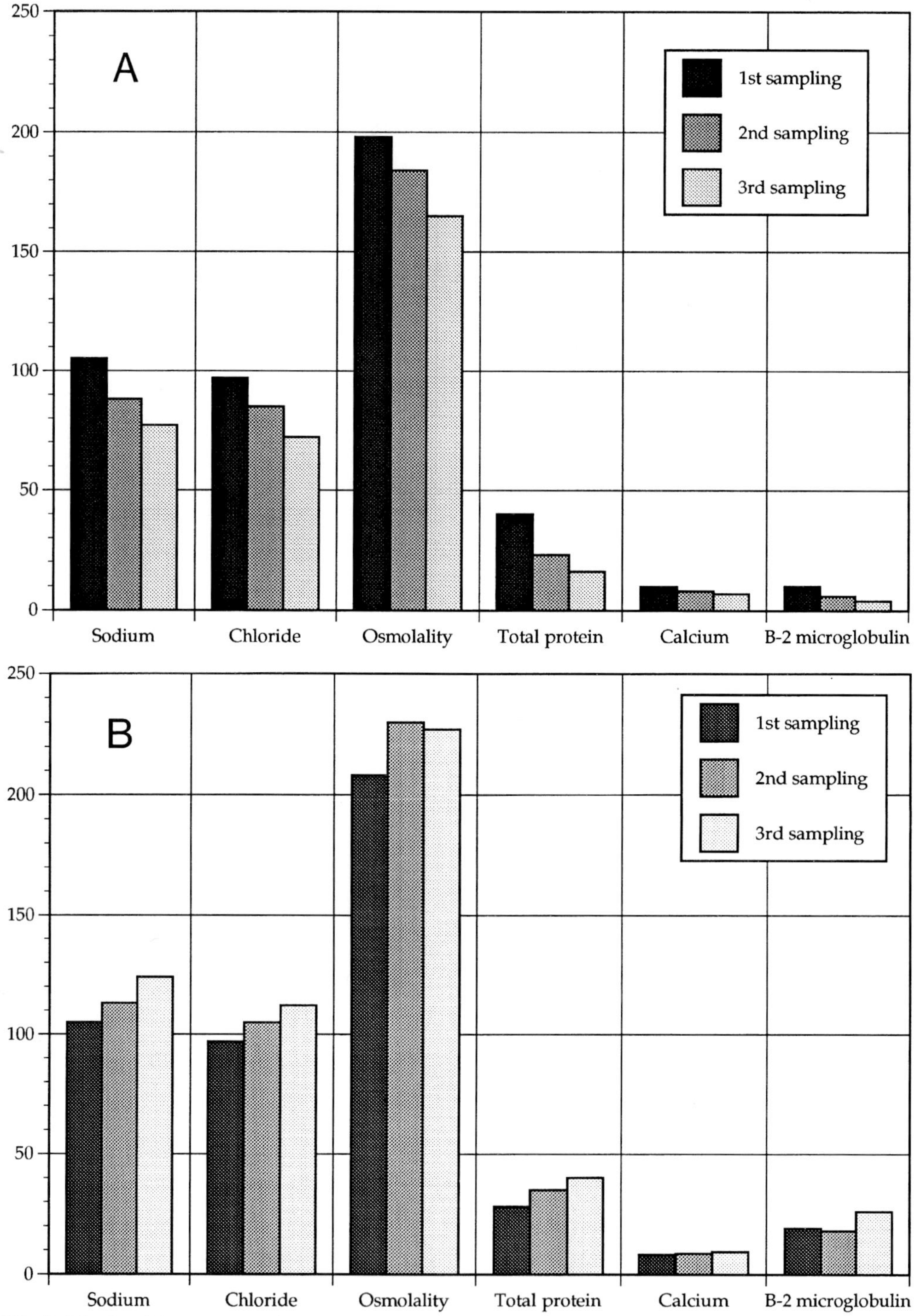


**FIG. 5–20.** Graphic representation of urine analysis based on serial vesicocenteses in the evaluation of renal damage. (A) Stepwise improvement in parameters with each of three bladder assignations and final values well below cut-off thresholds, representing absence of significant renal damage and a good candidate for in utero intervention. (B) Progressive worsening in urinary parameters with values above thresholds in a fetus subsequently shown to have advanced fiberocystic damage to the kidneys.

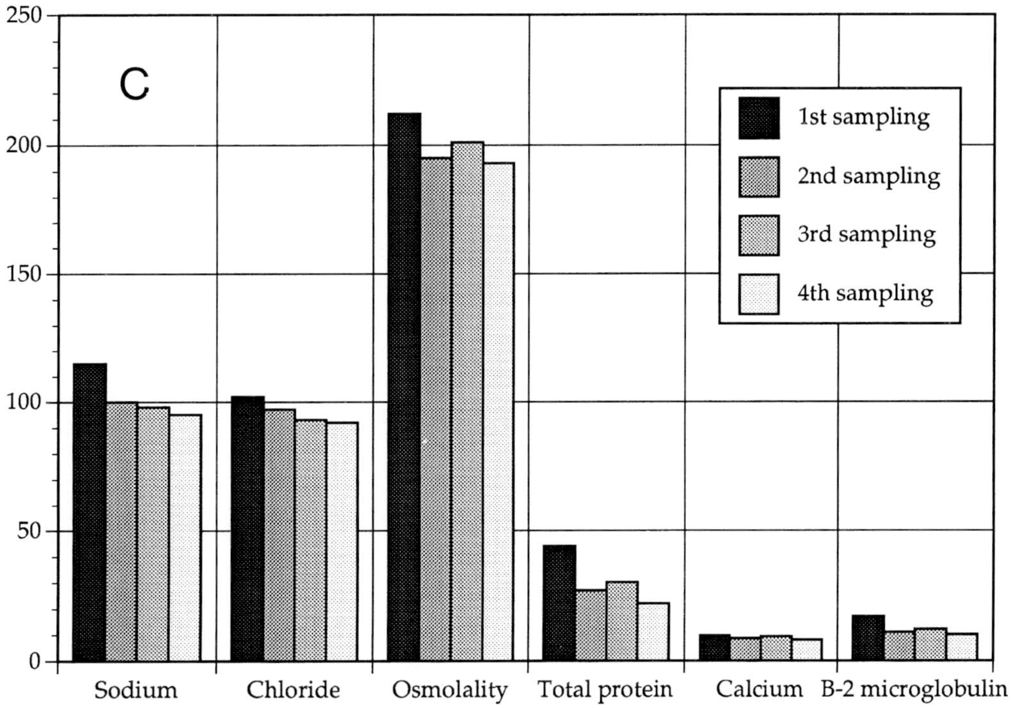


**FIG. 5–20.** *(continued)* (C) Intermediate prognostic values that show minimal improvement on serial samplings and hover near the cut-off thresholds for each urine parameter. Such patterns have been shown to represent the presence of moderate fiberoptic damage within the kidneys and presence of moderate renal insufficiency in infants born following successful in utero shunt therapy.

have renal insufficiency, may require early dialysis, and would likely require early renal transplant if it survives the neonatal period. As with any invasive procedure, the patient must have a clear understanding of the potential risks of the procedure itself to both the mother and fetus, the level of experience of the operator, as well as the possible complications which may occur later in the pregnancy.

## TECHNIQUE

Vesicoamniotic shunting represents a temporary therapeutic intervention allowing simple diversion of fetal urine from the obstructed bladder into the amniotic space (Fig. 5–21). It is essential that patients understand that such therapy is not curative but is, in essence, preventative in nature and the infant will require further evaluation and treatment for the obstruction following birth. Pregnancies complicated by severe oligohydramnios present a sonographic challenge in which visualization is significantly impaired. As such, we routinely utilize amnioinfusion at the time of initiation of our evaluation protocol to restore amniotic fluid volume to assist in sonographic visualization. Because amnioinfusion may carry an increased risk for chorioamnionitis in such cases, we routinely give the patient a loading dose and begin a 10-day course of oral antibiotics for prophylaxis. Amnioinfusion is done under continuous ultrasound guidance, using warmed lactated ringer solution and a 20-gauge spinal needle inserted as high in the fundus as possible to decrease the risk of fluid leakage. One must be exceedingly careful and utilize color-flow Doppler to identify and avoid the umbilical cord that always inhabits the small apparent fluid pockets present in these cases. We use a closed, sterile system consisting of a warmed IV bag of lactated Ringer's solution connected to a sterile set of IV tubing, a 3-way stopcock with a 20 cc syringe attached, and IV extension tubing connected to the infusion needle. The syringe and stopcock are used to intermittently draw fluid from the IV bag and then infuse fluid into the amniotic space to restore volume levels to low normal.

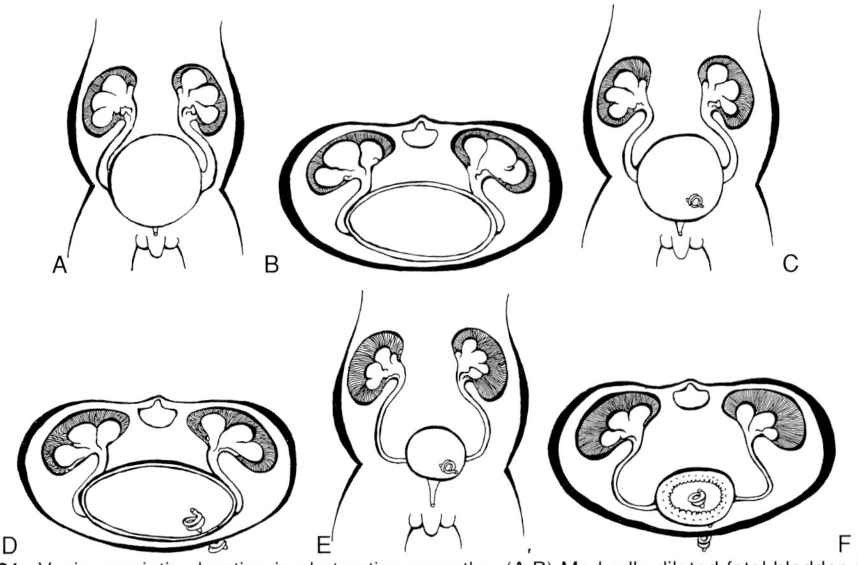


**FIG. 5–21.** Vesicoamniotic shunting in obstructive uropathy. (A,B) Markedly dilated fetal bladder, bilateral hydronephrosis, and hydroureters. (C,D) Initial placement of a vesicoamniotic shunt. Note the placement is suprapubic and just lateral to the midline. (E,F) Resolution of bladder displacement and reduction in ureteral distention, pylectasis, and hydronephrosis. Note proper shunt placement, which ensures good function after initial phase of bladder drainage has occurred.

Vesicocentesis is performed under continuous ultrasound guidance to ensure appropriate needle position throughout. Using a 22-gauge needle, the fetal abdomen is approached just above the pubic rami and lateral to midline. Before entering the bladder, color-flow Doppler is used to ensure that the potential needle track does not pass through the umbilical vessels that course laterally about the bladder (Fig. 5–22). The needle is then passed into the lower bladder and the urine completely emptied while constantly maintaining needle-tip placement within the cavity of the shrinking bladder (Fig. 5–23). Needle placement too high in the megacystis will not allow complete drainage as the bladder drains downward into the fetal

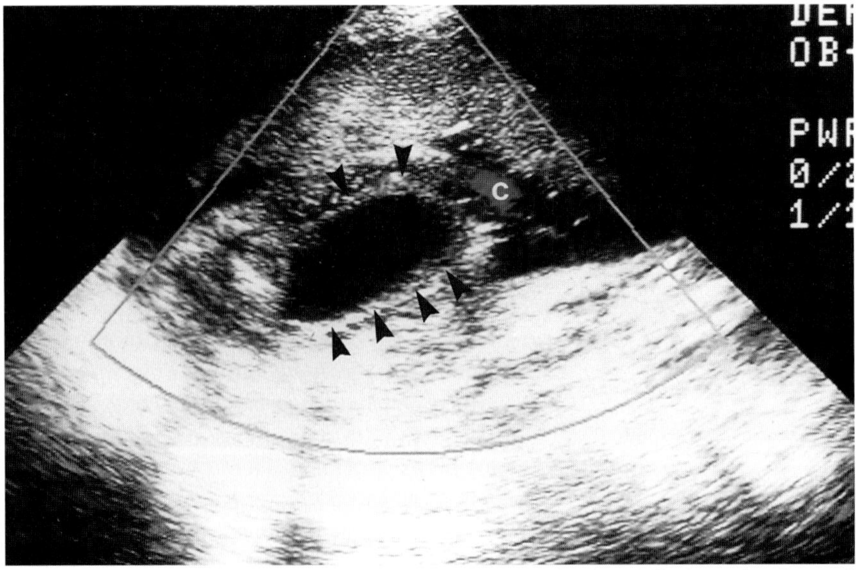


**FIG. 5–22.** Sonographic Doppler flow image showing path of umbilical arteries (arrows) around the dilated fetal bladder, which may be damaged during shunt placement, in a fetus with posterior urethral valves (c = insertion of umbilical cord).

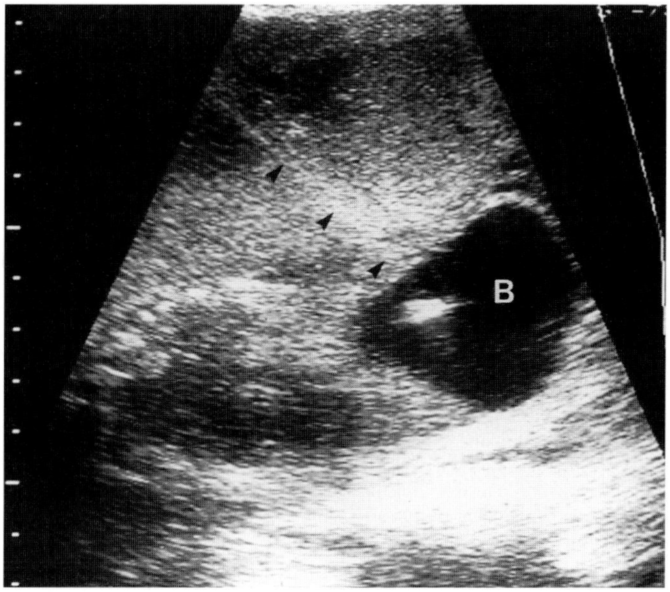


**FIG. 5–23.** Sonographic image of a fine-needle vesicocentesis. Note needle tip (arrows) is directed into lower bladder near proximal urethra to allow maximum drainage of the distended bladder (B). Also note absence of amniotic fluid prior to amnioinfusion.

pelvis. We do not paralyze the fetus with IM pancuronium prior to the vesicocentesis or vesicoamniotic shunt placement procedures.

Careful sonographic evaluation prior to attempted shunt placement is essential to identify the location and position of the fetus and placenta. It is preferable if the fetus can be approached without having to pass the shunt trocar through the placenta, although we have done so without subsequent problems in most cases. If a transplacental approach is unavoidable, one must traverse the placenta in a single smooth motion, keeping lateral motion of the trocar to a minimum, utilizing color-flow Doppler prior to passage through the chorionic plate to identify surface vessels that must be avoided. If possible, the fetus should be in the back down, vertex position, allowing a straight approach as high in the fundus as possible. This will significantly reduce the risk of post-procedure fluid leakage. If the fetus is uncooperative, we have walked the patient for several minutes to encourage position changes, postponed the procedure until the following day, and externally manipulated the fetus into the vertex position. If these measures fail and the only approach is through the lower uterine segment, then strict bed rest is recommended for at least 72 hours as our experience indicates the risk of fluid leakage is quite high. If shunt placement is undertaken, we continue oral antibiotic prophylaxis for an additional 5–7 days.

Once the appropriate approach is chosen, the maternal skin is anesthetised with 1% lidocaine and a small 3–5 mm stab wound made to allow easy passage of the shunt trocar. The shunt trocar is then carefully introduced into the amniotic space near the lower fetal abdomen. An adequate pocket of amniotic fluid needs to be present in which to drop the distal end of the vesicoamniotic shunt on exiting the fetal abdomen. If no such space is present, amnioinfusion to create such a fluid pocket can be done through the trocar or its sideport. We routinely use the shunt apparatus offered by Rocket of London, as well as their Rodeck vesicoamniotic shunt catheters (Fig. 5–24). The tip of the trocar is positioned in the same manner as the vesicocentesis needle and color-flow Doppler used to confirm the absence of umbilical vessels at that position. The trocar is then quickly inserted into the bladder and positioned into a central location (Fig. 5–25). At this point, the operative assistant should have carefully and gently straightened the vesicoamniotic catheter. The catheter is partially threaded into the trocar sheath prior to removal of the internal stylet wire as noted earlier. If the wire is removed prior to threading the catheter, difficulty with kinking and directing the catheter down the shaft of the trocar sheath may be encountered. Once in place, a short push rod is

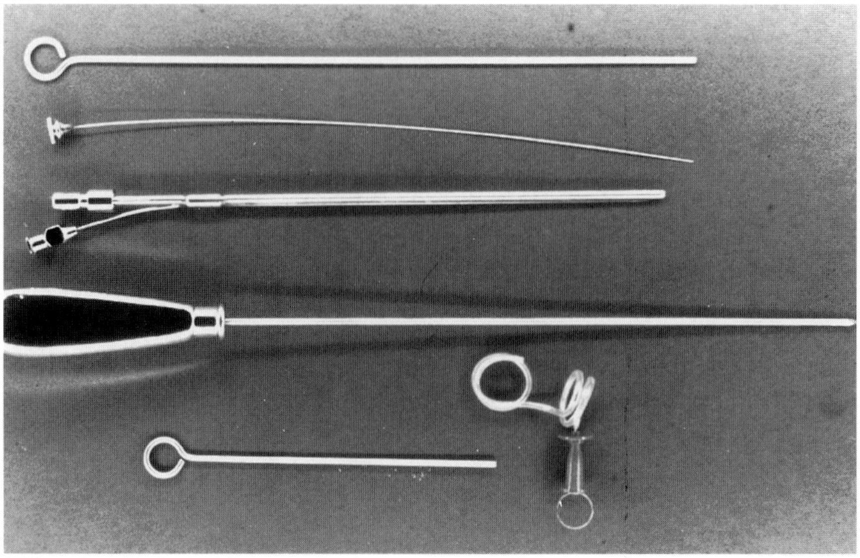

**FIG. 5–24.** Rocket vesicoamniotic shunt apparatus. Rodeck style double pigtail shunt is shown at lower right.

introduced and used to push the proximal segment of the catheter into the fetal bladder. This is then removed and a long push rod gently introduced until it comes in contact with the distal end of the shunt within the trocar sheath. The push rod is then held at this position while the shaft of the trocar sheath is slowly pulled back approximately 1 cm. At this point, the trocar sheath should lie just outside of the fetal abdomen, with the straight segment of the shunt catheter traversing the region between the bladder and amniotic space. Failure to properly perform this maneuver may result in partial displacement of the proximal end of the catheter and increased risk for shunt displacement.

The trocar sheath is now gently directed slightly away from the insertion site and the long push rod advanced to displace the distal end of the catheter into the amniotic space. Positioning of the proximal and distal segments of the catheter as well as bladder drainage is

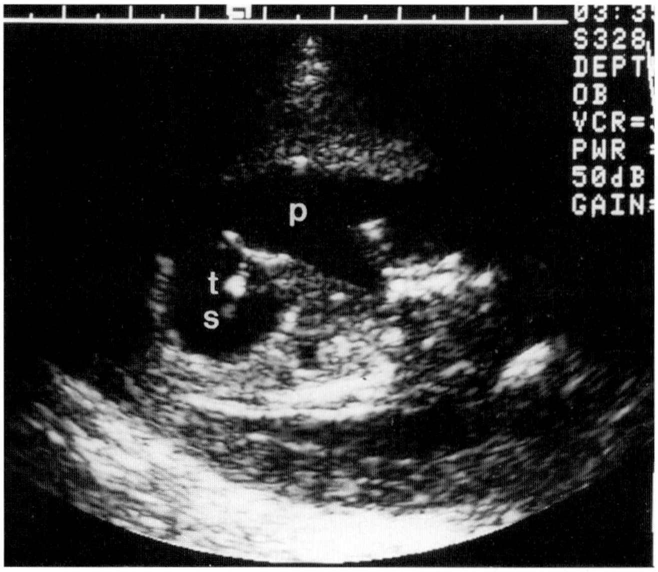


**FIG. 5–25.** Sonographic image showing a vesicoamniotic shunt. Shunt trocar (t) is within fetal bladder and the proximal bladder portion of the shunt (s) is seen protruding out the end of the trocar. Also, note large pocket (p) of amniotic fluid following amnioinfusion into which the distal amniotic portion of the shunt will be dropped.

A

B

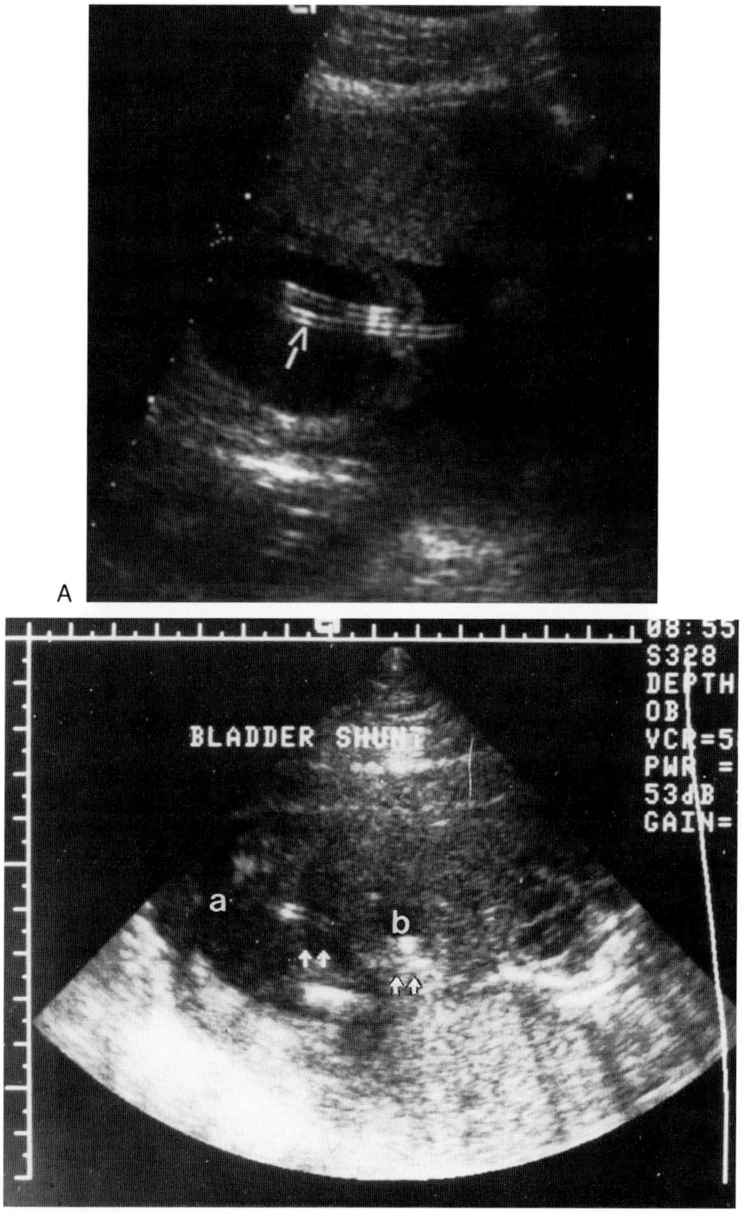


**FIG. 5–26.** (A) Sonographic image of proximal segment of Rodeck shunt (arrow) shortly after placement within a distended fetal bladder. Note catheter has begun to resume its original coiled shape; straight segment of catheter can be seen coursing through the abdominal wall into the amniotic space. (B) Sonographic image of indwelling shunt (double arrows) several minutes after placement into a distended fetal bladder (b). Note resolution of bladder distention, tight coiling of the proximal segment of the catheter within the bladder, and the straight segment of the catheter transversing the fetal abdominal wall into the amniotic space (a).

confirmed sonographically (Fig. 5–26). The patient is then placed on external fetal/uterine monitoring for approximately 2 hours. Any indication of uterine irritability is aggressively treated with intravenous fluids and tocolytic medications.

## *COMPLICATIONS*

Counseling of the patient prior to embarking on a course of prenatal evaluation includes discussions of potential complications of any invasive needle procedure such as subsequent chorioamnionitis, premature rupture of fetal membranes, direct trauma to the fetus, and intraplacental

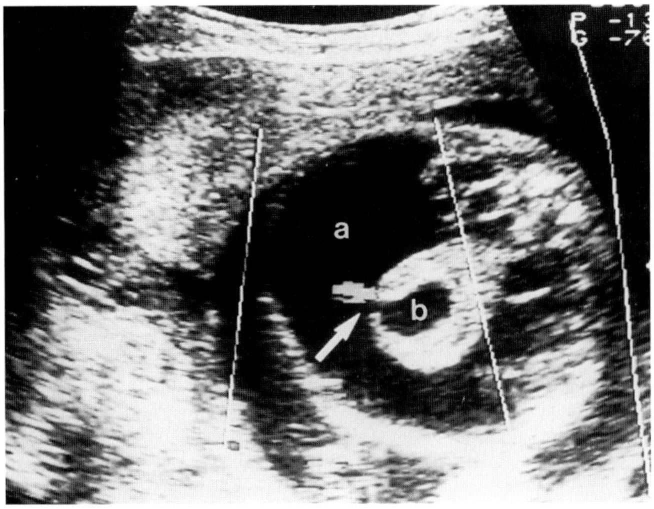


**FIG. 5–27.** Sonographic image of transient vesicoamniotic defect following catheter displacement into the amniotic space. Note the asymmetrically thickened bladder (b) wall, fetal ascites, and Doppler flow imaging of actual urine flow (arrow) from bladder to peritoneal space. Such defects generally close in 10–14 days.

bleeding and possible associated onset of preterm labor if transplacental approaches become necessary.

Transient vesicoperitoneal fistulas occasionally occur following vesicocentesis, resulting in urinary ascites (Fig. 5–27). Such fistulas spontaneously close in 10–14 days followed by redevelopment of megacystis. If the urinary ascites results in massive distention of the abdomen, drainage can be accomplished by placement of a peritoneal-amniotic shunt (Fig. 5–28). These can be easily placed into either of the lower abdominal quadrants, although care must be taken to avoid traumatic damage to the viscera from the shunt trocar. Once placed, the urinary ascites can be easily diverted to the amniotic cavity until fistula closure is complete.

Shunt displacement is also a fairly common complication, occurring in approximately 30% of cases in our series. Despite the fact that the Rodeck catheter is designed such that the distal end curls to lie flat against the fetal abdomen, it may become dislodged, necessitating replacement with recurrence of the megacystis (Fig. 5–29).

As noted earlier, if the catheter is placed too high within the megacystis, it may be placed under tension as the bladder shrinks with drainage, and eventually be displaced and pulled within the fetal abdomen (Fig. 5–30), resulting in loss of function.

We have observed one case in which a shunt was successfully placed following which the markedly thick-walled bladder completely drained. Unfortunately, because of apparent histologic changes at the ureterovesicle angles, this fetus developed bilateral ureteral obstructions, massive megaureters, and eventual renal failure.

Also, we have seen two cases of successful shunt placement at 19 and 20 weeks' gestation, in which catheter placement and function was optimal with decreasing hydronephrosis and maintenance of good amniotic fluid volumes. Unfortunately, in both cases, at 28–29 weeks' gestation the amniotic fluid volume began to slowly decrease, the renal parenchyma became increasingly echodense, and renal growth as measured from superior to inferior pole stopped and actually regressed over time. One fetus was stillborn and the other was a neonatal death. On autopsy, both demonstrated severe microcystic dysplasia and fibrosis, and in each case the catheter was noted to be patent and appropriately positioned within the fetal bladder.

## FOLLOW-UP

Following a vesicoamniotic shunt procedure, we perform a follow-up sonographic evaluation 24–48 hours later to confirm catheter placement and function. Weekly evaluations are recommended for at least the next 4–6 weeks to confirm catheter placement and function, amniotic fluid volume, and progressive resolution of the bilateral hydronephrosis. At that point, evaluations may be spaced to every 10–14 days, depending on maintenance of amniotic fluid volume.

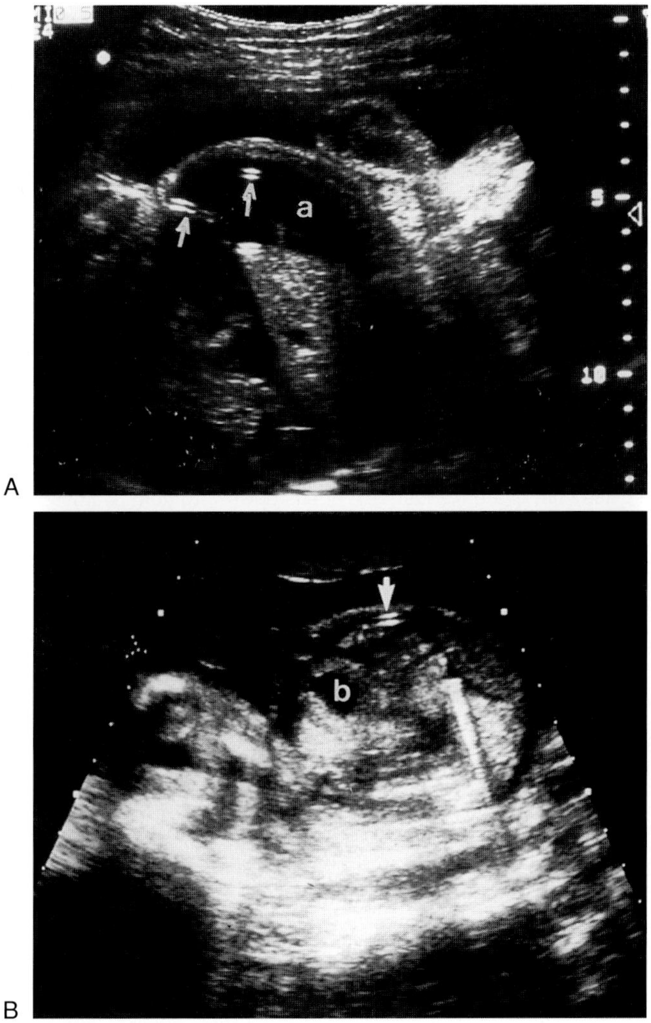


**FIG. 5–28.** Sonographic image of peritoneal-amniotic shunt placement. (A) Catheter shown shortly after placement into urinary ascites (a). Note catheter (arrows) has begun to resume its coiled shape within the peritoneal space. (B) Catheter (arrow) shown within peritoneal space with significant reduction in urinary ascites. Note thick-walled bladder (b) with open defect in dome allowing drainage of urine into the abdominal cavity.

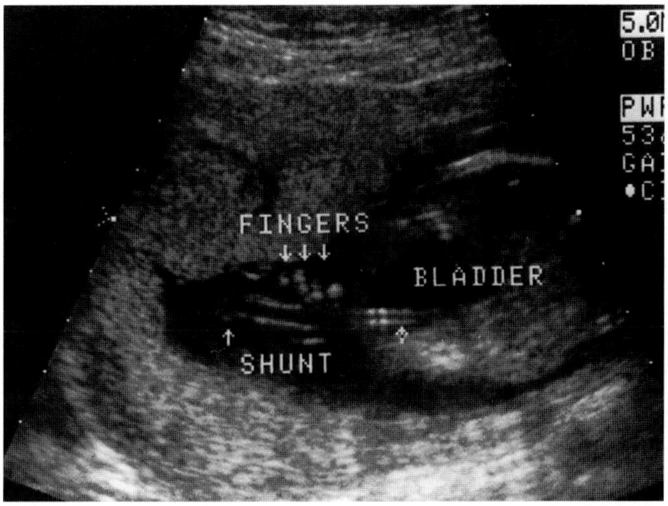


**FIG. 5–29.** Sonographic image of a well-placed vesicoamniotic shunt just before its displacement out of the fetal bladder and into the amniotic space. Note presence of inquisitive fetus at shunt site, implicating likely mechanism of shunt displacement.

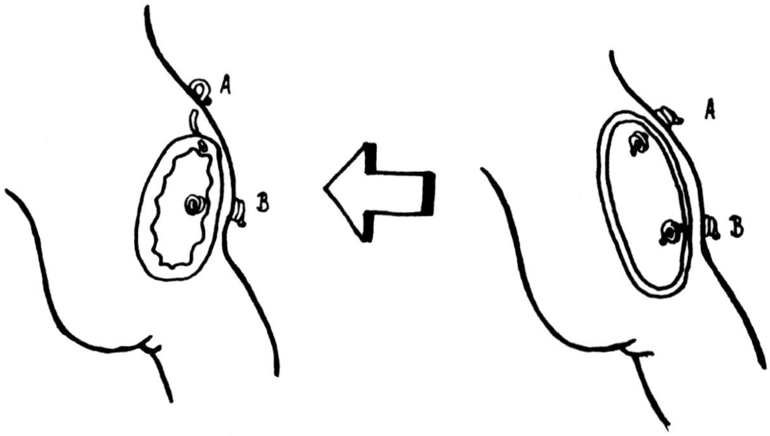


**FIG. 5–30.** Illustration of proper and poor positioning of vesicoamniotic shunt. Catheter A has been placed too high into the dome of the bladder (right), so that it becomes displaced out of the bladder as it drains downward (left). Catheter B is properly positioned low within the bladder, so that it maintains good function despite drainage of the fetal bladder.

Consultation with the pediatric urologist and neonatologist who will care for the child after birth is recommended so that postnatal management and treatment options can be discussed, a plan formulated, and a relationship established between the family and the postnatal team. This greatly facilitates communication and understanding of postnatal management, significantly reduces family anxiety, and fosters a trusting relationship between the family and medical team.

Route of delivery should be dictated by routine obstetrical indications and not influenced by the presence of an indwelling catheter. Pregnancies that have undergone shunting in our clinical series[7] have experienced spontaneous rupture of membranes and vaginal delivery at 33–35 weeks' gestation; the patient should be counseled about this possibility.

Following delivery, a bag can be placed on the abdomen to catch the urine, which can then be used for renal function studies. Also, the pediatric urologists at our center use the catheter for retrograde dye studies of the urinary tract prior to simply pulling the catheter once it is no longer necessary for urinary diversion.

## SUMMARY

The era of fetal medicine has become a reality as we have developed methodologies to medically and surgically treat fetuses in utero. Advances in diagnostic technology have improved our capacity to evaluate selectively fetuses with genetic disorders. In many such cases, fetuses who had previously faced a dismal prognosis can now be considered potential candidates for therapeutic intervention. The key to success in such interventions is an appreciation of the diversity of underlying etiologies and pathologic processes, as well as a thorough understanding of the appropriate detailed prenatal evaluation necessary for patient selection. Only then can one reliably predict which fetuses will truly benefit from invasive intervention, and prevent unnecessary procedures in cases where such intervention will not alter the eventual outcome and only serve to place the mother at unnecessary risk for complications.

## REFERENCES

1. Weiner C. Umbilical pressure measurement in the evaluation of nonimmune hydrops fetalis. Am J Obstet Gynecol 1993;168:817–823.

2. Freedman AL, Qureshi F, Shapiro E, Lepor H, Jacques SM, Evans MI, Smith CA, Gonzalez R, Johnson MP. Smooth muscle development in obstructed fetal bladder. Urology (submitted).
3. Freedman AL, Bukowski TP, Smith CA, Evans MI, Gonzalez R, Johnson MP. Fetal therapy for obstructive uropathy: diagnosis specific outcomes. Urology (submitted).
4. Quintero RA, Johnson MP, Romero R, Smith C, Arias F, Guevara-Zuloaga F, Cotton DB, Evans MI. In utero percutaneous cystoscopy in the management of fetal lower obstructive uropathy. Lancet 1995;346:537–540.
5. Inselman LS, Mellins RB. Growth and development of the lung. J Pediatrics 1981;98(1): 1–15.
6. Johnson MP, Corsi P, Bradfield W, Hume RF, Smith C, Flake AW, Qureshi F, Evans MI: Sequential fetal urine analysis provides greater precision in the evaluation of fetal obstructive uropathy. Am J Obstet Gynecol 1995;173:59–65.
7. Johnson MP, Bukowski TP, Reitleman C, Isada NB, Pryde PG, Evans MI: In utero surgical treatment of fetal obstructive uropathy: a new comprehensive approach to identify appropriate candidates for vesicoamniotic shunt therapy. Am J Obstet Gynecol 1994;170(6): 1770–1779.
8. Qureshi F, Jacques SM, Seifman B, Quintero R, Evans MI, Smith C, Johnson MP. In utero fetal urine analysis and renal histology do correlate with outcome in fetal obstructive uropathies. Fetal Diagn Ther (submitted).
9. Johnson MP, Hume R, Quintero R, Freedman A, Kithier K, Smith C, Cejka J, Qureshi F, Flake AW, Gonzalez R, Evans MI. In utero analysis of fetal proteinuria in obstructive uropathy. International Fetal Medicine & Surgery Society, 14th Annual Meeting, Newport, RI, May 3–6, 1995.

*Invasive Outpatient Procedures in Reproductive Medicine,* edited by Mark I. Evans, et al. Lippincott–Raven Publishers, Philadelphia © 1997.

# 6 Selective Termination

Mark I. Evans, Roderick F. Hume Jr, Avihai Reichler, Nelson B. Isada, Mark P. Johnson

The commonly recognized incidence of major birth defects in 1 in 30 babies does not apply to twins. The incidence in a twin pregnancy is more than just twice that of a singleton pregnancy. In monozygotic twins the risk of a significant birth defect approaches 10% and is mostly a function of the timing of the embryonic split.[1–3] The later the split of the embryo into two halves, the greater the chance of defects of laterality. In dizygotic twins, which are more common, the incidence of various birth defects is also increased. Monozygotic twins have the same risk for chromosomal abnormalities as a singleton because they came from the same embryo, but in dizygotic twins the risks are double that of the age incidence (Tables 6–1 and 6–2).[4]

When confronted with a twin pregnancy in which one twin has a serious fetal anomaly, counseling can be particularly difficult (Fig. 6–1). Until the past decade, couples have been left with the unenviable choice of either keeping both fetuses, one of whom will have significant problems, or terminating both fetuses, one of whom was believed to be normal. In 1978, Aberg was the first to perform selective termination for an abnormal twin.[4] In 1981, Kerenyi et al reported on selective termination for a fetus with Down syndrome.[5] Throughout the early 1980s, there were a few selected reports on attempted selective terminations, most of which did not have happy endings.[5–8] Many of the cases involved monozygotic twins with a shared placenta; termination of one fetus led to coagulation products diffusing across the placenta into the other fetus, with resultant damage and death.

Evaluation of the performance of selective termination in the second trimester for dizygotic twins has been much more promising. Recently, we have shown that the procedure can be technically successful in virtually 100% of cases and results in a live born singleton in approximately 85% of cases.[9] Furthermore, we know now that there is a correlation between favorable outcome and when in gestation the procedure is done (*i.e.,* the earlier the better) and that the use of potassium chloride is a less risky agent than air embolization (Fig. 6–2).

## INDICATIONS

When a patient with a twin pregnancy has been diagnosed as having one fetus with an abnormality, and the gestational age is within the framework for a legally permissible termination, the patient should be counseled as to the expected outcomes in her situation, as well as all of her available options. These options, of course, include keeping the pregnancy, terminating the pregnancy, or attempting a selective termination procedure.

There will always be considerable debate about what severity of anomaly justifies performing selective termination. There is no one acceptable answer. Conclusions vary among people, religious practices and beliefs, and cultural ideologies. In certain jurisdictions, particu-

**TABLE 6–1. INCIDENCE (%) OF MALFORMATIONS IN MONOZYGOTIC AND DIZYGOTIC TWINS AND IN SINGLETONS**

| Twins | | | | | |
|---|---|---|---|---|---|
| Monozygotic | | Dizygotic | | Singletons | |
| *Major* | *Minor* | *Major* | *Minor* | *Major* | *Minor* |
| 10.72 | 10.99 | 7.78 | 5.51 | 7.10 | 7.26 |

**TABLE 6–2. INCIDENCE OF CHROMOSOMAL ABNORMALITIES IN AT LEAST ONE FETUS IN A MULTIFETAL GESTATION**

| Maternal Age | Singleton | Twin | Triplet |
|---|---|---|---|
| 20 | 1/526 | 1/263 ≈ age 34 | 1/175 ≈ age 36 |
| 25 | 1/476 | 1/238 ≈ age 34 | 1/150 ≈ age 36 |
| 30 | 1/385 | 1/192 ≈ age 35 | 1/128 ≈ age 37 |
| 35 | 1/192 | 1/96 ≈ age 38 | 1/64 ≈ age 40 |
| 40 | 1/66 | 1/33 ≈ age 43 | 1/22 ≈ age 45 |

larly outside of the United States, termination of abnormal pregnancies is legally permissible at almost any gestational age.

## TECHNIQUE

Careful evaluation of fetal anatomy and placental position are crucial to the safe performance of selective termination. The first main concern is to ensure that the correct fetus is being terminated. While advances in ultrasound have made it rare that an abnormal fetus, even one with a chromosomal abnormality, has no detectable morphologic anomalies, occasionally such is still the case. Under these circumstances it is critical to ensure that the documentation from the laboratory and from the first ultrasound under which the amniocenteses or chorionic villus samplings (CVS) were performed is consistent with what is observed. Second, placental posi-

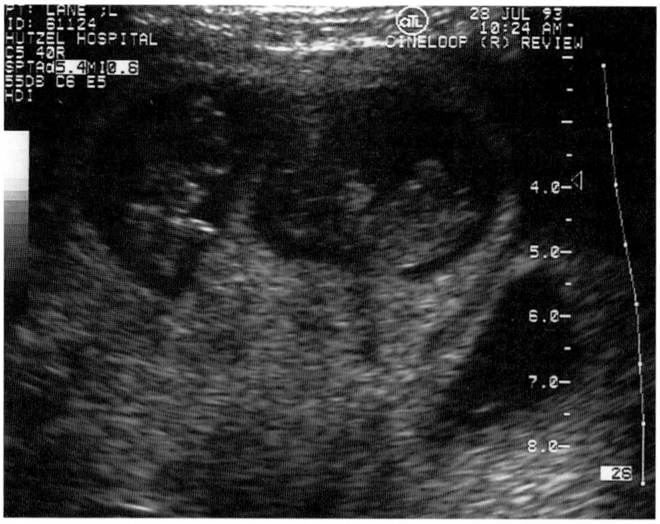


**FIG. 6–1.** Twin pregnancy at twelve weeks, showing fetus on right with omphalocele. Fetus was subsequently shown to have trisomy 13.

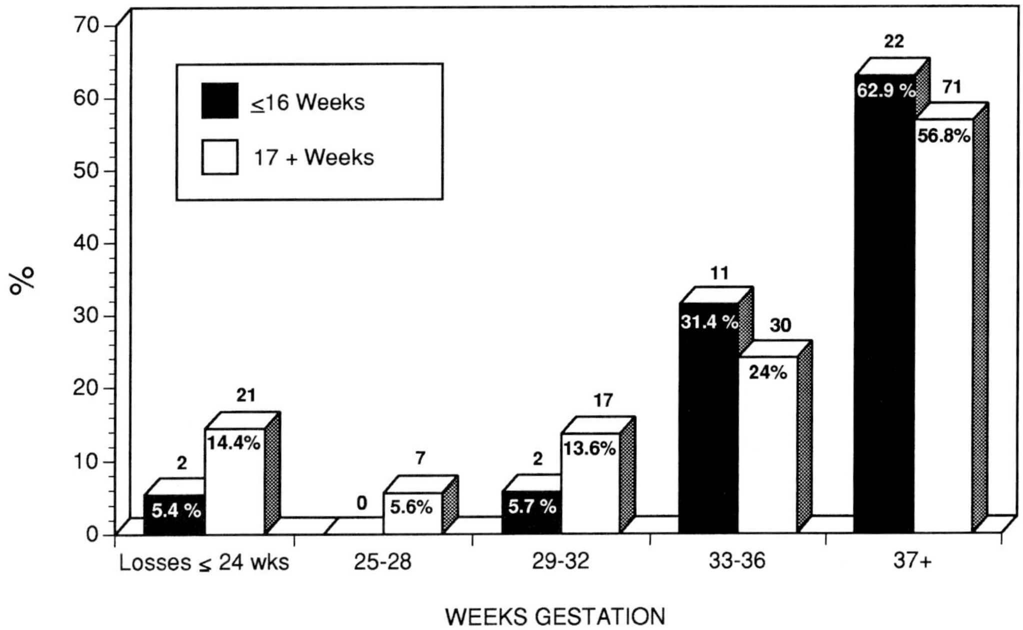


**FIG. 6–2.** Incidence of losses and deliveries as a function of when selective termination was performed.

tion must be observed (Fig. 6–3) and a demarcation made between the placentas to reduce the likelihood of either the injected potassium chloride (KCL) or coagulation products affecting the other twin. Very often, demarcation will be seen naturally between placentas, even when they are abutting, and in our experience this has been sufficient to suggest safety (Fig. 6–4). In most cases, we use a 20-gauge needle inserted transabdominally directly over the fetal thorax after appropriate prepping and draping (Figs. 6–5 and 6–6A,B). The needle must be placed directly into the fetal cardiac chamber with return of blood documented (Fig. 6–7A,B). Once the needle has been correctly positioned, approximately 2 cc of potassium chloride is injected over 30–45 seconds. This will usually produce cardiac slow-down, if not cessation.

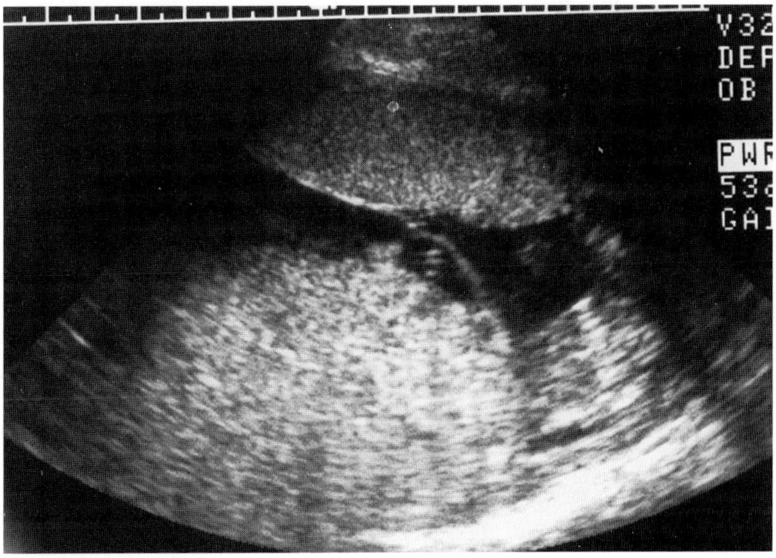

**FIG. 6–3.** Twin gestation with placentas on anterior and posterior walls, minimizing chance of any vascular communication.

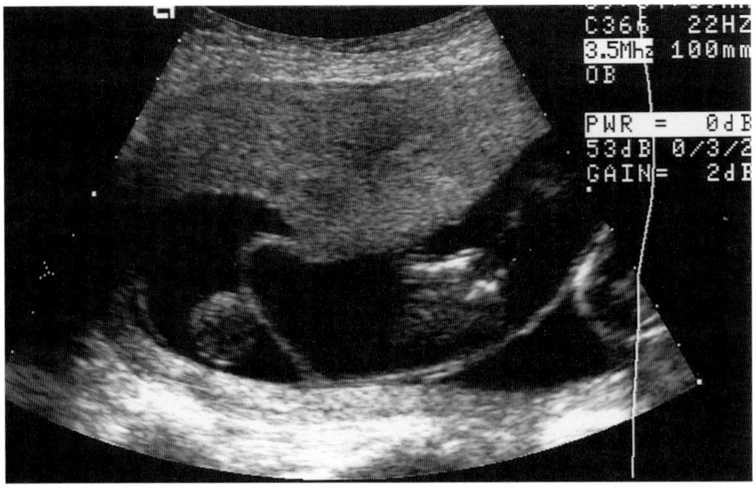


**FIG. 6–4.** Twin pregnancy with both placentas anterior but with area of decreased echogenicity just above membrane, suggesting lower likelihood of vascular communication.

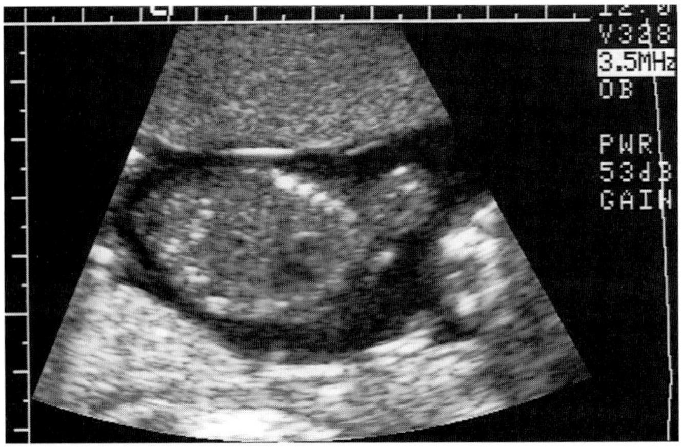


**FIG. 6–5.** Longitudinal view of twin fetus at level of cardiac chamber.

A

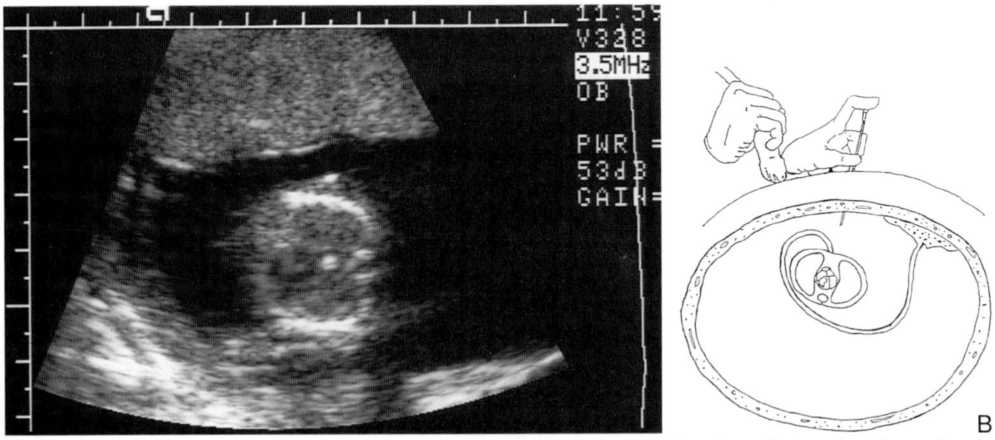


B

**FIG. 6–6A, B.** Transverse view of same fetus at level of cardiac chamber. Tip of needle is poised immediately above thorax.

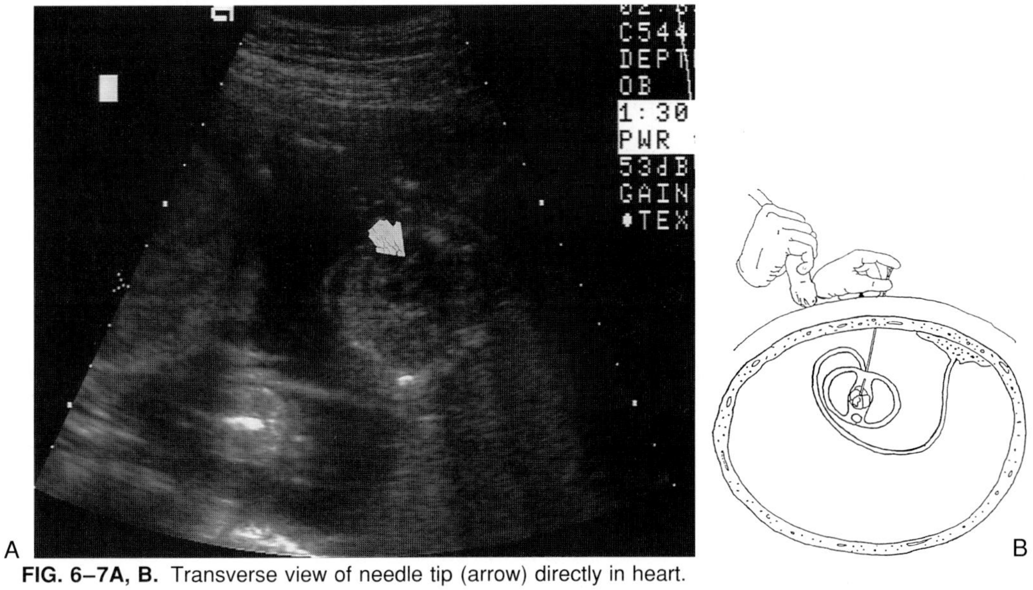

**FIG. 6–7A, B.** Transverse view of needle tip (arrow) directly in heart.

Then, depending on the gestational age, another 1–7 cc may sometimes be necessary. The needle should not be removed until confirmation of cardiac cessation is confirmed.

## CONTRAINDICATIONS

The safety of selective termination depends on lack of communication between the fetuses. It has been well appreciated for many years that the death of one monozygotic twin often leads to the death of the other. There have been documented instances of disseminated intravascular coagulation and sequelae of thromboemboli resulting in, for example, porencephalic cysts in surviving monozygotic twins. The literature suggests an approximately 80% fetal demise rate when one monozygotic twin dies either naturally or iatrogenically.[8] Consequently, the technique described above is not appropriate when there is one placenta with apparent vascular communication between the two fetuses. In such circumstances, a number of other techniques have been used, including open fetal surgery with a hysterotomy and removal of one fetus, injection into the umbilical cord of material to occlude it, and, lastly, fetoscopic or ultrasound visualization used to tie off the umbilical cord of an abnormal fetus.[11] The latter seems to be the most promising of these techniques, but a thorough discussion of this approach is beyond the scope of this book, although we and others have reported on them in the literature.

## CONCLUSIONS

Selective termination of an abnormal twin in fetal anomalies has become an important part of the armamentarium when multiple gestations are being evaluated and treated. Collaborative data suggest that selective termination procedures can be done safely and effectively, with an overall fetal loss rate of approximately 5% when the procedure is done at less than 17 weeks gestation, and 15% thereafter. Increasing experience will further refine the risks and probably lower them, which should allow for more appropriate counseling to parents in this very difficult situation.

## REFERENCES


1. Luke B. Monozygotic twinning as a congenital defect and congenital defects in monozygotic twins. Fetal Diagn Ther 1990;5:61–69.
2. Evans MI, Johnson MP, Isada NB, Holzgreve W. Selective termination. In: Brock DJH, Rodeck CH, Ferguson-Smith MA (eds). Prenatal diagnosis and screening. New York: Churchill Livingstone, 1992;689–697.
3. Drugan A, Johnson MP, Krivchenia EL, Evans MI. Genetics and genetic counseling of multiple gestation. In: Gall SA et al (eds). Multiple pregnancy and delivery. St. Louis: CV Mosby (in press).
4. Aberg A, Metelman F, Cantz M, Gehler J. Cardiac puncture of fetus with Hurler's disease avoiding abortion of unaffected co-twin. Lancet 1978;ii:990–999.
5. Kerenyi T, Chitkara U. Selective birth in twin pregnancy with discordancy for Down's syndrome. N Engl J Med 1978;304:1525–1527.
6. Rodeck C. Fetoscopy in the management of twin pregnancies discordant for a severe abnormality. Acta Genet Med Gemellol 1984;33:57–60.
7. Rodeck C, Mibashan R, Abramowicz J, Campbell S. Selective feticide of the affected twin by fetoscopic air embolization. Prenat Diagn 1982;2:189–194.
8. Golbus MS, Cunningham N, Goldberg JD, Anderson R, Filly R, Callen P. Selective termination of multiple gestations. Am J Med Genet 1988;31:339–348.
9. Evans MI, Goldberg JD, Dommergues M, Wapner RJ, Lynch L, Dock BS, Horenstein J, Golbus MS, Rodeck CH, Dumez Y, Holzgreve W, Timor-Tritsch I, Johnson MP, Isada NB, Monteagudo A, Berkowitz RL. Efficacy of second-trimester selective termination for fetal abnormalities: international collaborative experience among the world's largest centers. Am J Obstet Gynecol 1994;171:90–94.
10. Ginsburg NA, Appelbaum M, Rabin SA, et al. Term birth after midtrimester hysterotomy and selective delivery of an acardiac twin. Am J Obstet Gynecol 1992;167:33–37.
11. Quintero RA, Reich H, Puder KS, Bardicef M, Evans MI, Cotton DB, Romero R. Brief report: umbilical-cord ligation of an acardiac twin by fetoscopy at 19 weeks of gestation. N Engl J Med 1994;330(7):469–471.

*Invasive Outpatient Procedures in Reproductive Medicine,* edited by Mark I. Evans, et al. Lippincott–Raven Publishers, Philadelphia © 1997.

# 7 Multifetal Pregnancy Reduction

Mark I. Evans, Linda Littman, Lori St. Louis, Laura Blessed,
Jeanne Grager, Ivan E. Zador

## INTRODUCTION

Increasingly aggressive therapies for infertility, including ovulation stimulating drugs such as Clomiphene, human menopausal gonadotropin (Pergonal), Metrodin, and newer assisted reproductive technologies such as in vitro fertilization (IVF), gamete intrafallopian tube (GIFT), and zygote intrafallopian transfer (ZIFT), have allowed thousands of previously infertile couples to have their own children. As a noted side effect, however, there has been a concomitant dramatic increase in the number of multifetal pregnancies created under such circumstances. For example, during the 1980s, while the number of singleton deliveries per year rose approximately 20%, the number of triplets born in the United States increased over 100%.[1] Despite considerable increases in the improvement in the care of multiple pregnancies and, particularly, in the neonatal salvage of such babies, multifetal pregnancies make up a disproportionate contributor to overall perinatal morbidity and mortality. It has been estimated that for quadruplet babies who deliver at an average of 28 weeks, there is a 6% mortality per quadruplet baby and over a 25% chance of long-term morbidity[2] (Table 7–1). The costs of multifetal pregnancies have also been shown to be dramatically higher than just the singleton figure multiplied by the number of fetuses. A Boston-based study showed the total cost for singletons to be $9,845, but triplets $109,765.[3]

In the face of such daunting statistics combined with the ever-increasing generation of such pregnancies, a limited number of investigators in the mid-1980s developed a surgical response (*i.e.*, multifetal pregnancy reduction) to reduce in the first trimester the number of embryos to a more manageable number, usually twins. Collaborative data from centers with the most experience in the world have shown that multifetal pregnancy reduction (MFPR) can be performed with essentially a 100% technical success rate, and that there is considerably improved survival and decreased morbidity of fetuses after reduction than there would have been in higher-order multiple pregnancies without reduction.[3–9] Data over the past 8 years show an approximate 88% chance of reaching viability, with only approximately 5% of patients delivering with extremely early prematurity (*i.e.*, 25–28 weeks) (Fig. 7–1). Further delineation of the data shows that there has been a steep learning curve, and that outcomes have improved steadily over the past several years with increasing experience.

Two main techniques have emerged—transabdominal needle insertion for injection of intrathoracic potassium chloride and transvaginal or transcervical aspiration or mechanical disruption of the embryo. Analyses of the comparative data suggest that there probably is not much difference in outcomes when each procedure is performed by physicians trained in its

**TABLE 7–1. ESTIMATED RISKS OF MULTIFETAL PREGNANCIES**

| Number of Babies | Loss* | Gestational Age at delivery (weeks) | Neonatal** mortality | Neonatal morbidity |
|---|---|---|---|---|
| 5+ | 50% | 27–28 | 20% | 30% per baby |
| 4 | 25% | 29–30 | 6% | 27% per baby |
| 3 | 15% | 33 | 3% | 15% total |
| 2 | 8–10% | 36 | 2% | 7–8% total |
| 1 | 2–4% | 40 | 1% | 2–4% total |

* Through 24 weeks for first-trimester diagnosed pregnancies

**per baby

use. As an overgeneralization, those physicians who come from a transvaginal sonography and, commonly, IVF background may have more facility performing the procedure transvaginally. Most physicians, however, who perform MFPR come from a genetics or maternal-fetal medicine background for whom transabdominal procedures have been more prevalent and, therefore, safer. In this chapter, the transabdominal approach is described.

## INDICATIONS

When MFPR was first developed in the mid-1980s, the risks of the procedure were unknown and potential side effects to surviving fetuses had not been determined. Most investigators, therefore, believed that a very conservative approach was most appropriate. Twins were deemed

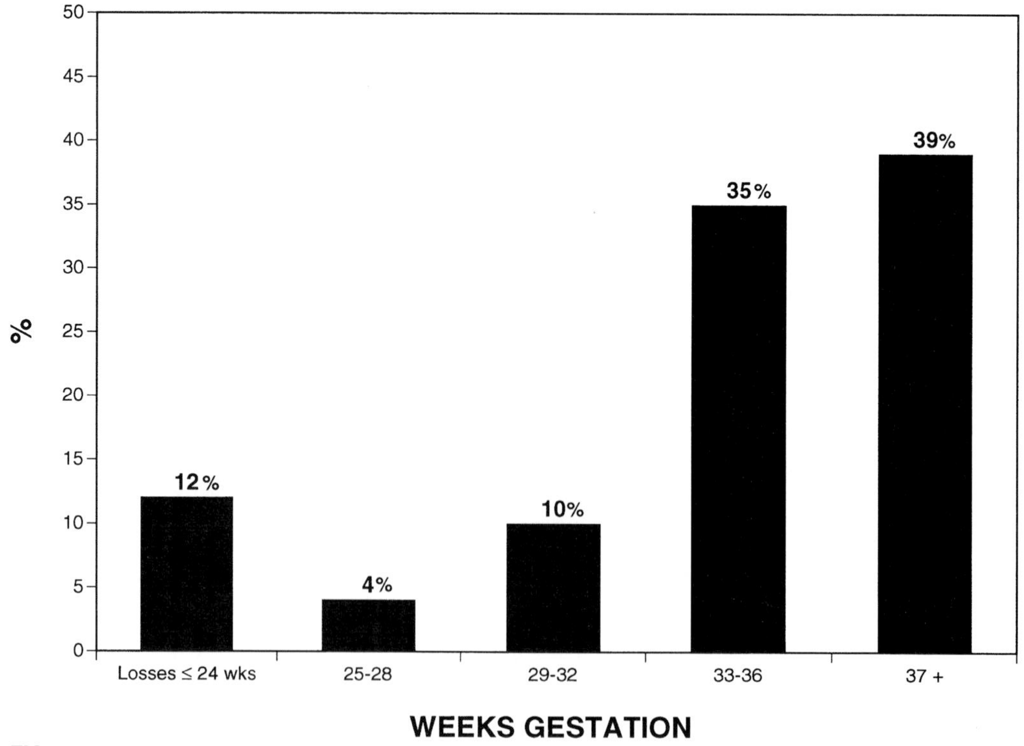


**FIG. 7–1.** Histogram detailing pregnancy outcome in 2,000 multifetal pregnancies treated by transabdominal multifetal pregnancy reduction.

to be the appropriate stopping number except under extraordinary circumstances. It was argued and generally agreed that twins were the most appropriate stopping number because[4]

1. every obstetrician knew how to care for twins
2. the perinatal outcome with twins, while not quite as good as for singletons, was generally felt to be an acceptable risk
3. virtually all of the patients coming for this procedure were infertility patients for whom bearing two children would get them that much closer to their family planning desires
4. there were unknown and potentially dangerous risks to their surviving fetuses, so that if only one fetus were left and it would be lost, no children would be had, whereas if two fetuses were left and one were lost, there would still be one baby to take home
5. there were ethical concerns about performing a procedure ''frivolously'' and the potential for abuse of the procedure; for example, its use for sex selection.

There was relatively little disagreement that with quadruplets or more, because the natural history of the outcome was so poor, virtually any attempt to reduce the number to a more manageable gestation was likely to be an improvement. Triplets were felt to be an arguably debatable gray zone in which reasonable and informed physicians staked out diametrically opposing conclusions. Patterns of support in opposition to MFPR did not directly follow traditional pro-choice or right-to-life patterns. Many observers who ordinarily considered themselves pro-choice had difficulty with the concept of partial reduction, and many who normally considered themselves pro-life found it difficult to argue against trying to reduce the enormous risks of, for example, a sextuplet or octuplet pregnancy in which realistically there would otherwise be no hope for survival.

## TECHNIQUE

As with all procedures that significantly affect pregnancy, proper counseling prior to any attempt is critical for the patient to understand the relevant risks and benefits involved. Over the past several years, fortunately, experience suggests that the vast majority of patients undergoing infertility therapies are at least being made aware of the possibility of a multifetal pregnancy. Such was not the case in earlier years. A thorough ultrasound examination is required to document proper fetal number (Fig. 7–2). Sonographers who do not have considerable experi-

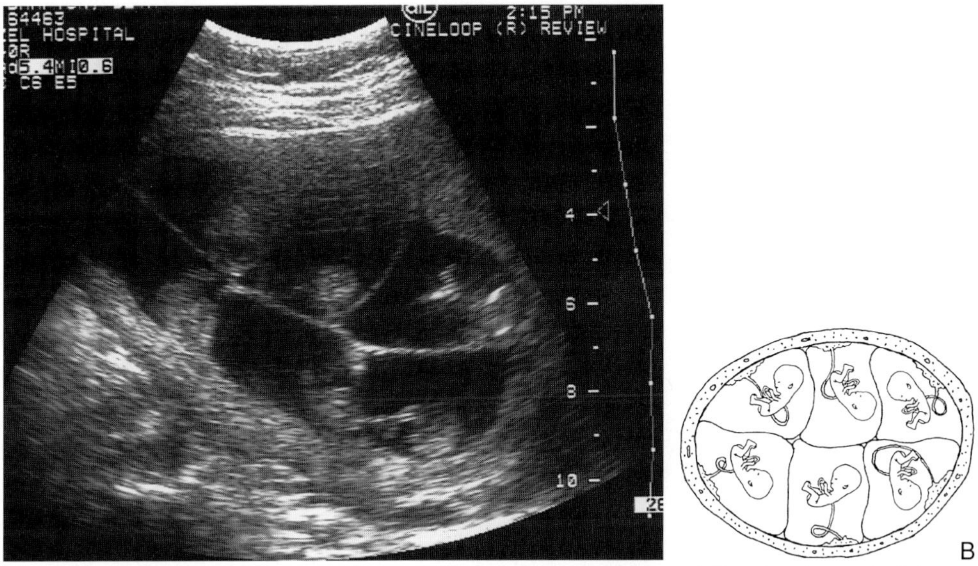


A B

**FIG. 7–2.** Transabdominal ultrasound (A) and schematic (B) at 10 weeks gestation showing sextuplet pregnancy.

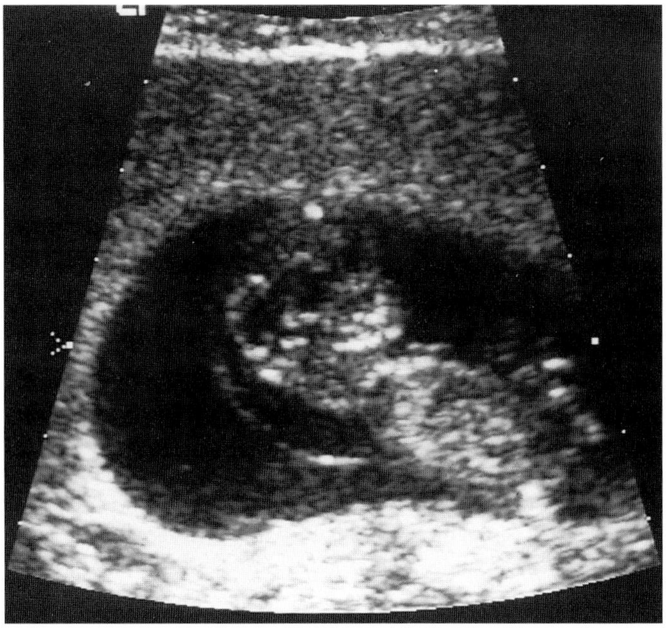

FIG. 7–3. Large posterior nuchal membrane extends from top of head to thorax. Depending on maternal age, this finding increases risk of embryo being aneuploid to as much as 50%.

ence in multiple pregnancies can make an error in assessment of the number of fetuses relatively easily. With experience, this problem has also decreased over the years but, particularly with higher order multiples, it is still a considerable risk today. Ultrasound examination should also, even in the first trimester, look for fetal anomalies. The appearance of a cystic hygroma or considerable size discrepancy between one embryo and the others can suggest a vastly increased risk of congenital abnormalities, and would dictate that that embryo be one chosen for reduction (Fig. 7–3). In the authors' experience, an embryo with an obvious abnormality or size discrepancy will be found in about 5% of cases. In the remaining 95% of cases, the embryo(s) selected for reduction will be based strictly on technical issues (*i.e.*, which ones can be reached by the easiest and, therefore, the safest method) (Fig. 7–4). In practice, using the transabdominal

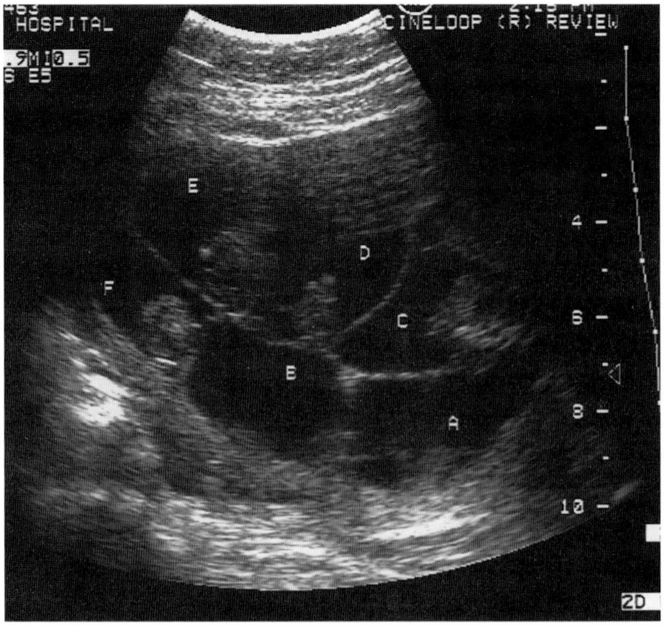


FIG. 7–4. Sextuplet pregnancy. Choice of embryo is based on position, if there are no anomalies. In this case, C, D, E, and F would be most likely chosen for reduction. Depending on exact angles, E and F could be done with a single needle insertion.

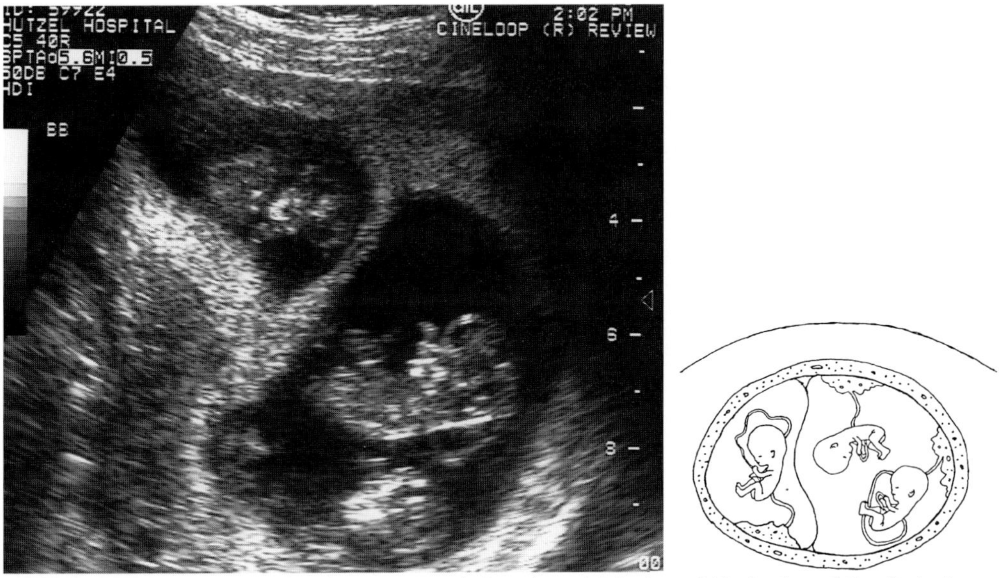


**FIG. 7–5.** Triplet pregnancy showing monoamniotic pair and "singleton." Reduction of the "twins" was accomplished with one needle.

route, embryos closer to the fundus tend to be easier to reach. For those physicians who do the procedure transvaginally, the opposite is true. Other relevant factors in the determination of which embryos to select include the appearance of a presumed monozygotic twin pair, particularly if monoamniotic (Fig. 7–5). On the basis of the known increased risk of congenital malformations in identical twin pairs, we prefer to reduce such twins in preference to other embryos. It would not make sense to reduce only one of the twin pair; the disruption of a shared vasculature has been shown, at least in later pregnancy, to have significant adverse sequelae.

The abdomen is washed and prepped in the usual manner and covered in sterile drapes. Using ultrasound, a spot on the abdomen directly above the sac to be entered is chosen, and a needle—generally a 22-gauge, 3.5-inch spinal needle, is inserted through the abdominal wall in a directly vertical approach (Fig. 7–6). Experience has shown that significant angulation of the needle is far more painful than a downward entry. In the vast majority of cases when multiple embryos need to be reduced, it is less painful for the patient to have separate needle entries than to try to significantly redirect the needle from one area to another. With experience, positioning of the needle into the appropriate sac becomes straightforward. However, for the physician inexperienced in the procedure, practicing the same routine with precise localization on amniocentesis procedures would be a reasonable practice methodology.

Once the needle is in the appropriate sac, it needs to be maneuvered directly over the embryonic thorax (Fig. 7–7A,B). In the authors' experience the attempt to insert the needle into the thorax is best done with a transverse ultrasonographic view; attempting to do it with a longitudinal view allows, in too many instances, the direction of the needle thrust to be off course and to miss laterally (Fig. 7–8). With the transverse view, the needle should be lined up in an exactly perpendicular plane to the thorax, so that there is no opportunity for it to roll (Fig. 7–9). The insertion of the needle must be done briskly; if the needle is pushed slowly and tentatively, the embryo will merely be pushed out of the way. Once the needle is inserted, then the best view is to return to the longitudinal plane so that the position of the needle can be checked, vis-à-vis the diaphragm (Fig. 7–10). In the first trimester, positioning of the needle above the diaphragm is sufficient, and direct intracardiac placement is not easily achieved and rarely necessary. At 9 weeks' gestation or less, the embryonic tissue provides minimal resistance, and it is very easy to go completely through the embryo and beyond. At 10–11 weeks,

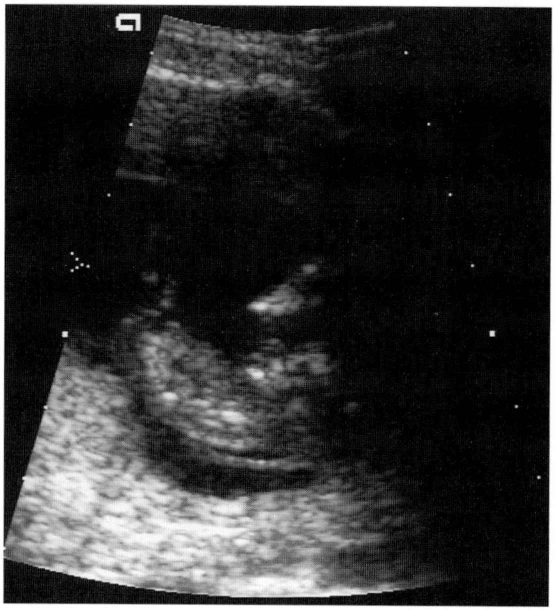

**FIG. 7–6.** Needle insertion into amniotic sac over fetal thorax as shown in longitudinal view. Embryo has small nuchal membrane.

there is relatively little embryonic movement but reasonable resistance to the needle, allowing for a firm entry to remain as placed. Beyond 12 weeks it is more common for the embryo to roll if the placement is not perfect.

Once the needle is appropriately inside the embryonic thorax, the stylet is removed and a 3 cc syringe is attached to the end of the needle. Aspiration is performed to show that there is negative pressure (*i.e.*, no fluid is being returned), confirming that the needle is appropriately placed into tissue. Then, using a 1 cc insulin syringe, KCl is injected very slowly. Injection that is too rapid will actually push the embryo off the tip of the needle. If the position of the needle is in fact above the diaphragm, a pleural effusion, occasionally a pericardial effusion and pleural or cardiac silhouette will be seen following the injection of as little as 0.3 cc (Fig. 7–11). Generally, between 0.5 and 1 cc is injected to ensure cardiac standstill. The needle

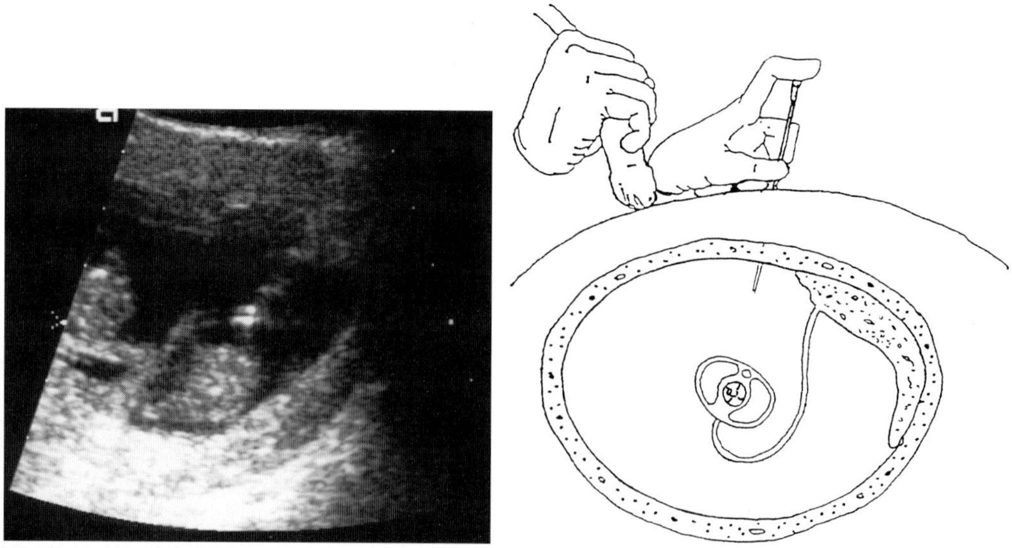

**FIG. 7–7.** Needle is inserted into sac and is hovered directly over thorax, which is seen in transverse view. Needle must enter thorax at 90° in center or it may "roll" off to side.

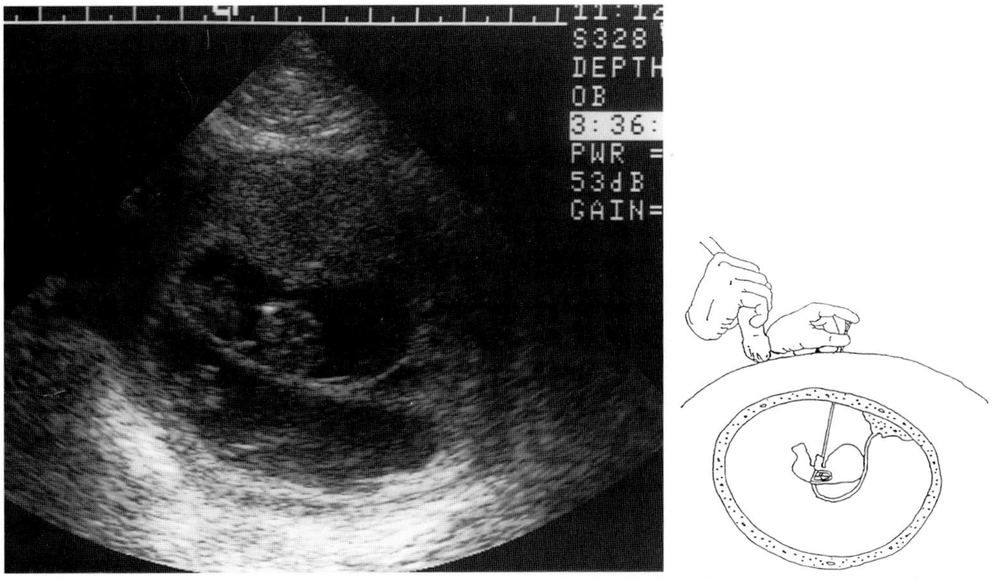


**FIG. 7–8.** Needle inserted into thorax under transverse view. Needle is "off course" and enters thorax at glancing angle.

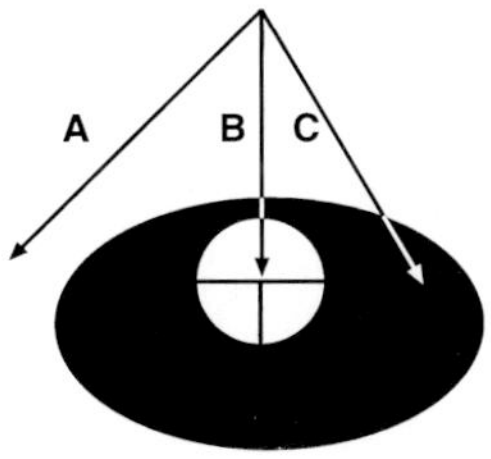


**FIG. 7–9.** Needle approach must be at center of embryo on transverse view (B) or the embryo will "roll" away (A, C). Once inserted, the direct approach enters the cardiac area. If the angle is off, the entire embryo may be missed (A) or only partially entered (C).

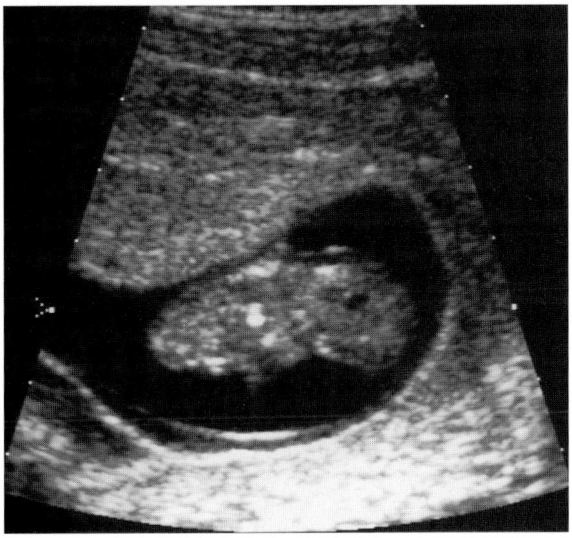

**FIG. 7–10.** Needle tip (bright spot) positioned in embryonic thorax at level of pericardium above diaphragm.

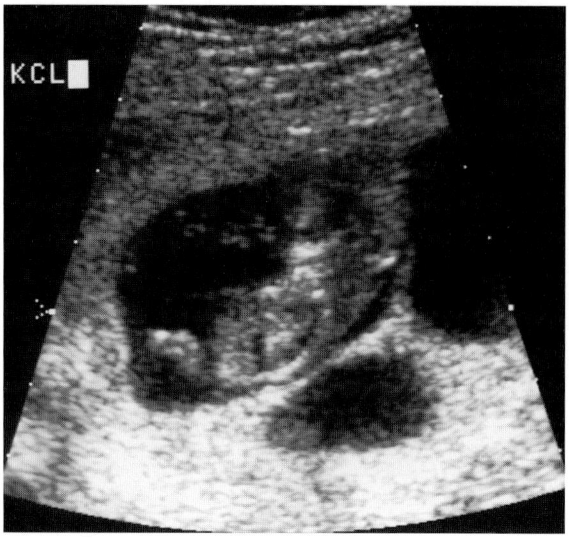


**FIG. 7–11.** Pulmonary silhouette is visible following injection of KCL into fetal thorax of same fetus as in Figure 7–10. Cardiac activity should cease with minimal delay.

should be kept in place for at least a couple of minutes to make sure that there is not re-initiation of cardiac activity.

If the needle is within the fetus but not properly placed, maneuvering can often achieve better placement. If this is not successful with relative ease, it is better to pull the needle back so that the embryo falls off, then reposition and reenter.

If the next embryo to be reduced is directly below or at only a minor angular deviation, the same needle can be used. However, in the vast majority of cases, it is better to use a clean needle with a separate insertion.

## CONTRAINDICATIONS

There are no specific surgical contraindications to the procedure. However, as outlined above, reducing only one of a monozygotic twin pair would not seem appropriate, and the authors have significant ethical problems with the use of fetal reduction for eugenic purposes such as sex selection. Collaborative data suggest that reduction to a singleton pregnancy from triplets or more generally has a worse outcome than stopping at twins.[8,9] However, these data are somewhat confounded by the fact that because most of the investigators involved in this endeavor have generally not ''liked'' to reduce to singletons, the vast majority of cases in which pregnancies were reduced to singleton were because of other serious complications associated with the pregnancy that would make a twin pregnancy particularly dangerous. Under such circumstances it is not surprising, given the high risk nature of the group, that there would be a higher loss rate. However, of those pregnancies that were not lost, the pattern of gestation was consistent with the singleton pregnancy, and had a slightly longer term of gestation that those cases reduced to twins.

## CONCLUSIONS

Multifetal pregnancy reduction has significantly improved the outcome of higher order multiple pregnancies and has allowed increasingly aggressive therapy for patients resistant to ovulation stimulating drugs to have their own babies. At the same time, however, there has been a laxness in the care of some patients, resulting in a tremendous increase in the number of multiple pregnancies, many of which may not have been necessary given more vigilant infertility treatments.

## REFERENCES


1. Luke B. The changing pattern of multiple births in the United States: maternal and infant characteristics, 1973 and 1990. Obstet Gynecol 1994;84:101–106.
2. Versmold H. Multifetal pregnancy outcome. Singapore; FIGO, 1992.
3. Callahan TL, Hall JE, Ettner SL, Christiansen CL, Greene MF, Crowley WF, Jr. The economic impact of multiple-gestation pregnancies and the contribution of assisted-reproduction techniques to their incidence. N Engl J Med 1994;331:244–249.
4. Evans MI, Fletcher JC, Zador IE, Newton BW, Quigg MH, Struyk CD. Selective first trimester termination in octuplet and quadruplet pregnancies clinical and ethical issues. Obstet Gynecol 1988;71:289–296.
5. Berkowitz RL, Lynch L, Chitkara U, et al. Selective reduction of multiple pregnancies in the first trimester. N Engl J Med 1988;318:1043.
6. Evans MI, Dommergues M, Wapner RJ, Lynch L, Dumez Y, Goldberg JD, Zador IE, Nicolaides KH, Johnson MP, Golbus MS, Boulot P, Berkowitz RL. Efficacy of transabdominal multifetal pregnancy reduction: collaborative experience among the world's largest centers. Obstet Gynecol 1993;82(1):61–66.
7. Timor-Tritsch IE, Peisner DB, Monteagudo A, Lercner JP, Sharma S. Multifetal pregnancy reduction by transvaginal puncture: evaluation of the technique used in 134 cases. Am J Obstet Gynecol 1993;168:799–804.
8. Evans MI, Dommergues M, Timor-Tritsch I, Zador IE, Wapner RJ, Lynch L, Dumez Y, Goldberg JD, Nicolaides KH, Johnson MP, Golbus MS, Boulot P, Aknin AJ, Monteagudo A, Berkowitz RL. Transabdominal versus transcervical and transvaginal multifetal pregnancy reduction: international collaborative experience of more than one thousand cases. Am J Obstet Gynecol 1994;170:902–909.
9. Evans MI, Dommergues M, Wapner RJ, Goldberg JD, Lynch L, Zador IE, Carpenter R, Timor-Tritsch I, Brambati B, Nicolaides KH, Dumez Y, Monteagudo A, Johnson MP, Golbus MS, Brambati L, Polak SM, Berkowitz RL. International collaborative experience of 1789 patients having multifetal pregnancy reduction: a plateauing of risks and outcomes. JSGI 3(1):20–22, 1996.

# II GYNECOLOGIC PROCEDURES

*Invasive Outpatient Procedures in Reproductive Medicine*, edited by Mark I. Evans, et al. Lippincott–Raven Publishers, Philadelphia © 1997.

# 8 Breast Biopsy

Bruce H. Drukker

## INTRODUCTION AND INDICATIONS

Excisional breast biopsy remains the ultimate procedure for determining histologic characteristics of certain breast masses. Of note, however, is the ever-increasing utilization of direct-needle biopsy, fine-needle aspiration cytologic examination (FNAC), and stereotaxic aspiration or tissue biopsy to assess breast histology. The over-riding concept, which must be followed when treating a breast problem, is the need for a tissue diagnosis or a precise, unrefutable diagnosis of a benign characteristic when imaging is utilized to evaluate a breast mass.

The indications for excisional breast biopsy are distinct and include:

- A distinct, persistent palpable mass, which may or may not be mammographically suspicious or which may or may not be seen on mammographic imaging.
- A mammographically identifiable mass, which is nonpalpable but has suspicious characteristics for malignancy.
- A mammographically detected, nonpalpable lesion that is increasing in size.
- A cystic mass with septations of the cyst wall, invaginations of the cyst wall, or suspicious cytology on fine-needle aspiration (FNA).
- A cystic mass that recurs on two occasions following aspiration, which had previously demonstrated benign cellular changes.
- Suspicious calcifications or densities noted on mammography that are nonpalpable and require needle localization technique.

Historically, some lesions of the breast, particularly large lesions, were initially evaluated by incisional biopsy. With increasing breast awareness by women and utilization of screening mammography, early diagnosis has virtually eliminated the need for incisional biopsy. Excisional breast biopsy remains the gold standard.

## TECHNIQUE

This procedure can be carried out on an ambulatory basis in any setting suitable for a surgical procedure, including an office facility with the capabilities to do minor surgery, an ambulatory surgical setting, or a traditional hospital operating suite. The procedure can be carried out under local anesthesia or general anesthesia, when indicated. Obviously, the setting chosen for biopsy will dictate in part the type of anesthetic chosen for the procedure. In many situations, local anesthesia is an ideal choice and can be augmented with intravenous sedation, producing a very comfortable biopsy experience for the patient. A word of caution regarding local anesthesia—for smaller lesions, infiltration of a 8, 10, or perhaps 15 cc of anesthetic solution may distort the tissue sufficiently so that a small palpable lesion is no longer palpable and make

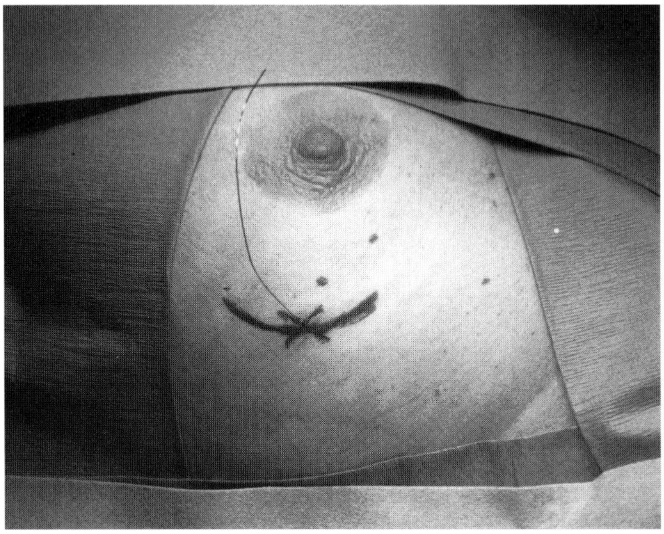

**FIG. 8–1.** Breast prepared and draped for breast biopsy, with localizing wire in place and incision marking completed.

localization difficult at the time of excisional biopsy. Also, in lesions located deep within the substance of the breast, particularly those adjacent to the pectoralis major muscle, local anesthesia may not be adequate to permit appropriate dissection without patient discomfort. Therefore, a variety of parameters, including size and location of mass, patient desire, and the facility chosen need to be considered when anesthesia requirements are evaluated.

At the actual time of breast biopsy it is important to observe the basic principles of cosmesis. All patients are concerned about pathology results of a breast biopsy, but they are also particularly concerned about the appearance of the breast following the surgical procedure. With this in mind, after the patient has been placed on the operating table, it is important for the patient to sit up to allow the breast to be carefully visualized, the mass palpated, and the site of needle insertion (if needle localization has been utilized) identified. With the patient in the sitting position, the normal position of the breast can be identified and an appropriate incision following Langer's lines can be planned.[1] Ideally, a sterile skin-marking pencil should be utilized to identify the incision line and anesthetic then injected (Figs. 8–1 and 8–2). In general, circumferential incisions can be made in the peri-areolar area or areas 3–4 cm or

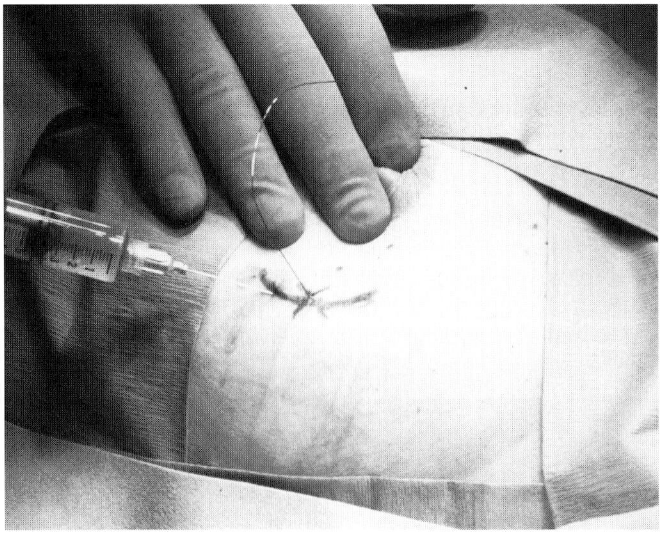

**FIG. 8–2.** Injection of local anesthesia.

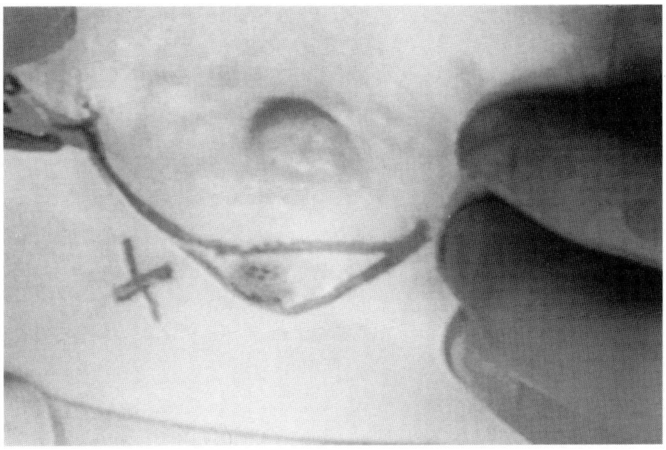

**FIG. 8–3.** Incision being made in skin. Localizing wire will be free and mobile.

more away from the areola. On the very inferior portions of the breast radial incisions can be made; however, these may be less cosmetic than radial incisions (Fig. 8–3). Prior to beginning the incision, the patient should be appropriately positioned so that the breast appears to be in a normal position. Slight elevation of the head and rotation of the operating table toward the side of the breast not being biopsied will produce a normal resting position of the breast, ensuring a good cosmetic result. The breast should be carefully prepared with a povidone iodine solution and draped in a standard fashion. After the initial skin incision has been made and the skin edges elevated, meticulous hemostasis is necessary, utilizing a pinpoint cautery or 3–0 absorbable suture. Delicate skin hooks and tissue forceps are ideal for handling the skin edges (Fig. 8–4). Once the substance of the breast has been entered, the mass must be identified. The tissue adjacent to the mass can often be grasped with an Allis clamp and then by sharp dissection, either with a scalpel or Metzenbaum scissors, the lesion can be totally excised (Figs. 8–5, 8–6, and 8–7). After the lesion has been excised, complete hemostasis is absolutely mandatory, again using pinpoint cautery and 3–0 absorbable suture material (Fig. 8–8). After hemostasis has been achieved, the operative site should be flushed with normal saline, removing any debris or old blood. The defect then can be closed. Few, if any, sutures

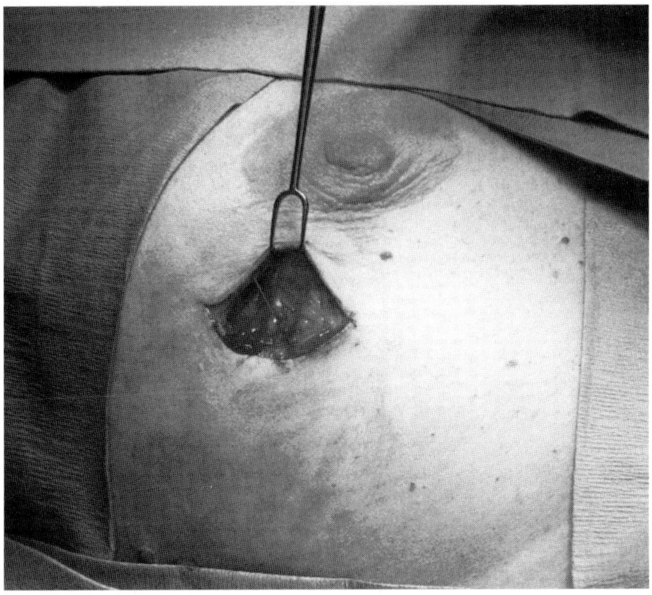

**FIG. 8–4.** Incision completed. Localizing wire clipped approximately three inches from skin.

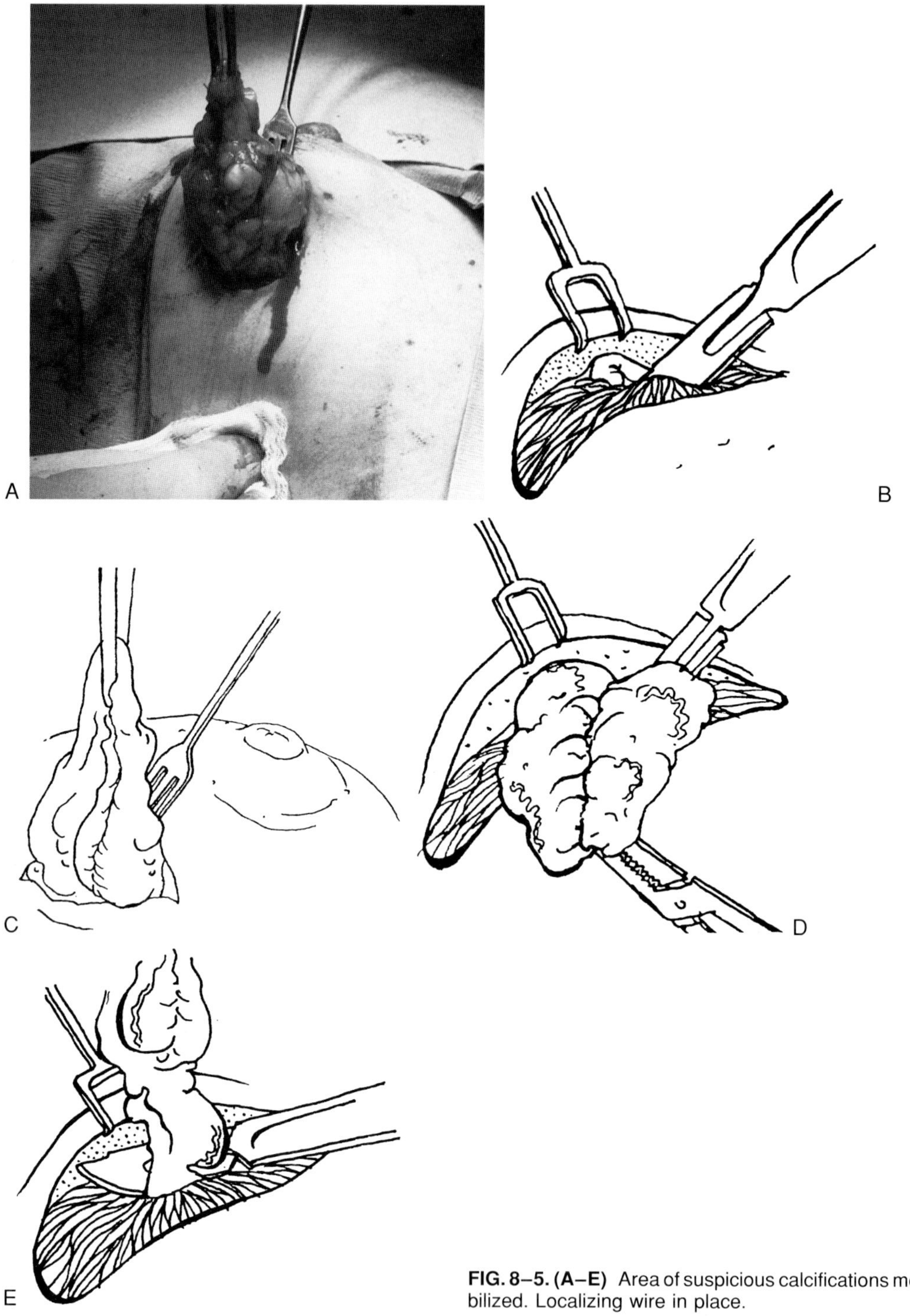


**FIG. 8–5. (A–E)** Area of suspicious calcifications mobilized. Localizing wire in place.

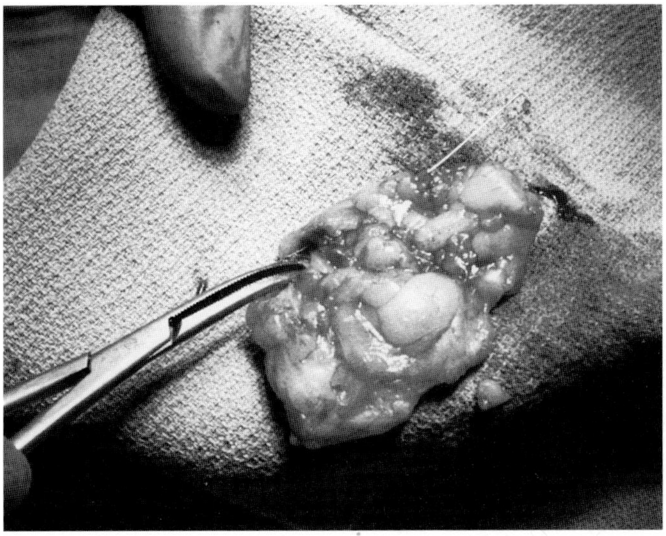

**FIG. 8–6.** Specimen removed. Localizing wire visible and in place.

are needed in the subcutaneous tissue. If the lesion is deep, the dead space can be occluded by one or two 3–0 absorbable sutures and the skin closed with fine 4–0 subcuticular absorbable sutures (Fig. 8–9). Very small incisions can be closed with steri strips (Fig. 8–10). After the biopsy has been completed, a small dry dressing, generally of telfa, and 4 × 4 gauze pads, can be applied (Fig. 8–11). Generally, the dressing should be left in place for 24 or 36 hours and during this period of time the patient is asked to wear a brassiere day and night. When the dressing is changed, the patient is given 4 × 4 gauze pads that she can use to put against the incision, merely for comfort, and, if steri strips have been utilized, these should be removed in seven days. The patient again is asked to wear a brassiere day and night for a seven-day period.

For a patient who is having an excisional biopsy following needle localization, the incision is made so that it closely circumvents the wire with a tiny portion of skin attached to the wire. In some situations, the incision can be constructed so that no piece of skin is attached

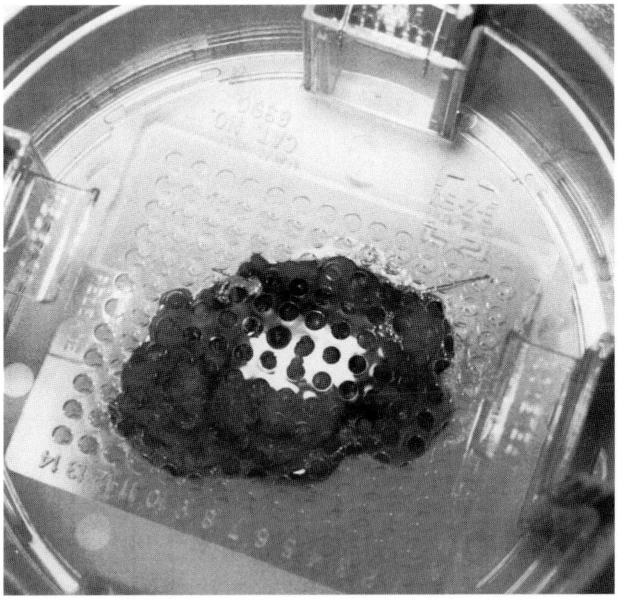

**FIG. 8–7.** Specimen with localizing wire in place in compression device to be submitted for radiographic confirmation of removal of suspicious calcifications.

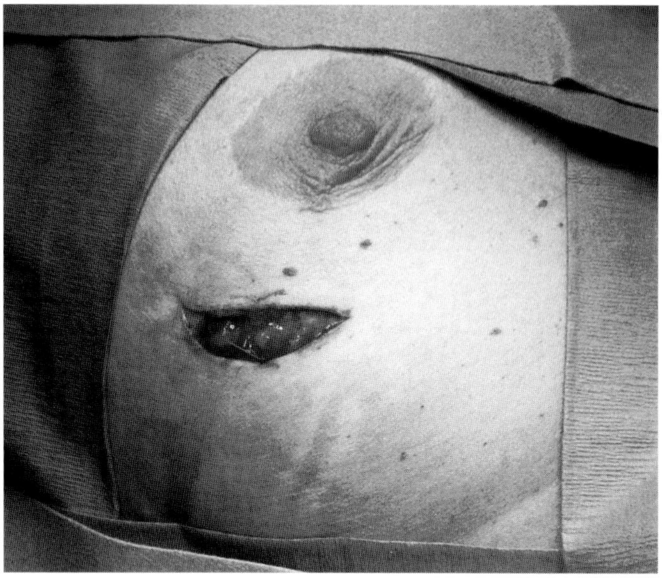

**FIG. 8–8.** Incision ready for closure. Note minimal to no visible defect in external contour of breast.

to the wire. After the skin incision is made, the procedure is similar to that described for excisional biopsy without wire localization; however, the tissue is followed down along the wire by sharp dissection until the terminal hook of the wire is noted. When one gets to this area, a substantial amount of tissue adjacent to the hook is removed, thus ensuring removal of the area on mammogram that had been the point of concern and for which localization was necessary. Prior to beginning an excisional biopsy with localization, it is absolutely important to have the needle localization mammograms in the operating area so that they can be visualized and to have knowledge of the length of the wire utilized for localization to allow one to know how far the dissection will have to go below the skin. After the wire and the tissue that surrounds the hooked end have been removed, it must be radiographed if calcifications have been noted to ensure that the calcifications have been removed. If one finds that the calcifications have been missed, additional tissue can be obtained at the operative site and x-rayed

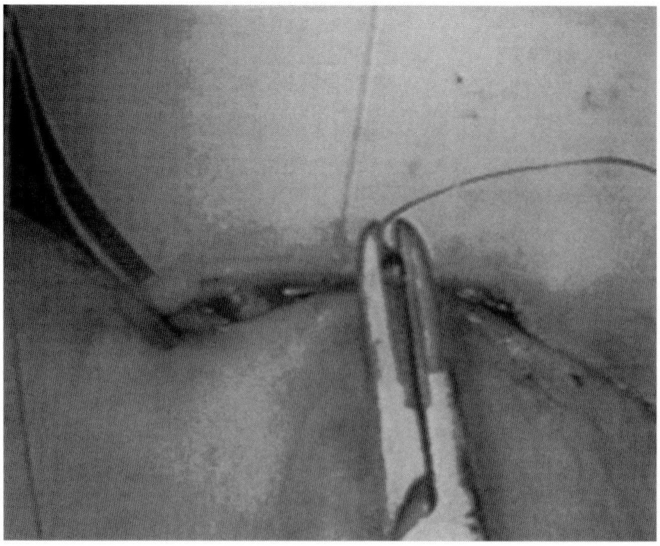

**FIG. 8–9.** Suturing of incision.

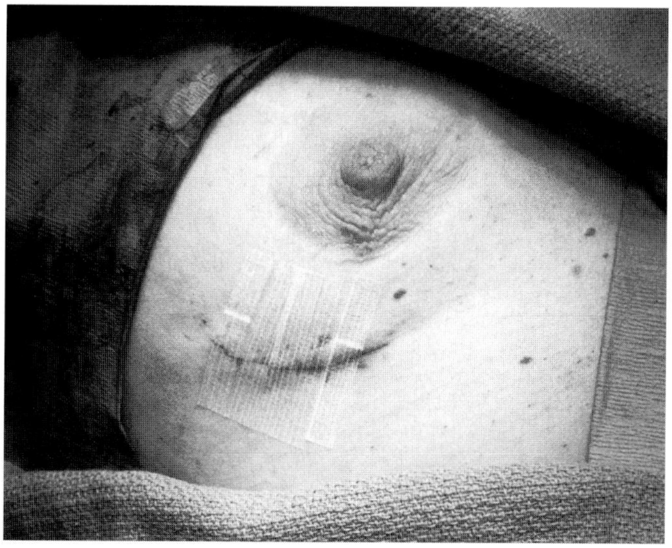

**FIG. 8–10.** Incision closed and ready for dressing.

again. However, if after the second try the calcifications are not present, it becomes of greater concern to continue resecting breast tissue in a blind fashion. In some situations it may be more appropriate to close the incision according to acceptable standards and to have the patient re-localized and repeat the operative procedure approximately six weeks later. The use of a sterile dressing for wire localization excisional biopsies is similar for other breast biopsies.

Occasionally, nipple biopsy because of discharge, redness, or erosion is necessary. Nipple discharges are of concern, particularly if bloody, serosanguinous, or merely serous. Although only approximately 12% of breast cancers present with concomitant nipple discharge,[2] these conditions should be evaluated by mammography, duct injection when possible, nipple secretion cytology, and often biopsy of the nipple surface or a portion of the ductal system below the areola or adjacent to the areola. Biopsy of the nipple surface can be accomplished under local anesthesia with a minimal wedge of tissue taken. The wedge should be very small,

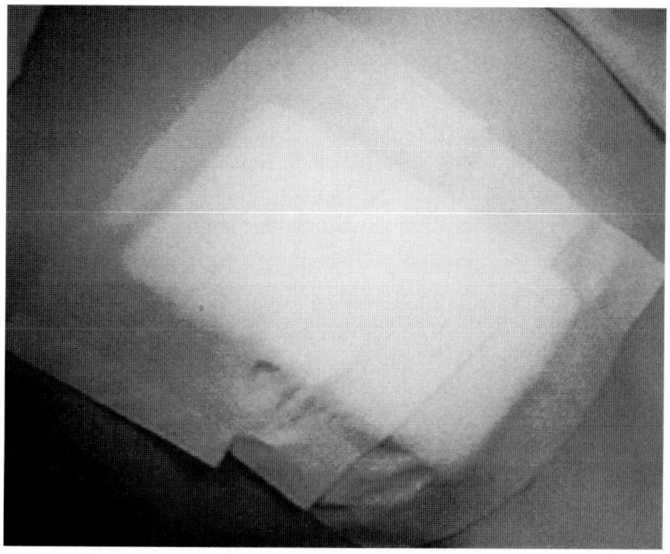

**FIG. 8–11.** Telfa dressing covering incision.

containing just enough tissue for appropriate histologic preparation. This small defect can be repaired with 4–0 or 5–0 absorbable sutures. A dry, sterile dressing should be placed over the nipple. The breast, of course, should be supported. Excision of the ductal components, if papillomas are of concern, can be accomplished also with local anesthesia. After appropriate preparation of the breast, a circumferential incision is made at the areolar margin over the area of the duct in question. Then, by sharp dissection, the portion of the ductal system involved can be removed. This defect is closed in the same manner as previously described.

## RESULTS AND INTERPRETATION

The outcome of breast biopsy is dependent on an adequate, properly prepared specimen with clear margins. Although cosmesis is a prime concern during breast biopsy, this should not preclude obtaining a sharply dissected biopsy specimen. Following the basic tenets of breast biopsy will permit appropriate histologic evaluation with multiple stains as needed, leading to an accurate diagnosis. Interpretation is generally straightforward and only impeded by an inadequate specimen or poor preparation. The results of breast biopsy should be excellent in virtually all situations.

## CONTRAINDICATIONS

There are few contraindications to breast biopsy, assuming the patient is in good health. However, the physician should consider the following relative considerations. First, a large, easily palpable mass, particularly if suspicious for carcinoma, can readily be assessed using a needle biopsy. This will reduce to a degree some of the morbidity associated with the excision of a large breast mass. Second, if there is a substantial inflammatory condition in the breast, every attempt should be made to have this controlled prior to a breast biopsy. On the other hand, if inflammatory carcinoma of the breast is suspected, biopsies should be obtained in order to demonstrate histologic confirmation and permit rapid institution of appropriate therapy.

## COMPLICATIONS

Complications following excisional biopsy should be minimal, particularly if one adheres to the rigid criteria of impeccable hemostasis. Occasionally a patient may develop a hematoma or seroma. Should this occur, needle aspiration generally resolves the problem. If a hematoma does not reabsorb, incision and drainage may be required. Occasionally, a delayed hematoma may form 2–4 weeks following biopsy. This infrequent occurrence seems to be related to suture slippage or dissolution of cautery eschar, concomitant with poor breast support or extremely vigorous physical activity, such as jogging, which will permit substantial breast mobility in the poorly supported breast. These patients will complain of pain and swelling and develop some ecchymoses, which clearly suggests the presence of a delayed hematoma. On the other hand, if there has been ductal contamination or if preparation of the skin is inappropriate or other factors present, infection may occur. It should be emphasized again to the patient, however, that all of these complications occur very infrequently. Breast biopsy is the gold standard for final diagnosis of equivocal or perplexing breast lesions. It is a procedure that is certainly within the realm of the gynecologic surgeon and, when a surgeon demonstrates appropriate education, the procedure can be carried out with facility and expertise, providing a definitive resolution to many breast problems.

## REFERENCES

1. Nichols DH. The role of the gynecologist in the diagnosis and management of breast cancer. In: Hindle WH (ed.). *Breast disease for gynecologists.* East Norwalk;Appleton and Lange, 1990.
2. Rothenberg RE. The nipple in breast cancer. In: Arcel IM, Cleary JB (eds.). *Breast cancer.* New York;McGraw-Hill, 1987.

The photographs utilized were taken from an instructional videotape, ''The Evaluations of Conditions of the Breast,'' produced by Ciné-Med, Woodbury, Connecticut, 06798

*Invasive Outpatient Procedures in Reproductive Medicine,* edited by Mark I. Evans, et al. Lippincott–Raven Publishers, Philadelphia © 1997.

# 9 Colposcopy and Cervical Biopsy

John M. Malone, Jr.

## INTRODUCTION AND INDICATIONS

Cervical cancer in the United States, although declining in frequency, still represents a major health problem occurring approximately 13,500 times per year.[1] Cervical cancer is unique among the gynecologic malignancies in that, with appropriate screening, major reductions in incidence and mortality are achievable.

Although the exact cause is as yet unknown its natural history and risk factors are fairly well known. Our knowledge extends through its precursor lesions and continues through its development and further progress.

Since the early part of the twentieth century attempts have been made to screen for cervical cancer. Hinselmann[2] first described the colposcope in 1925 and advocated its use as the primary method of screening for cervical cancer. Initially, colposcopy was not widely accepted because of relatively poor optics and light sources and because of a misleading understanding of cervical cancer's natural history.

In the 1940s, Papanicolaou[3] published his pioneering work on the use of cytology in the diagnosis of cancer; with experience it became apparent that the Papanicolaou (Pap) smear could not only diagnose cancer but was also able to identify its precursor lesions, thereby allowing for the identification of women truly at risk for cervical cancer. With this knowledge precursor lesions could be treated and, hopefully, invasive cancer prevented.

When faced with an abnormal pap smear it is incumbent on the treating physician to explain the abnormality. In the past, to do so gynecologists resorted to either blind biopsies or cone biopsies of the cervix. Colposcopy has reemerged but, instead of being the primary screening tool for cervical cancer, it has now become an adjunct to cytology. It provides the practitioner with a technique to assess the cervix more accurately. Used this way colposcopy allows for directed biopsies and more precise treatment of preinvasive lesions. Along with cytology and histology, colposcopy is now considered to be part of the triad utilized to screen women for cervical cancer.

## TECHNIQUE

The colposcope (Fig. 9–1) consists of a stereoscopic, binocular microscope that magnifies the cervix 3–10 times. The colposcope should be equipped with a green filter, which filters out red and thereby enhances the vascular appearance of the cervix by making the vessels dark.

Before starting a colposcopic examination it is important that conditions be optimal. The patient should be positioned in such a way that it will facilitate the examination and allow the

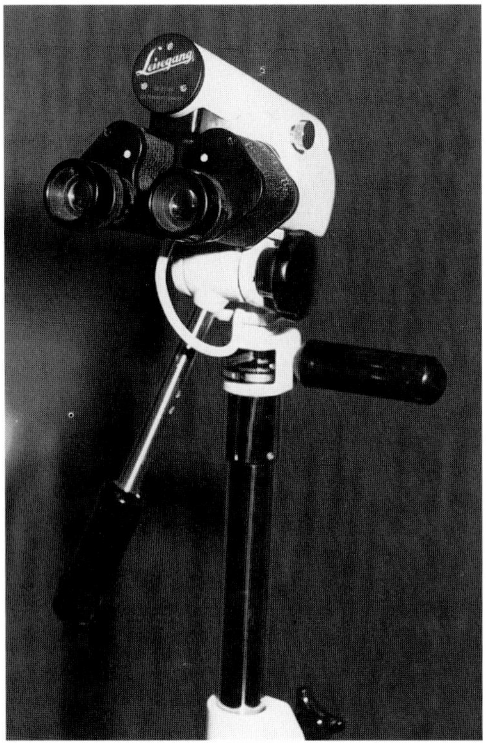

**FIG. 9–1.** Colposcope with binocular lenses, control for focus, and retractable green filter.

examiner to perform the procedure comfortably and without physical contortion. Ideally, the cervix should be at eye level and the plane of the cervix at right angles to the beam of the colposcope. All instruments and supplies needed for the examination should be at hand (Fig. 9–2, Table 9–1).

After the patient has been positioned, any vaginal discharge should be collected and prepared for saline and KOH wet mounts. The cervix should then be liberally washed with 2% acetic acid. Acetic acid dehydrates the cells by causing a transient coagulation of cytoplasmic proteins in the superficial cells and allows for easier identification of epithelial and

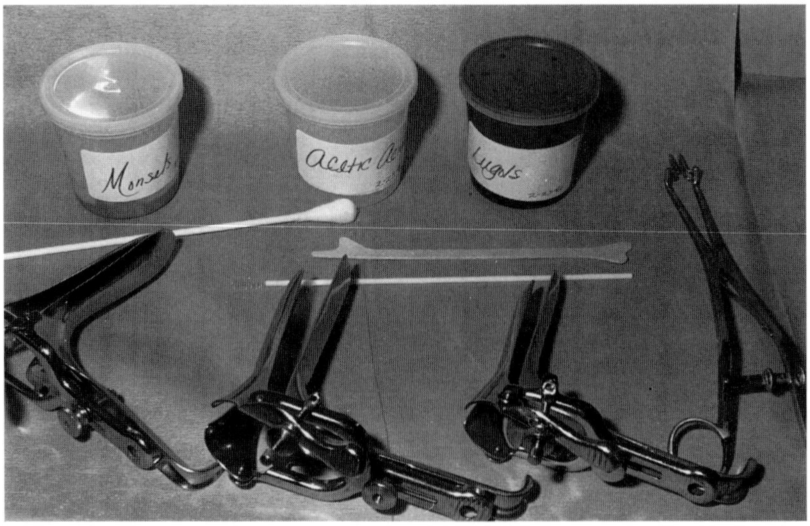


**FIG. 9–2.** Colposcopy tray. Supplies include variously sized speculums, endocervical speculum cytobrush, Ayre spatula, Lugol's solution, acetic acid, and Monsel's solution.

**TABLE 9–1. SUPPLIES NEEDED FOR A COLPOSCOPIC EXAMINATION**

| | |
|---|---|
| Speculum, assorted sizes | Cytobrush |
| Ayre spatula | Cytofixative |
| Tenaculum | Endocervical curette |
| 2% Acetic acid | Lygol's solution |
| Cotton swabs | Endocervical speculum |
| Biopsy instruments | Monsel's solution |
| Condoms or lateral wall retractors for the speculum | |

vascular abnormalities. While the acetic acid is dehydrating the cervix, the wet mounts should be examined.

Frequently, in either pregnant or obese patients it is difficult to visualize the cervix secondary to the vaginal walls collapsing in on the axis of the colposcope. This can be prevented by either sheathing the speculum with a condom or using a speculum with lateral wall retractors. The cervix is then examined colposcopically. First, the speculum needs to be properly positioned to allow complete visualization of the cervix. The cervical transformation zone is then visualized (Fig. 9–3). The cervical transformation zone (TZ) corresponds to that area of the cervix which was covered with columnar epithelium at the time of birth and later undergoes a process of squamous metaplasia. The TZ is bounded on the outside by the original squamocolumnar junction (OSCJ) and its inner margin is the active squamocolumnar junction (ASCJ). The surface of the TZ is characterized by having a white sheen, minute blood vessels, and frequently gland openings are seen. This dynamic zone is where dysplasia and subsequent malignancies are thought to start. Once identified, the TZ needs to be evaluated for the presence of vascular and epithelial abnormalities. The green filter is then used to highlight vascular abnormalities. If needed, Lugol's solution can be applied. This iodine-based solution stains the glycogenated vagina. Areas poor in glycogen (*i.e.*, columnar epithelium or regenerative epithelium) will not stain (Fig. 9–4, Color Fig. 11). An endocervical speculum (Fig. 9–5) can be used to ''open'' the cervical os when there is cervical stenosis or atrophy, making it difficult to fully evaluate the ASCJ. If indicated, a directed biopsy is done. Various instruments have been utilized (Fig. 9–6), all of which have the ability to reach the designated spot without blocking the view of the colposcopist. In addition to ectocervical biopsies, scrapings or biopsies from the endocervix are also warranted to rule out endocervical disease. The Kervorkian

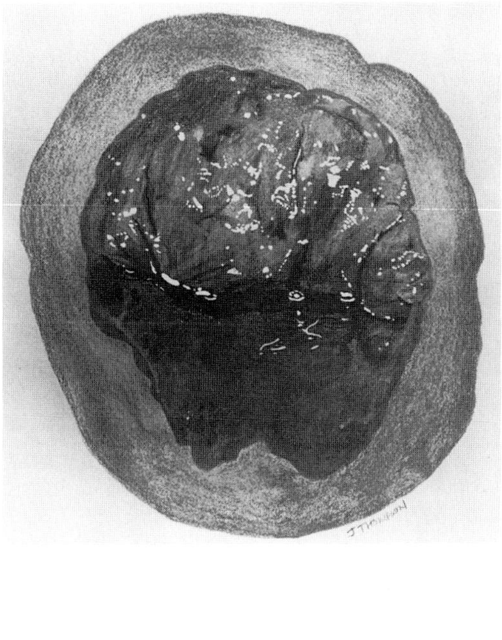

**FIG. 9–3.** Adequate colposcopy showing entire cervical transformation. There are wide areas of immature metaplasia.

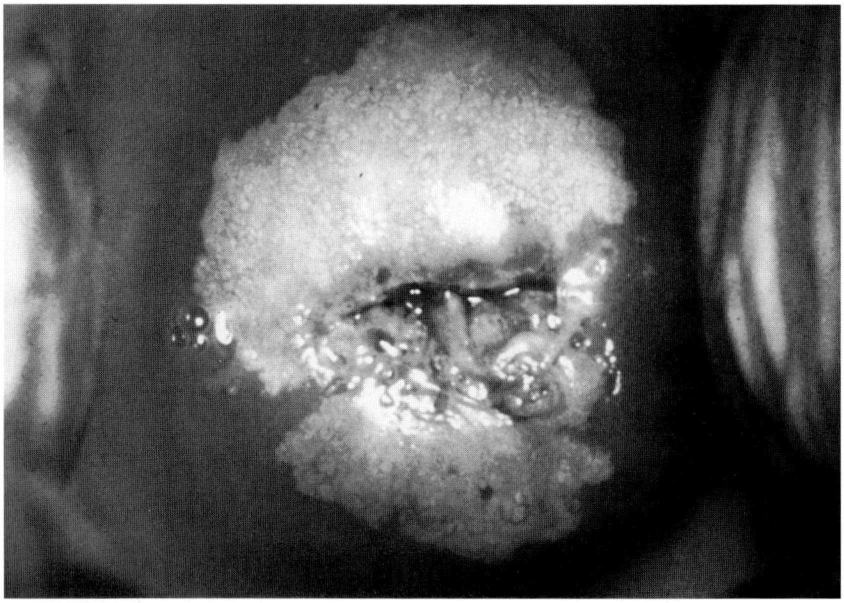

**FIG. 9–4.** Colpophotograph showing the characteristic yellow staining reaction seen with quarter strength Lugol's iodine. See Color Fig. 11.

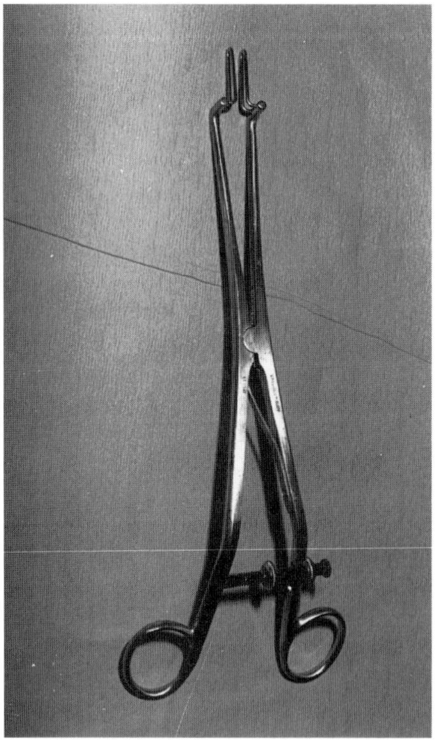

**FIG. 9–5.** Endocervical speculum.

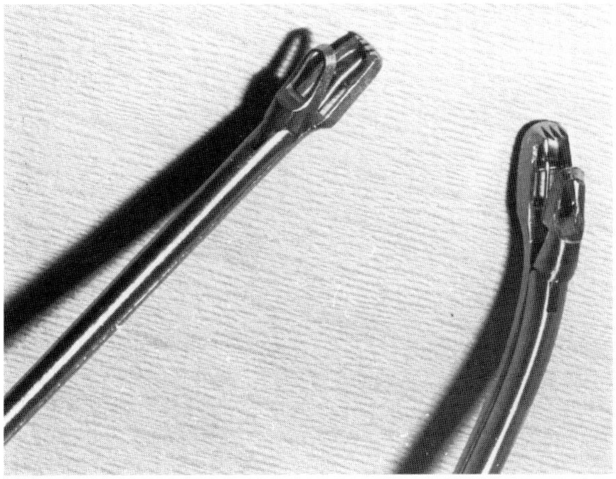

**FIG. 9–6.** Cervical biopsy instruments.

endocervical curette (Fig. 9–7) is ideally suited for the purpose. Following the biopsy, areas of cervical bleeding can be controlled by using Monsel's solution (ferric subsulfate solution). Finally, it is a good idea to draw a picture of what was seen, including boundaries, abnormal areas, and sites of biopsy.

## INTERPRETATION OF RESULTS

Colposcopy is pattern recognition and in itself is not diagnostic. The examiner needs to be able to completely visualize the TZ and recognize normal versus abnormal. By making that distinction the examiner can then selectively biopsy the abnormal. Formal diagnosis only occurs after the biopsy specimen has been examined histologically.

Ideally, colposcopic findings, cytology, and histologic results correlate. When they do, the next step is usually obvious. The problem arises, however, when there are discrepancies. In a simplistic sense, the major question in regard to a discrepancy is whether or not there is either an undiagnosed cancer, an underdiagnosed dysplastic process, or a falsely positive Pap smear.

In order for a colposcopic examination to be considered adequate, the following criteria must be met: the entire TZ must be seen, any lesion must be seen in its entirety, and there

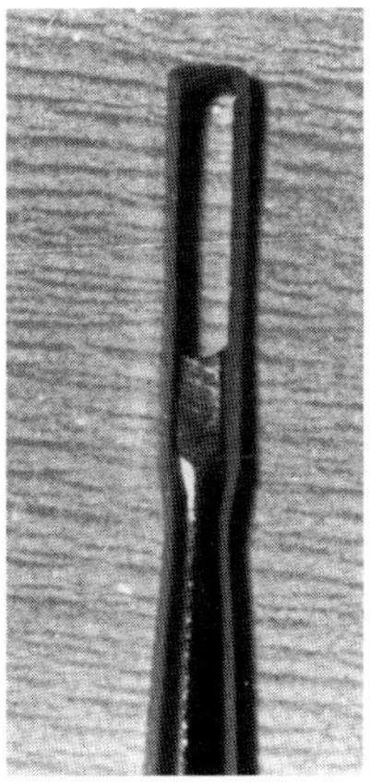

**FIG. 9–7.** Kervorkian endocervical curette.

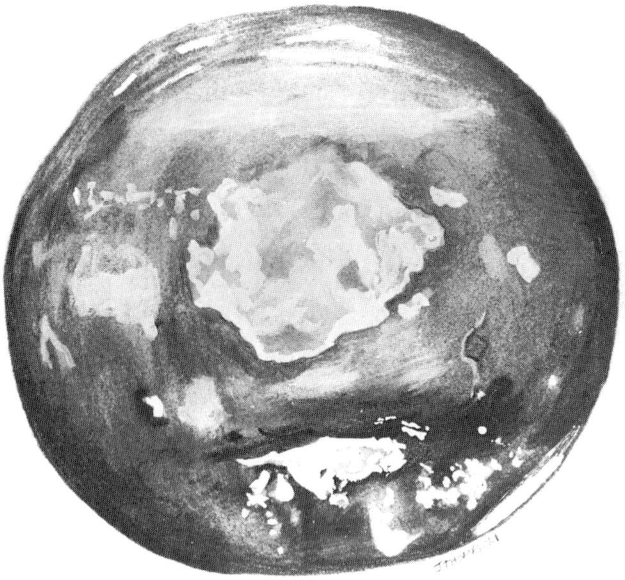

**FIG. 9–8.** Adequate colposcopic examination. The entire TZ is seen, there is a well-circumscribed epithelial abnormality on the posterior lip of the cervix.

should be no lesions extending into the endocervical canal (Figs. 9–3 and 9–8). An inadequate (Fig. 9–9, Color Fig. 12) examination would represent a failure to accomplish the above. Abnormal vascular patterns represent neovascularization of the surface epithelium; normal cervical squamous epithelium is virtually devoid of blood vessels. With neoplasia new vessels develop that extend into the surface epithelium. When the course of these vessels runs parallel to the surface of the epithelium it takes on the appearance of a mosaic (Fig. 9–10, Color Fig. 13). If the vessels grow perpendicularly to the plane of the epithelium they will appear as small dots, so-called punctation (Fig. 9–11). Haphazard vascular growth with multiple branches is called atypical vascularity (Fig. 9–12); abnormal epithelium takes on a white color, which

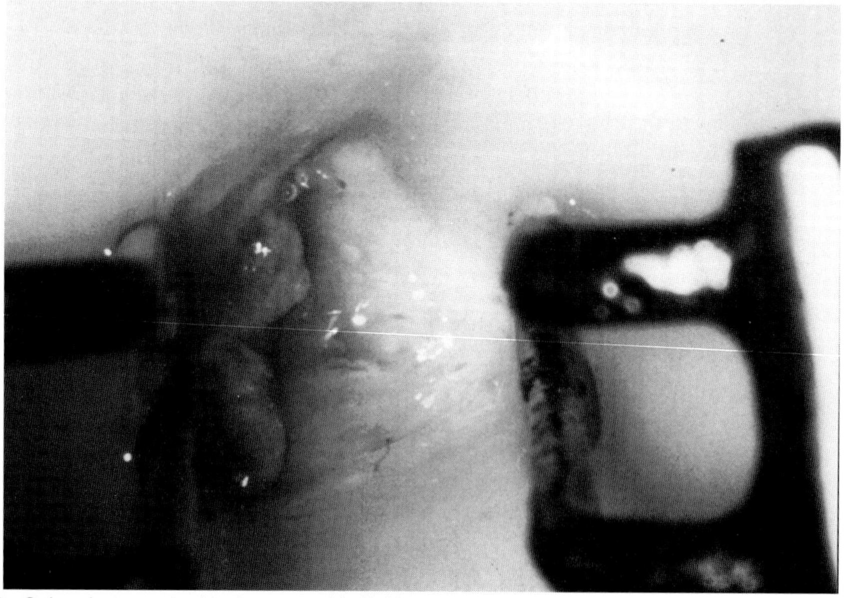

**FIG. 9–9.** Colpophotograph showing an epithelial lesion extending into the endocervical canal, well out of colposcopic range; an inadequate examination. See Color Fig. 12.

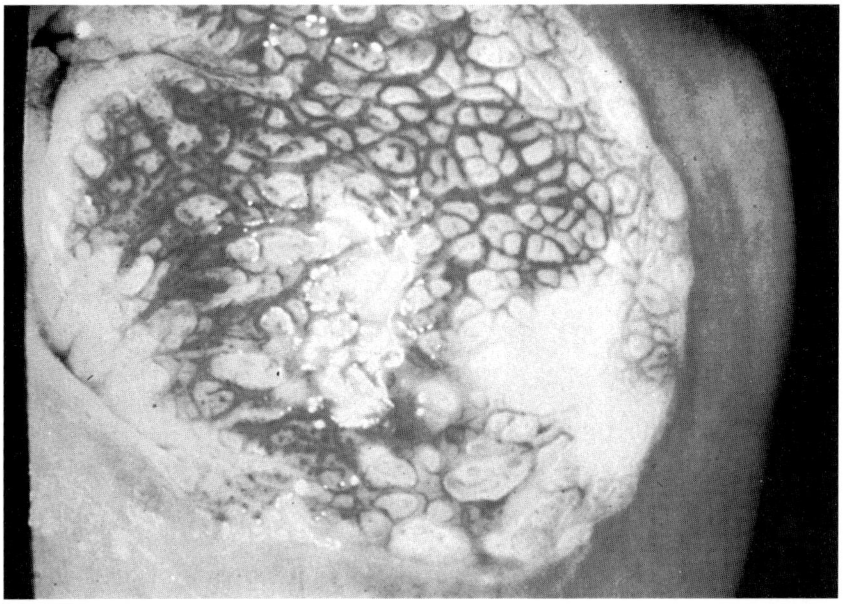

**FIG. 9–10.** Colpophotograph showing white epithelium and vascular mosaicism. See Color Fig. 13.

results from a decrease in tissue translucency. This is caused by either keratin deposition on the epithelial surface or an increase in the number of cells in the epithelium making the tissue denser (Fig. 9–13, Color Fig. 14). In addition, there can be multiple abnormalities seen, combining both epithelial and vascular changes (Fig. 9–10 and 9–14, Color Fig. 15).

There are a number of conditions that make adequate colposcopy difficult; pregnancy, obesity, vaginal atrophy, and cervical stenosis being the most common. With persistence and modifications in technique most of these difficult cervices can be adequately examined. With either menopause or previous radiation therapy the vaginal and cervical epithelium become atrophic and contracted. This distortion can lead to difficulties with colposcopy. With patience and the occasional use of pre-examination topical estrogen[4] the atrophy can be relieved and the transformation zone seen.

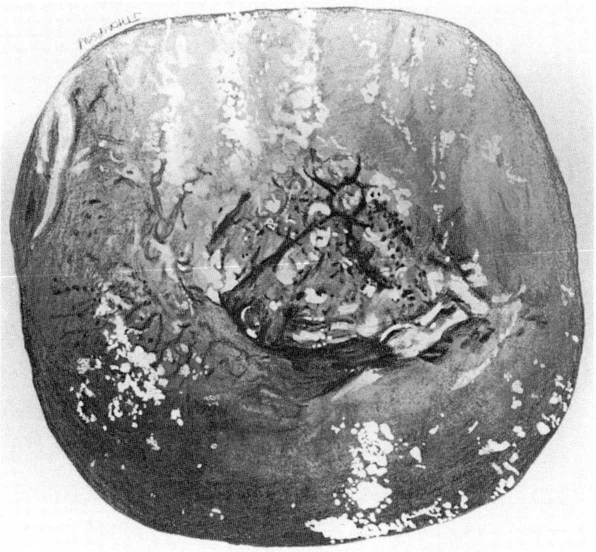

**FIG. 9–11.** Vascular abnormality: punctation. Vessels grow perpendicularly to the epithelial surface, thereby taking on a punctate appearance.

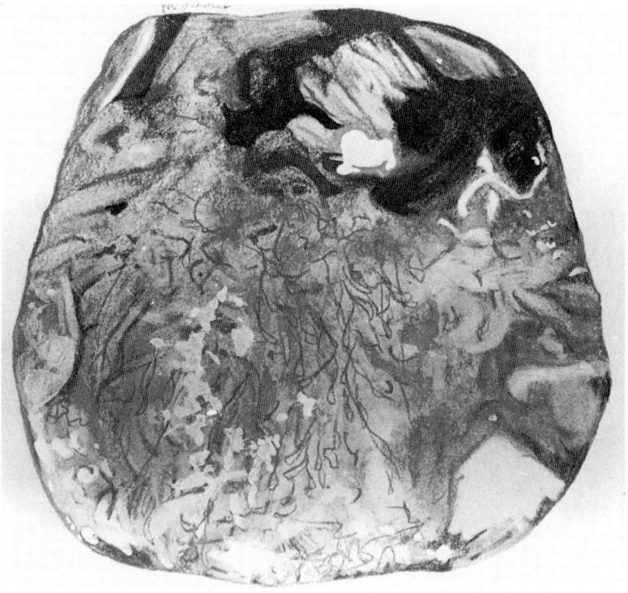

**FIG. 9–12.** Atypical vessels. Blood vessels have a haphazard course with multiple branches.

## CONTRAINDICATIONS

Colposcopy is a well-tolerated procedure that with patience and tenacity can be performed on virtually anyone. As the examiner becomes more experienced, the length of time for the procedure and discomfort to the patient should decrease.

There are few absolute contraindications to colposcopy and biopsy of the cervix. These would include the possibility of metastatic choriocarcinoma to the cervix and vagina, hemangioma of the cervix, and placenta previa. Otherwise, colposcopy can be done in most patients. Common sense would dictate, however, that the vigor with which the examination is pursued and the tenacity with which one goes after a biopsy should be tempered by underlying circumstances.

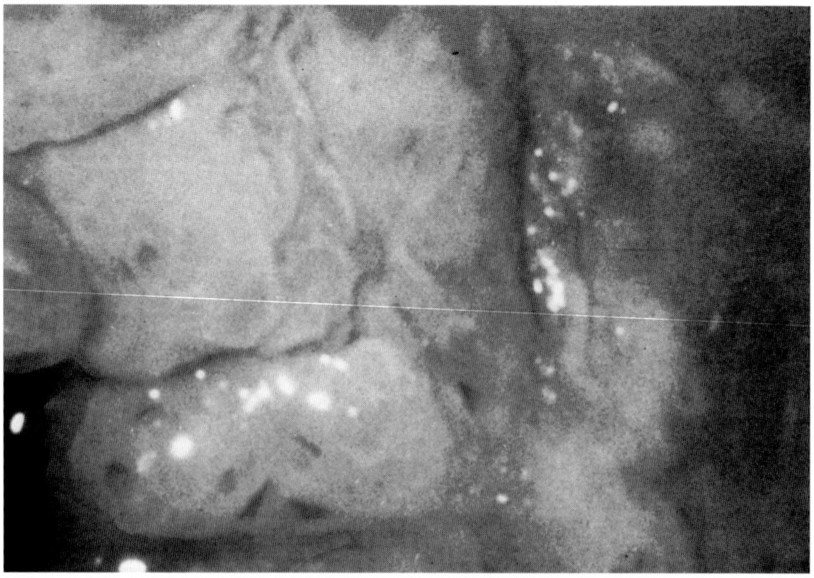

**FIG. 9–13.** Colpophotograph showing white epithelium encroaching on the endocervical canal. See Color Fig. 14.

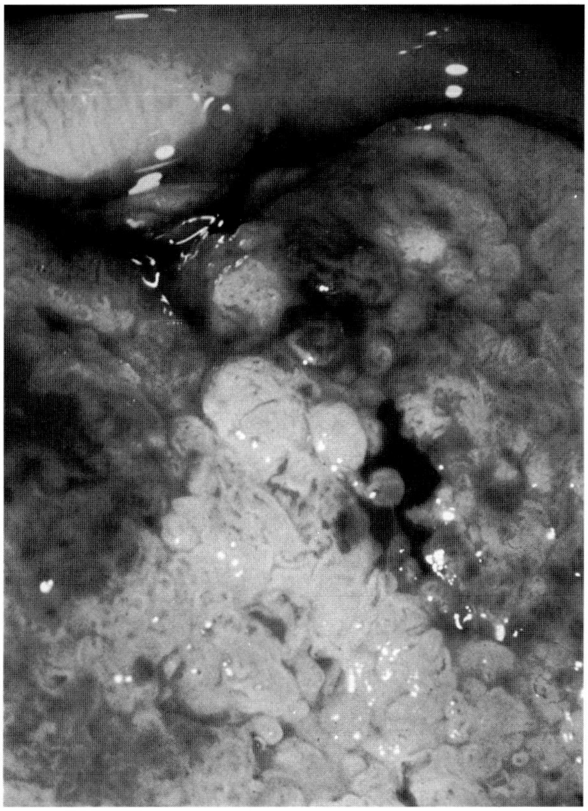

**FIG. 9–14.** Colpophotograph showing overt carcinoma, recognized by the blunt, exophytic excrescenses and horizontally running tumor vessels. See Color Fig. 15.

On occasion, an adequate examination cannot be done in the office. If warranted, the patient should then be examined under anesthesia.

## COMPLICATIONS

There are few major complications related to colposcopy. The two most frequently encountered are pain and bleeding. Patient discomfort is encountered frequently. Some of this can be allayed by explaining to the patient what the examination entails and how they may feel. It is rare to encounter a patient whose pain can not be adequately handled with either acetaminophen or one of the nosteroidal analgesic drugs. Bleeding is often unavoidable. In order to minimize it, care must be exerted to only biopsy the designated areas, to minimize the number of biopsies, and to have readily available gauze for packing, Monsel's solution, and, if needed, cautery devices.

## REFERENCES


1. American Cancer Society. Cancer Statistics 1993: A Cancer Journal for Clinicians, 1993; 43(1):18.
2. Hinselmann H. Verbesserung der inspektionsmoglich keiten von vulva, vagina und portio. Munchner Med Wochenschr 1925;72:1723.
3. Papanicolaou G, Traut HF. 1943. Diagnosis of uterine cancer by the vaginal smear. Commonwealth Fund New York, 1943.
4. Teaff NL, Malone JM, Ginsburg KA, Bartles LW, Halger BB. Cervical dysplasia in the postmenopausal female: diagnosis and treatment, Int J Gynecol Obstet, 1990;34:145–149.

*Invasive Outpatient Procedures in Reproductive Medicine,* edited by Mark I. Evans, et al. Lippincott–Raven Publishers, Philadelphia © 1997.

# 10 The Loop Electrosurgical Excision Procedure

Ralph Richert, Thomas C. Wright, Jr.

## INTRODUCTION AND INDICATIONS

The loop electrosurgical excision procedure (LEEP) was developed by Walter Prendiville[1] as an adaptation of the method originally described by Cartier.[2] LEEP can be applied to all portions of the lower male and female anogenital tract and to skin lesions on other parts of the body. It can be used for diagnostic excision, small biopsies, or ablations. LEEP has largely replaced the $CO_2$ laser for the diagnosis and treatment of HPV-related lesions of the anogenital tract.

LEEP is used principally to remove HPV-related lesions and has, as its principal advantage, the ability to produce a specimen for diagnosis and treatment at the same time. In contrast to ablative procedures such as cryotherapy or $CO_2$ laser ablation, LEEP removes the tissue intact and allows the entire specimen to be sectioned for diagnosis. This enormously reduces the risk of missing invasive cancers of the cervix and adenocarcinomas in situ when patients are triaged using colposcopically directed biopsies and endocervical curettage, and it reduces the risk that a patient will be treated for an intraepithelial lesion when she, in fact, has invasion.

LEEP is easy to teach, easy to learn, and easy to apply. It requires a colposcopic evaluation of the patient to determine what tissue should be removed and to determine the margins of excision. The procedure should not be used in the anogenital tract by individuals who are not skilled colposcopists. The procedure may be applied subsequent to colposcopically directed biopsies and endocervical curettage or, if a clear-cut lesion is present and is recognized by a skilled colposcopist, a ''see-and-treat'' approach may be used, in which the lesion is removed and the patient is treated at the first visit post abnormal Pap smear detection.

Following colposcopic evaluation, the technique of the LEEP excision and fulguration should be carried out using a modern electrosurgical generator with a foot switch and a series of loops and needles, which are carefully chosen to provide the most appropriate combination of widths and depths. For practical purposes, the 5 mm ball electrode is used for most electrofulguration procedures with some applications, particularly to external HPV-related lesions, appropriately using the macroneedle. The following photographs and diagrams illustrate LEEP for the cervix. Similar principles apply when using the procedure for external warts or flat lesions of the vagina, vulva, or anus with minor, but important, variations in technique. A text such as *Electrosurgery for HPV-Related Diseases of the Anogenital Tract*[3] should be consulted for a more detailed explanation of the procedure.

## TECHNIQUE

The Prendiville loop (Fig. 10–1) is made of fine, stainless steel wire, has an insulated cross bar, and is designed to fit in the standard electrosurgical ''pencil'' holder. This loop was

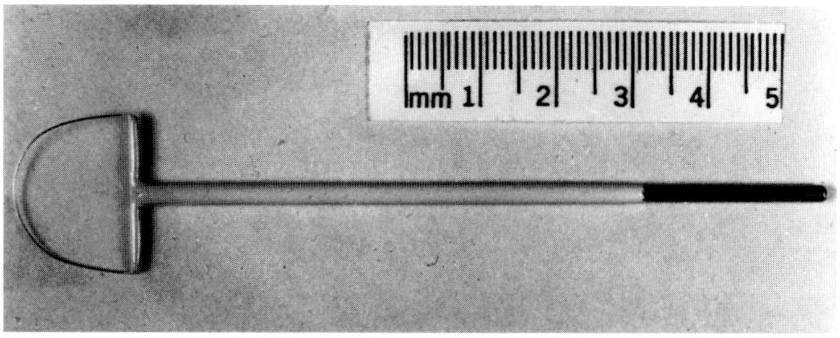

**FIG. 10–1.** The Prendiville loop.

originally the "standard." It measures 2 × 2 cm. It is not necessary to use a loop that can penetrate 2 cm deep into the tissues as there is no clinical need to remove this much tissue at a single pass. A loop of this size can remove too much tissue too fast, and its use has been associated with unintentional cervical amputations and other significant complications. Loops of this size should not be used except under very unusual circumstances.

The standard loops commonly used for cervical LEEP are shown in Figure 10–2. The loop on the right measures 2 cm across the base and 8 mm deep. The loop in the center is similar to the one on the right except that the vertical depth is 7 mm. Almost all cervical loop excisions can readily be accomplished using the 2 × 0.7 cm loop. As these loops are most commonly used to excise tissue from the exocervix, they are commonly referred to as "exoloops." The loop on the left measures 1 × 1 cm and is used principally to remove a cylinder of tissue from the endocervical canal. It is commonly referred to as an "endoloop." The endoloop shape may be curved, as illustrated here, or square. This is a matter of personal preference.

The standard ball electrode is illustrated in Figure 10–3. Although 3 mm- and 5 mm-diameter balls are commercially available, the 5 mm ball is preferable; it covers a wider area and can be used to fulgurate the base of excision rapidly.

The cervix is exposed using an insulated speculum and insulated lateral vaginal wall retractors (Fig. 10–4, Color Fig. 16). The built-in tube is connected to a smoke evacuator, which is used during the procedure. Placing a condom from which the tip has been amputated over the blades of the speculum is another method for excluding the vaginal side walls from view and preventing the inadvertent electroexcision of vaginal tissue at the beginning or end of a cervical LEEP.

Figure 10–5 shows a diagrammatic illustration of the steps in a standard cervical LEEP for cervical intraepithelial neoplasia (CIN), which is confined to the portio and does not extend into the canal. The lesion is identified colposcopically using acetic acid (a). Aqueous Lugol's is applied to the cervix to delineate the lesional tissue better (b) (Lugol's staining persists

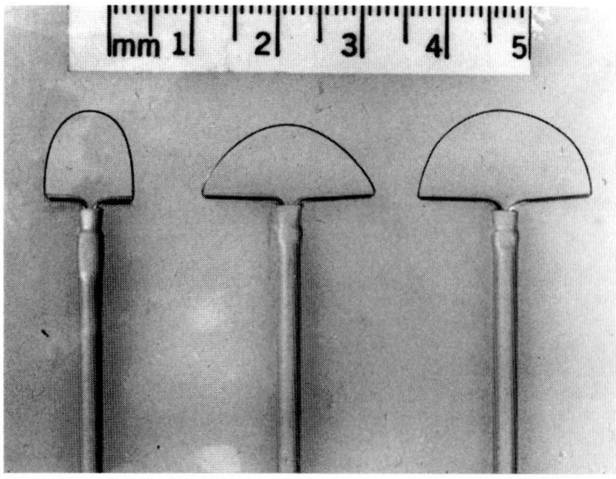

**FIG. 10–2.** Standard loop types used for LEEP.

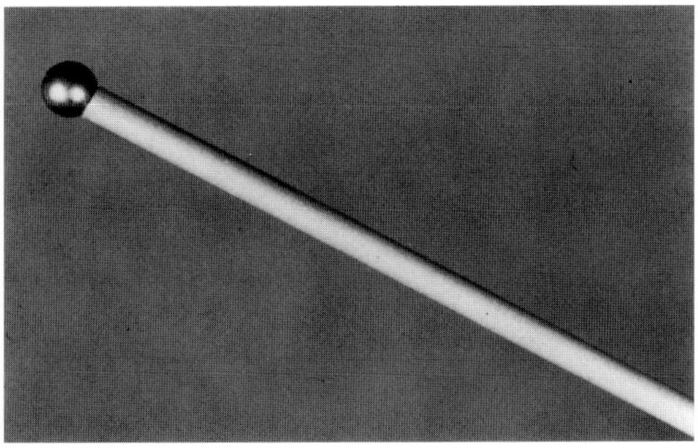

**FIG. 10–3.** Standard ball electrode used for LEEP.

longer than aceto-white epithelium). 2–4 mL of 2% xylocaine containing 1:100,000 units of epinephrine is injected 1–2 mm beneath the epithelium at 12, 3, 6, and 9 o'clock, using a dental syringe. If the cervix is particularly large, additional injections of local anesthetic can be used (c). The lesion is excised with a single pass of the 2 × 0.8 cm exoloop, which penetrates into the cervical stroma to a depth of approximately 6 mm (d). The excised tissue is removed and processed like a conization for histological examination (e). The crater is assessed colposcopically and, if no residual disease is evident on the portio or in the canal, an endocervical curettage is performed (f). The crater and any residual immature transformation zone is fulgurated using the 5 mm ball electrode (g). The crater is filled with Monsel's paste (ferric subsulphate) (h).

A diagrammatic illustration of the management of a patient in whom the cervical lesion extends beyond the area of tissue that can readily be removed by a single pass of the 2 × 0.7 cm exoloop electrode is given in Figure 10–6. Having completed the steps illustrated in Figure

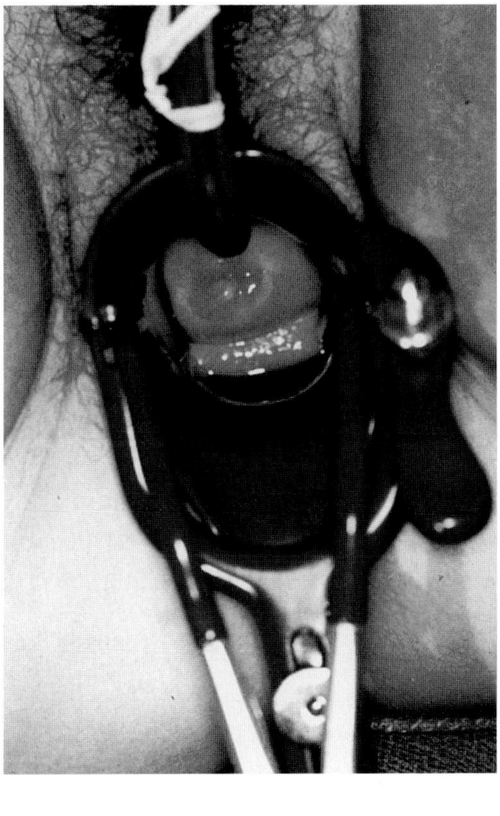

**FIG. 10–4.** Exposure of the cervix. See Color Fig. 16.

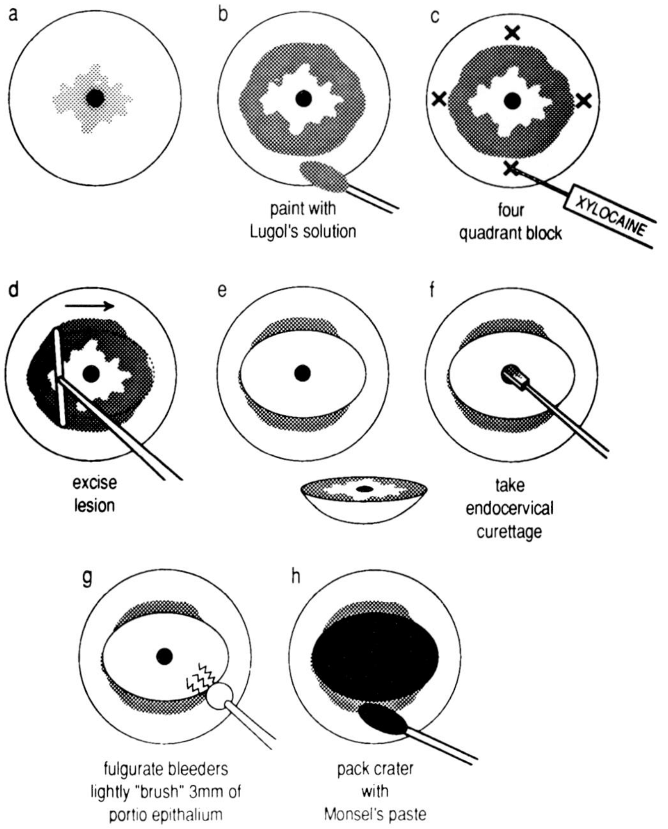


**FIG. 10–5.** Steps in a standard cervical LEEP procedure (see text for details).

10–5, a pass with the exoloop is made across the lesion such that the center of the exoloop passes through the endocervical canal and the depth of excision is greatest in the region of the endocervical canal (a). After removal of the excised tissue and reexamination with a colposcope, it is apparent that residual disease is present on the anterior and posterior lips (b). An additional pass with the exoloop is made to remove the lesion from the anterior lip (c). An additional pass with the exoloop is made to remove the residual CIN from the posterior lip (d). Note that neither of these excisions uses the full volume capacity of the exoloop. It is only necessary to excise widely enough and deep enough to remove the lesional tissue and the surrounding immature transformation zone (d). A diagram of the cervix after the three passes have been made (e). The three pieces of tissue are submitted for histological examination (f). The crater is treated in a fashion similar to that described in Figure 10–5.

If a cervical lesion extends well out on the portio epithelium and into the fornix and the distribution is such that it cannot readily be removed by the exoloop procedure, an alternative approach (Fig. 10–7) is to remove the majority of lesion with a single pass of the exoloop (a), following which the residual tissue (b) can be electrofulgerated (c, d). This procedure should only be used by expert colposcopists who can assure themselves that invasion is not present in the tissues which are to be fulgurated rather than excised.

A photograph of a cervix with an aceto-white, well-demarcated lesion consistent with high-grade CIN is given in Figure 10–8. The panel on the right shows the same cervix after the application of Lugol's solution. It is important always to use aqueous Lugol's, as alcoholic solutions or any other flammable liquid may be ignited by the loop procedure.

A dental syringe using an ampule containing 2% xylocaine with epinephrine in a concentration of 1 : 100,000 is used to apply local anesthetic to the cervix (Fig. 10–9, Color Fig. 17). The anesthesia should not be applied using a paracervical block as it is more time-consuming, painful, and not necessary. The extended needle is then placed immediately beneath the epithe-

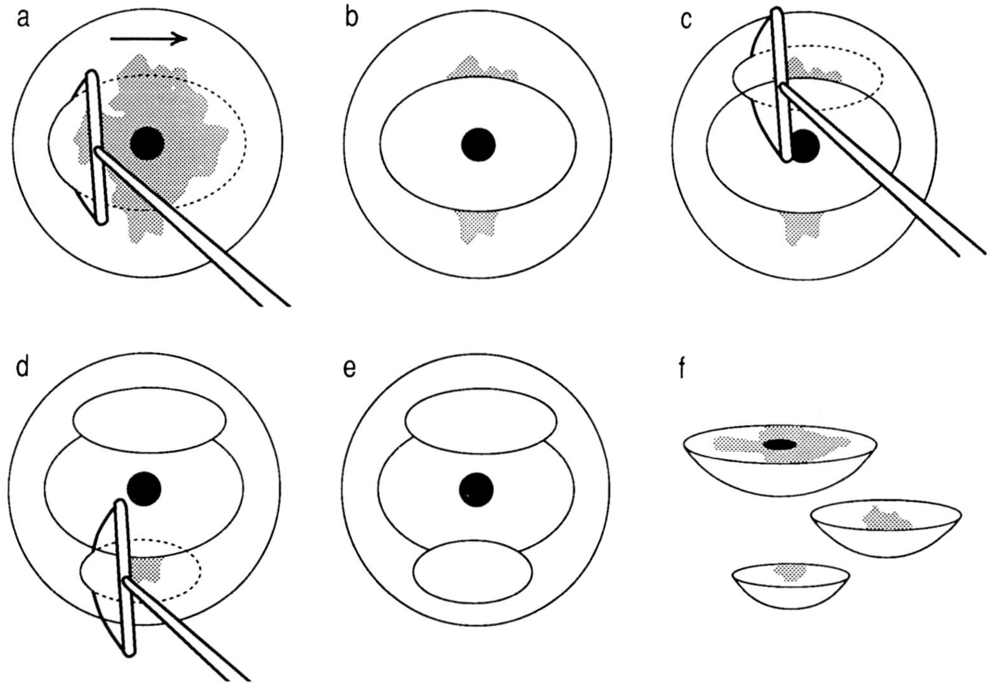


**FIG. 10–6.** Management of the patient with more extensive tissues involvement (see text for details).

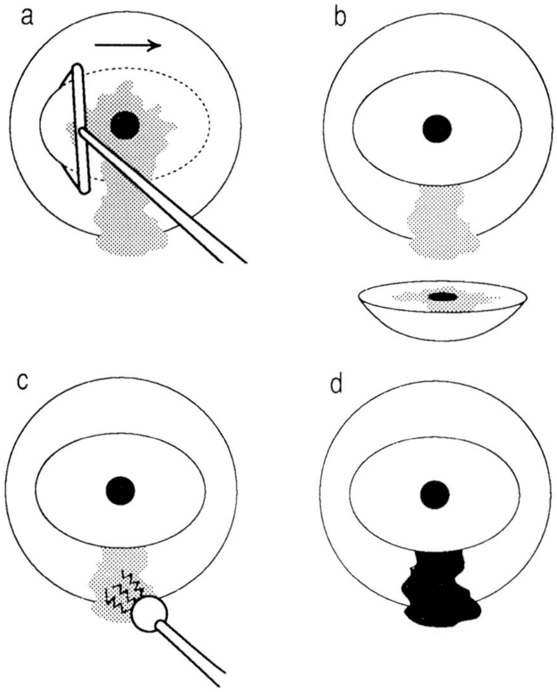


**FIG. 10–7.** Management of the patient with the exoloop procedure followed by electrofulgeration.

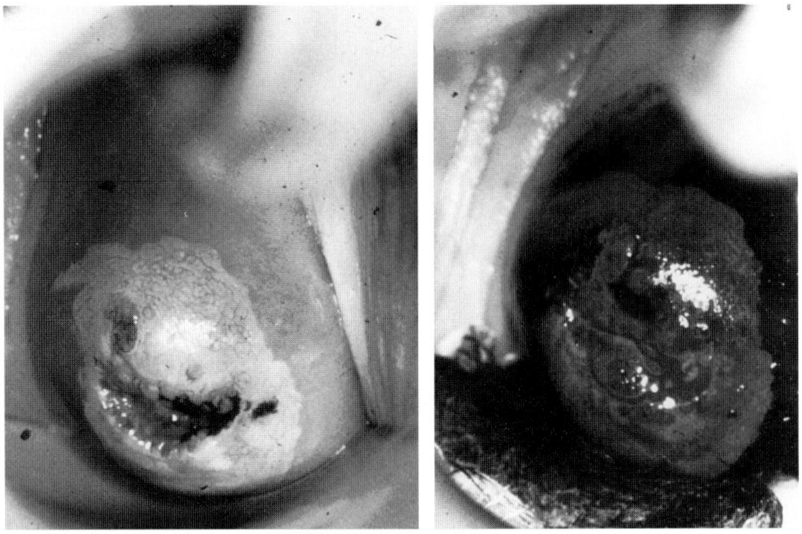

**FIG. 10–8.** Cervix with high-grade CIN (left). Same cervix after application of Lugol's solution (right).

lium at the 12 o'clock position (Fig. 10–10, Color Fig. 18). After the anesthetic is placed, several minutes should be allowed to elapse before the procedure is initiated. The 2 × 0.7 cm exoloop is passed into the cervical tissue vertically after the electrosurgical generator has been activated using a blend 1 current (Fig. 10–11, Color Fig. 19) The loop is then continuously, but slowly, passed through the tissue (right panel), gradually penetrating to its deepest point in the canal and then slowly brought through to the other side, diminishing the depth with lateral excursion. The passage of the loop through the cervical tissue should describe a hemisphere rather than a hemicylinder.

After the lesional tissue is excised the base should be reexamined with a colposcope as should the periphery of the excisional site (Fig. 10–12, Color Fig. 20). If additional lesional tissue is found at the periphery or in the base of the excisional crater, additional passes may be made with the loop to remove the tissue or persistent glands. In this case there is persistent bleeding, which will require electrofulguration. The 5 mm ball electrode is used to electrofulgurate the base of excision tissue in order to control the bleeding (Fig. 10–13, Color Fig. 21)

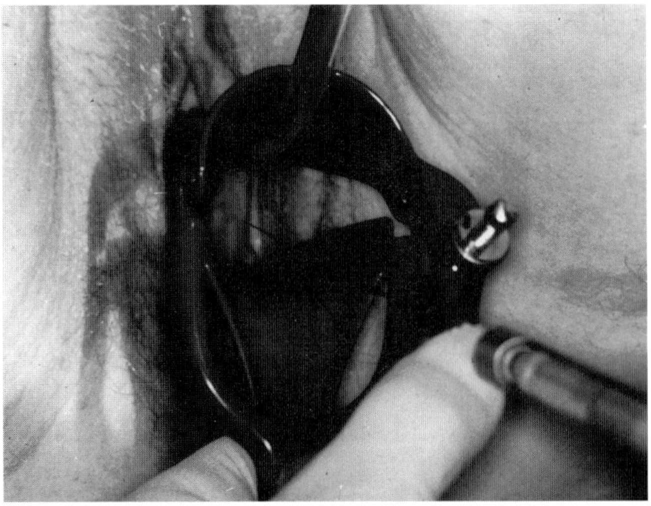

**FIG. 10–9.** Anesthetic application to the cervix. See Color Fig. 17.

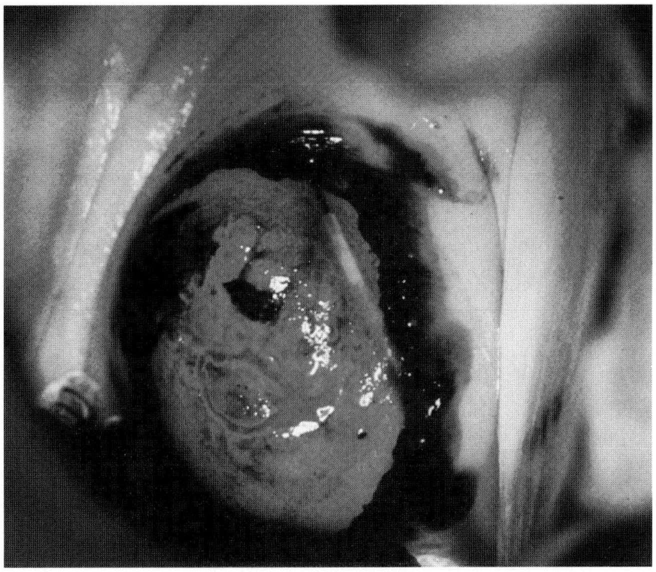

**FIG. 10–10.** Subepithelial anesthetic application. See Color Fig. 18.

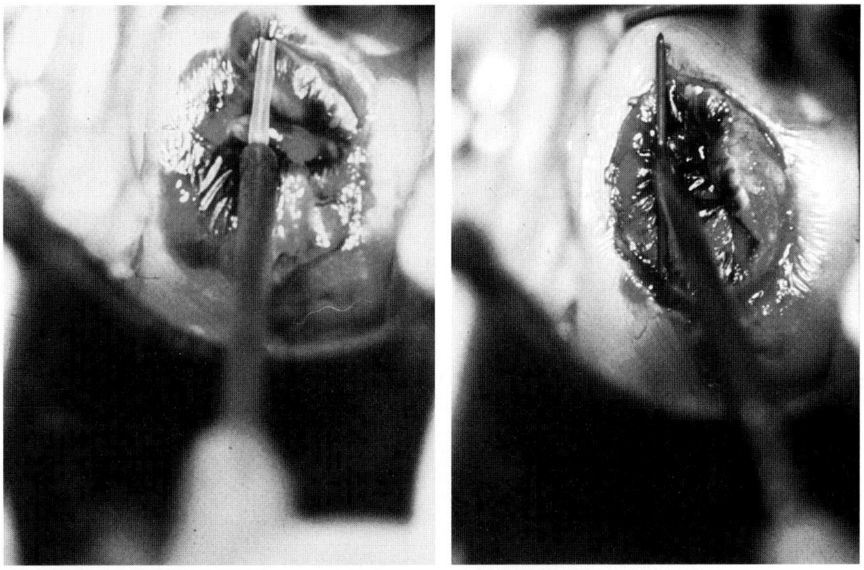

**FIG. 10–11.** Use of the exoloop (see text for details). See Color Fig. 19.

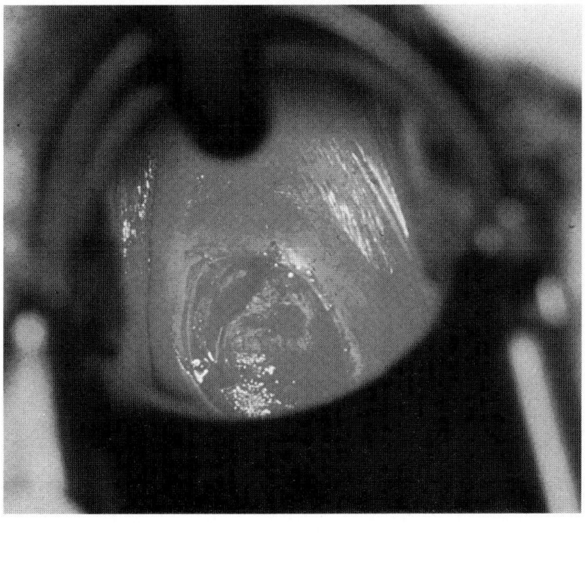

**FIG. 10–12.** Postexcision colposcopic examination. See Color Fig. 20.

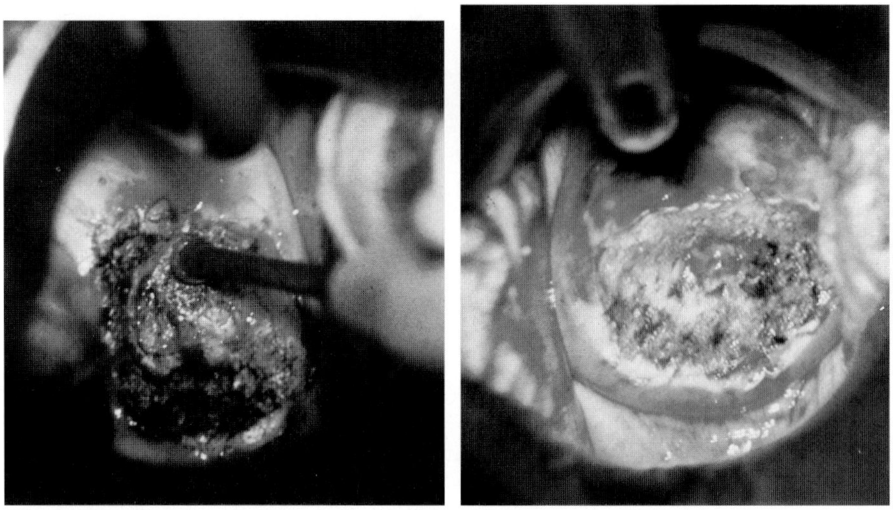

**FIG. 10–13.** Use of the ball electrode for electrofulguration. See Color Fig. 21.

(right panel). It is important that fulguration rather than electrodesiccation be used to minimize tissue damage. If any immature transformation zone is left behind, the 5 mm ball can be used to ablate that tissue as well as fulgurate the crater base. In the left panel, the base has been fully electrofulgurated, and there is no persistent bleeding. The crater is filled with Monsel's paste (Fig. 10–14, Color Fig. 22), a ferric subsulphate that has been evaporated to the consistency of molasses.

Figure 10–15 illustrates contrasting the approach to a purely exocervical lesion, which can be removed by a simple pass of the exoloop (left panel), and a lesion that extends deeply into the canal and requires deep excision using the electrosurgical conization, as popularized by Mor-Yosef et al.[4]

The therapeutic approach to a cervix in which there is lesional tissue on the portio, extending

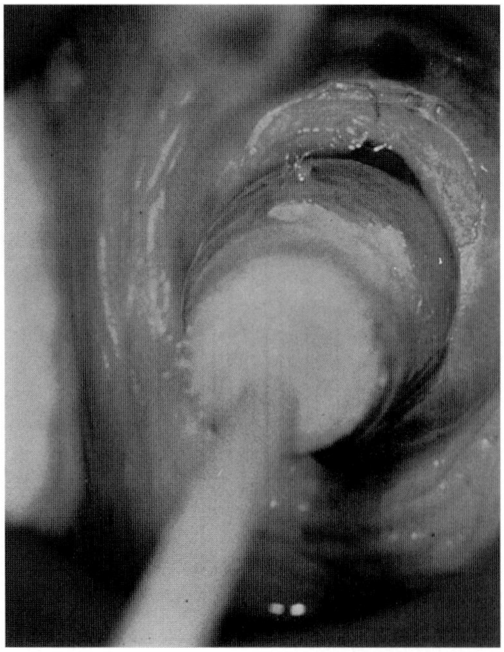

**FIG. 10–14.** The crater is filled with Monsel's paste. See Color Fig. 22.

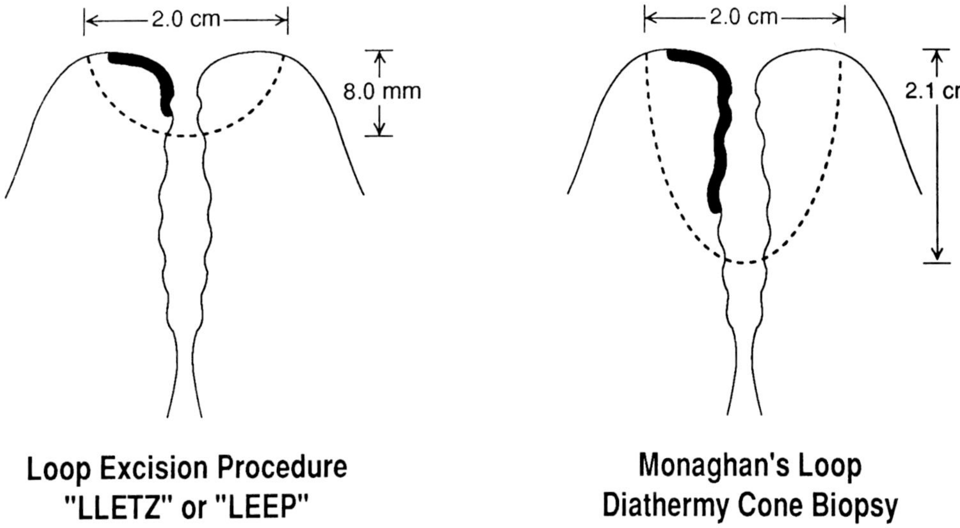


**FIG. 10–15.** Contrasting approaches to exo- and endocervical lesions.

into the endocervical canal, is illustrated in Figure 10–16. When there is both ectocervical and endocervical disease, it is necessary to use a combined procedure, which will generally result in an excision with a ''cowboy hat'' configuration. In the sequence labeled A, the endoloop is used to excise the endocervical canal to a depth of 1 cm prior to the portio lesion being removed by a single pass of the exoloop. The use of the endoloop prior to the exoloop is indicated in those patients in whom the disease extends more deeply into the canal. The object is to avoid cutting across significant disease if at all possible. As 95% of invasive cancers occur within one punch biopsy of the external os, it is most desirable to remove this area intact, without producing incidental thermal damage. In the sequence labeled B the exoloop excision is performed first, but if a small area of residual CIN is found in the canal colposcopically, then the exoloop can be used to excise that tissue with a margin of normal endocervix.

Figure 10–17 (Color Fig. 23) shows a cervix in which there is a large exocervical lesion that extends deeply into the canal. In the left panel the exoloop has been used to excise the portio lesion and the canal to a depth of 7 mm. In the right panel the crater remaining after

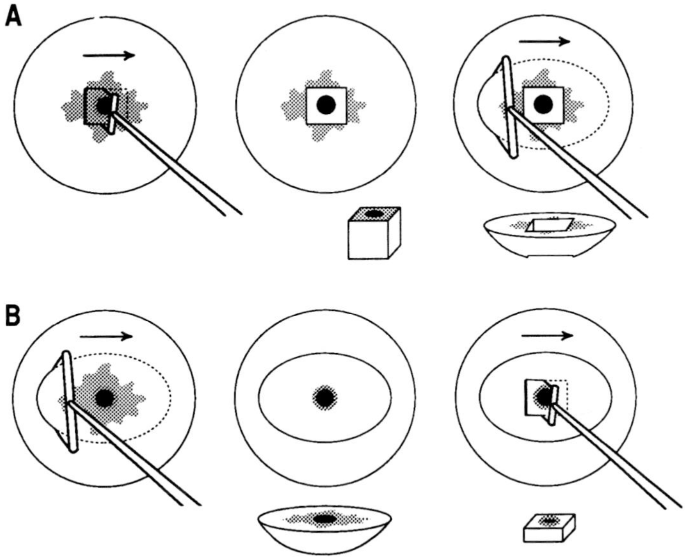


**FIG. 10–16.** Therapeutic approaches to lesions extending into the endocervical canal (see text for details).

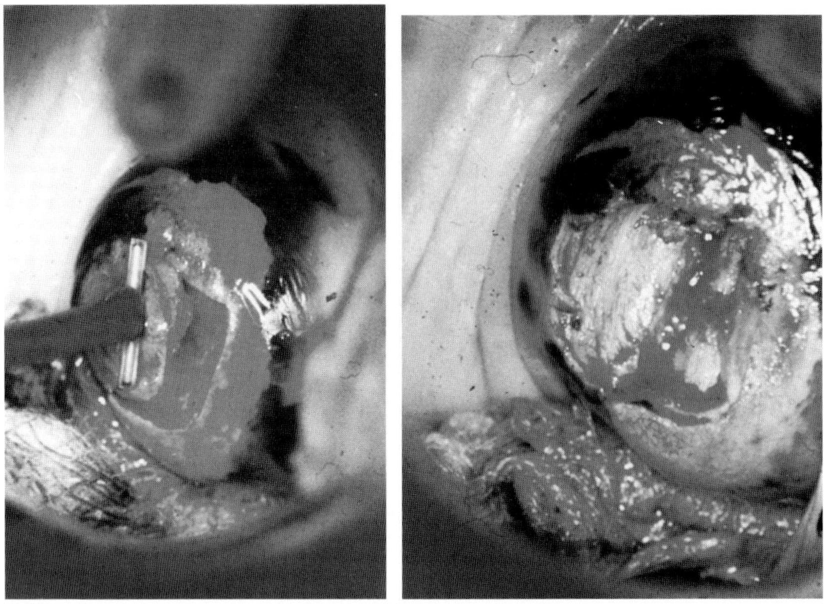

**FIG. 10–17.** Large exocervical lesion. See Color Fig. 23.

the tissue has been removed can be seen with some residual bleeding. In Figure 10–18 (Color Fig. 24) the endoloop is being used to excise additional endocervical canal to a depth of 1 cm. It is necessary to infiltrate the canal with the dental syringe with a long needle prior to an endoloop excision to provide additional anesthesia for the procedure. The left panel of Figure 10–19 (Color Fig. 25) shows the ''cowboy hat'' crater after the combined exo- and endoloop excision. In the right panel Monsel's paste has been placed in the crater. In this cervix no residual bleeding or oozing was noted after completion of the excisional procedures, and electrofulguration was not used. The exoloop and the endoloop excised tissues are submitted for pathologic examination in a plastic tissue-processing cassette to prevent twisting, curling, and tangential cutting (Fig. 10–20, Color Fig. 26). In a small proportion of patients residual

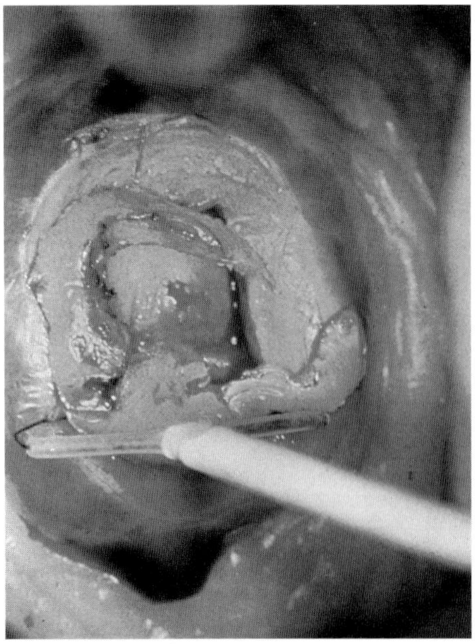

**FIG. 10–18.** Endoloop excising additional endocervical canal tissue. See Color Fig. 24.

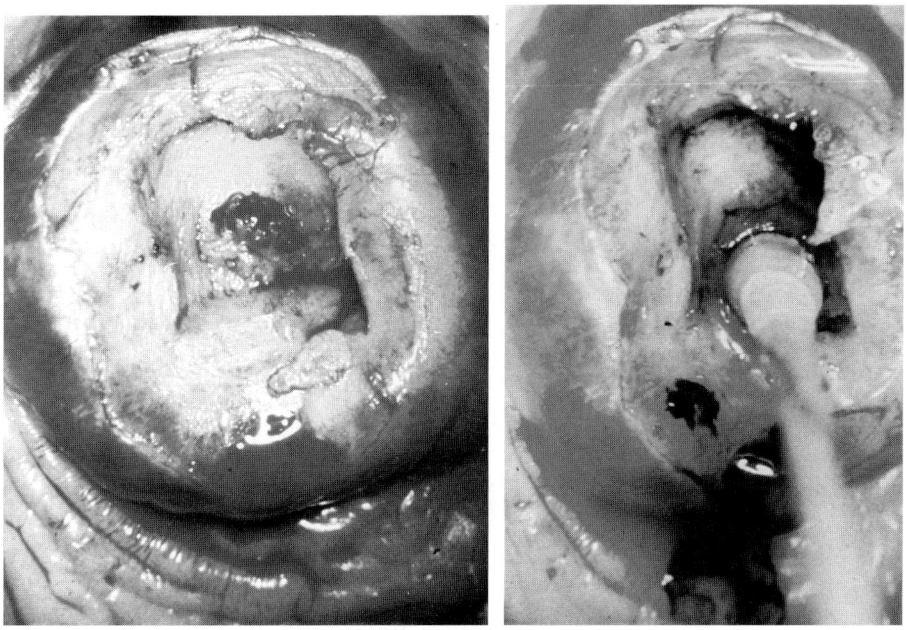

**FIG. 10–19.** "Cowboy hat" crater (left) and application of Monsel's paste (right). See Color Fig. 25.

bleeding will occur post LEEP. When such patients are examined, clotted blood will usually be found in the crater with oozing vessels or, sometimes when the clot is removed, a small bleeding vessel. These patients may readily be managed by electrofulguration of the base and a reapplication of Monsel's paste. It is extremely uncommon for the patient to have a reoccurrence of bleeding a second time (Fig. 10–21, Color Fig. 27).

## INTERPRETATION OF RESULTS

Most authors report a cure rate with a single loop procedure for CIN of approximately 95%.[5] This rate is comparable to ablation or excision with the $CO_2$ laser. The loop procedure has

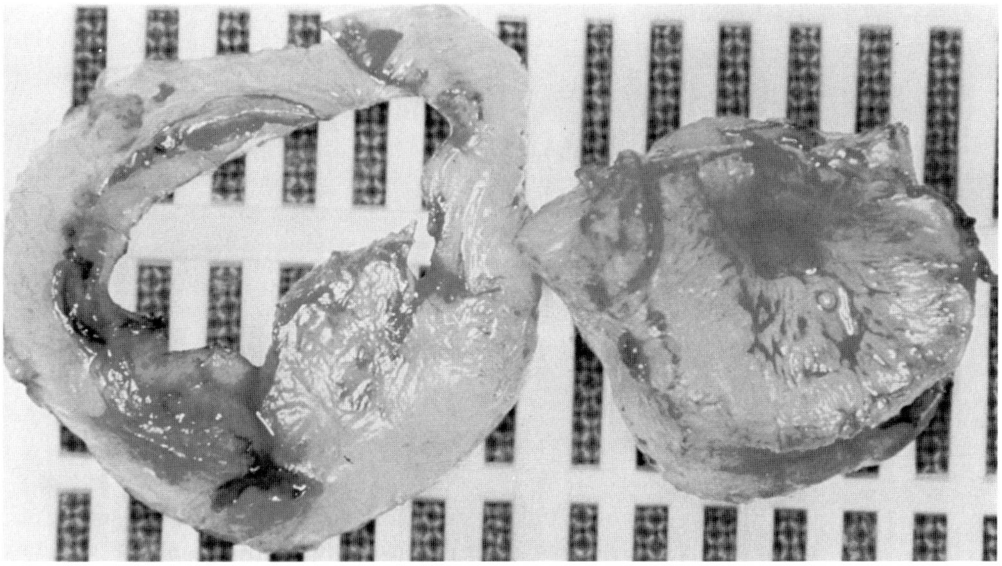

**FIG. 10–20.** Exo- and endoloop excised tissues prepared for pathologic examination. See Color Fig. 26.

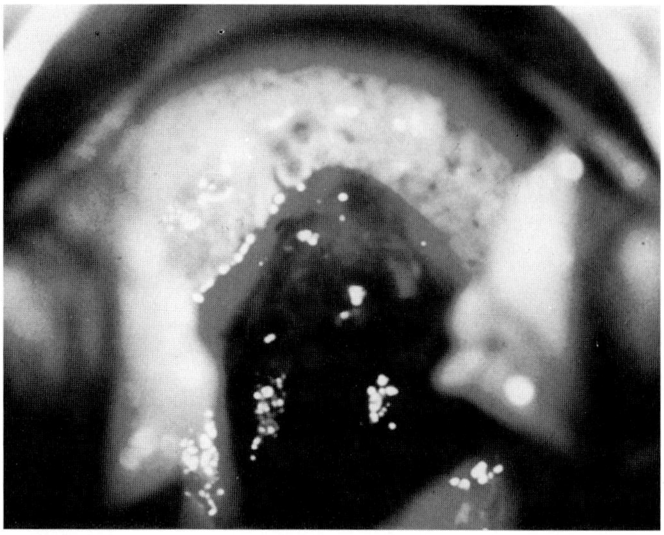

**FIG. 10–21.** Post-LEEP residual bleeding. See Color Fig. 27.

not been used for as long as laser conization and the number of reported patients is fewer, with less long-term follow-up. The published results with LEEP are virtually identical to those published over the past 15 years for $CO_2$ laser conization, and future results would be expected to parallel laser data. The only difference between the two procedures is the manner in which the energy is delivered. Healing post-LEEP is similar to healing post laser conization or post cold-knife conization, and generally occurs within a three-month period. The most important data relevant to LEEP are the consistent findings that in 4–6 patients per 1,000 undergoing a LEEP for CIN, a more severe lesion is found in the excised specimen. This ranges from microinvasive carcinoma and adenocarcinoma in situ to frankly invasive cancer. The use of an excisional procedure rather than an ablative procedure for patients with CIN is the major advantage of LEEP. Using LEEP, it is extremely unlikely that a significant lesion will be missed and hence extremely unlikely that a patient will be treated inappropriately for a low-grade lesion when a more significant lesion is present.

## CONTRAINDICATIONS

The contraindications to LEEP excision include a clinically apparent invasive carcinoma of the cervix, a bleeding disorder, pregnancy (except in highly experienced hands), breast feeding, equivocal cervical changes, diethylstilbestrol (DES)-exposed patient (except in highly experienced hands), and severe cervicitis. Of these, the most commonly violated contraindication is that of severe cervicitis. Just as with $CO_2$ laser ablation or conization, patients who have a highly inflamed cervix may have significant intraoperative bleeding when the cervix is excised. A patient with cervicitis should have that condition treated and the cervix restored to a non-inflamed state prior to the loop procedure being applied.

## COMPLICATIONS

Principal complications include perioperative bleeding, postoperative bleeding, cervical infection, and cervical stenosis. Perioperative bleeding occurs infrequently if patient selection is appropriate. The second most common cause of intraoperative bleeding is the insertion of the loop vertically into the cervix, well lateral to the os and cutting through the cervical branch of the uterine artery. The exoloop should be drawn through the cervix like an ice-cream scoop, and the lateral cuts should not be vertical.

The other source of intraoperative bleeding is the inadvertent extension of the loop excision into the vaginal wall. A deep wound in the lateral vaginal wall will commonly produce brisk bleeding. Postoperative bleeding is a relatively uncommon event occurring in 1–2% of patients, provided Monsel's paste is placed in the crater at the termination of the procedure. The rate of cervical stenosis is about 1% and occurs principally in women in the peri- or postmenopausal age group. Because stenosis is more common in this age group, older patients who are treated by this procedure should be seen in the early postoperative period and the cervix dilated if narrowing of the canal is occurring.

Overall, LEEP is a major advance in the technology of diagnosing and treating HPV-related lesions of the male and female anogenital tract. Because it is a simple procedure with little morbidity and few complications and because it virtually eliminates the inappropriate treatment of significant lesions as low-grade intraepithelial abnormalities, it has become the procedure of choice for most HPV-related lesions.

## REFERENCES

1. Prendiville W, Cullimore J, Norman S. Large loop excision of the transformation zone (LLETZ): a new method of management for women with cervical intraepitheliala neoplasia. Br J Obstet Gynaecol, 1989;96:1054–1060.
2. Cartier R. Practical colposcopy (2nd ed.). Paris: 1984.
3. Wright TC, Richart RM, Ferenczy AF. Electrosurgery for HPV-related lesions of the anogenital tract. New York: Arthur Vision, 1992.
4. Mor-Yosef S, Lopes A, Pearson S, Monaghan J. Loop diathermy cone biopsy. Obstet Gynecol 1990;75:173–178.
5. Wright TC, Cagnon MD, Richart RM, Ferenczy A. (1992). Treatment of cervical intraepithelial neoplasia using the loop electrosurgical excision procedure. Obstet Gynecol 1992;79: 173–178.

*Invasive Outpatient Procedures in Reproductive Medicine,* edited by Mark I. Evans, et al. Lippincott–Raven Publishers, Philadelphia © 1997.

# 11 Vulvar Examination and Biopsy

Raymond H. Kaufman

## INTRODUCTION

A basic concept related to disease involving any site of the body applies equally to vulvar diseases—prior to the institution of therapy, a correct diagnosis must be established. Unfortunately, by the time the gynecologist sees many patients with vulvar disease, the patient has been treated with a multiplicity of medications, which makes proper diagnosis difficult. A concept often expressed by the late Edward Fredrich was that the *telephone is not a diagnostic tool.* Treatment should rarely, if ever, be prescribed over the telephone prior to examining the patient.

## TECHNIQUE

### *EXAMINATION OF THE VULVA*

In most instances, visual examination of the vulva allows the gynecologist to define clearly the changes that are present. However, it is also advisable to enquire about and even inspect other areas of the body for the presence of dermatologic problems that may also involve the vulva. For example, the individual with erosive lichen planus of the vulva will often have lesions involving the buccal mucosa. Likewise, the changes of psoriasis that may be classical elsewhere on the body may be present in an atypical fashion when found on the vulva, because of the local environment of warmth and moisture. Of value is the use of a hand magnifying glass to allow the clinician to inspect the vulva in greater detail. The use of a colposcope is also of value, especially in defining possible changes related to papilloma virus infection. However, the hand magnifying glass suffices in most instances. Often, washing the vulva and vestibule with 3–5% acetic acid will highlight lesions, especially those related to papilloma virus infection and those lesions representing intraepithelial neoplasia. This is especially true on the mucosal surfaces of the vulva (*i.e*, the inner labia minora and vestibule).

In evaluating the patient seen primarily for complaints relative to the vulva, it is advisable to evaluate carefully the vagina and cervix for the presence of vaginitis or cervicitis. Often, the individual with a candidal infection of the vagina will have secondary manifestations present on the vulva or an associated candidal infection of the vulva. Likewise, the irritating discharge associated with a trichomoniasis will frequently result in secondary changes on the vulva. The diagnosis of vaginal infection is often easily made in the office on the basis of saline and potassium hydroxide wet-mount preparations obtained from vaginal secretions. This, associated with the determination of the vaginal pH utilizing pH ''strips,'' will allow one to make an accurate diagnosis in the vast majority of cases.

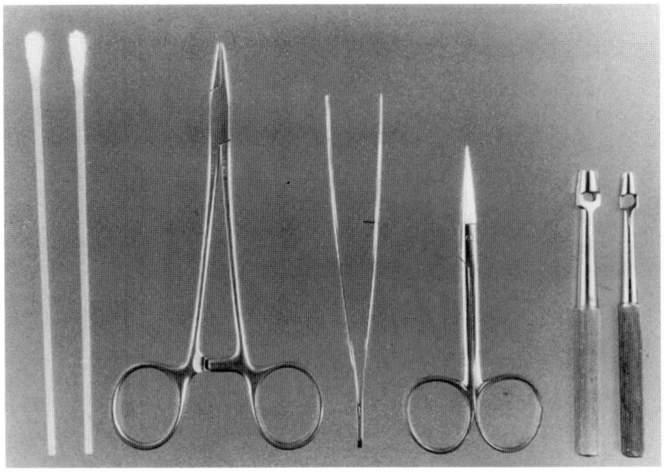

**FIG. 11–1.** Vulvar biopsy tray: 4 mm and 6 mm dermal punches are present on right.

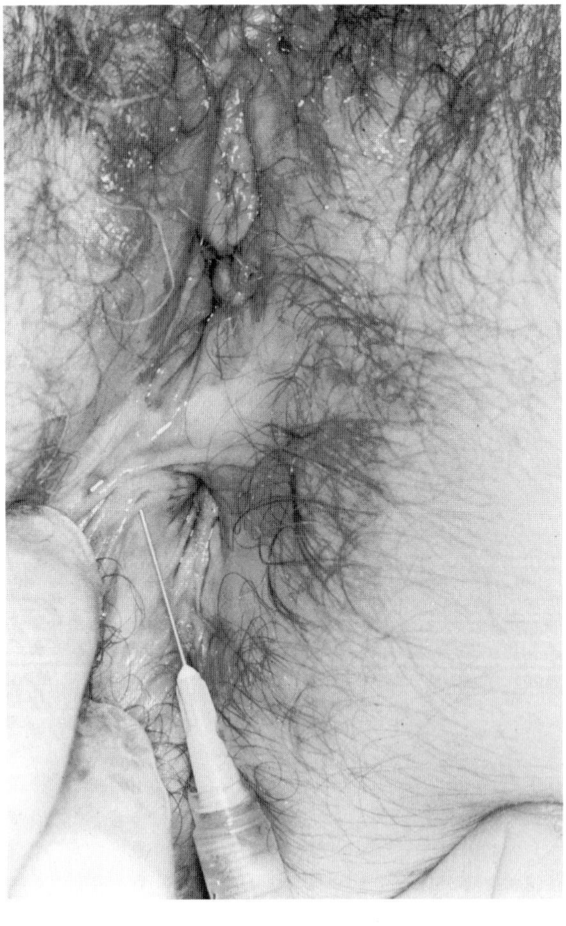

**FIG. 11–2.** A solution of 1% lidocaine is injected into the biopsy site. A 30-gauge needle is usually adequate.

*Invasive Outpatient Procedures in Reproductive Medicine,* edited by Mark I. Evans, et al. Lippincott–Raven Publishers, Philadelphia © 1997.

# Color Plate

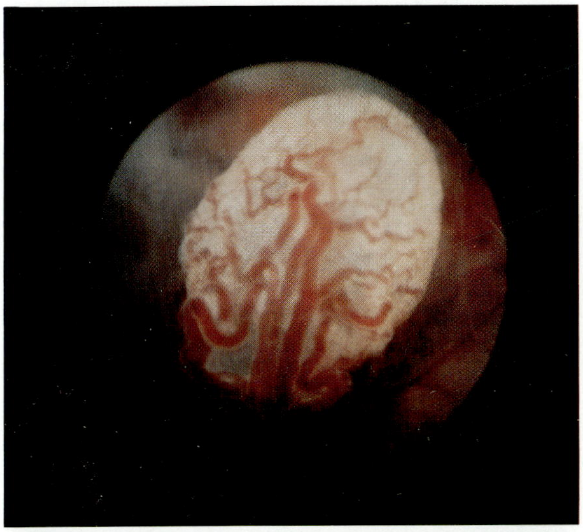

**Color Fig. 1 (Fig. 4–3).** Yolk sac with vascular network.

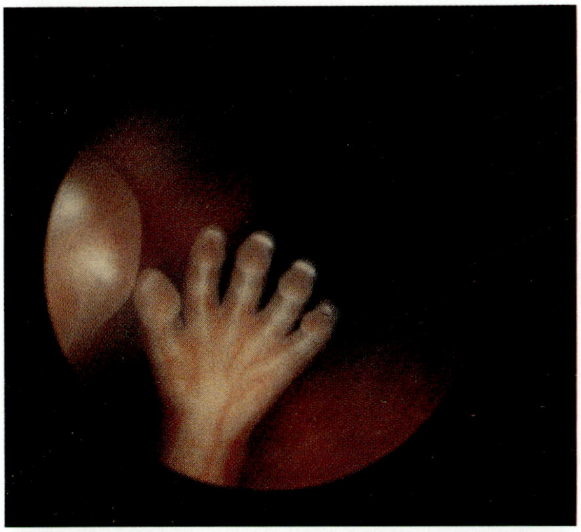

**Color Fig. 2 (Fig. 4–4).** Direct visualization of fetal hand at 9 weeks.

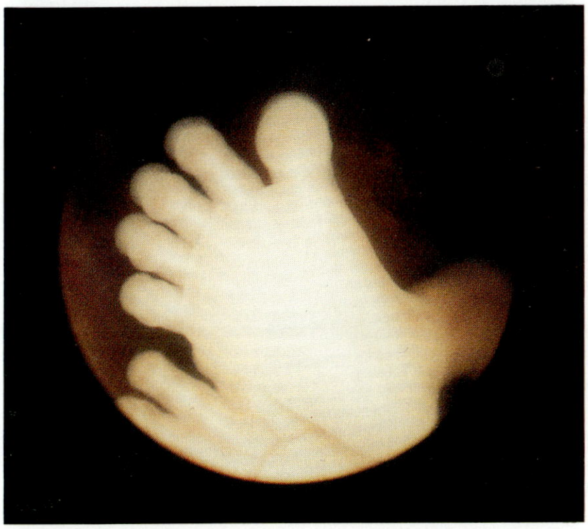

**Color Fig. 3 (Fig. 4–5).** Fetal toes at 9 weeks.

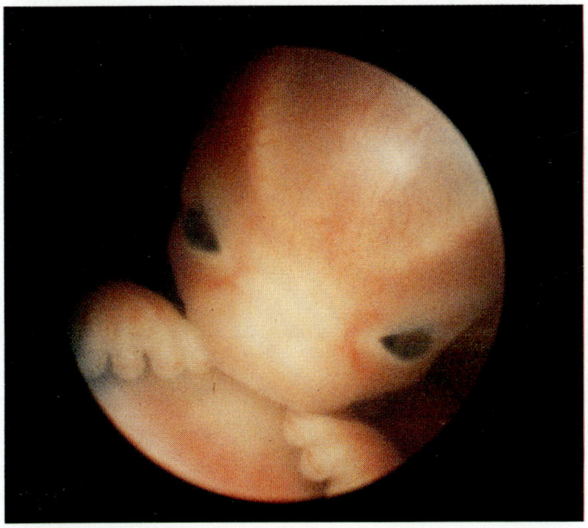

**Color Fig. 4 (Fig. 4–6).** Frontal view of face.

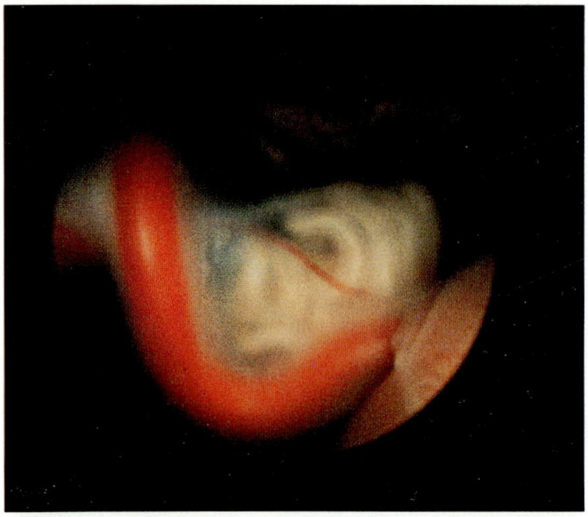

**Color Fig. 5 (Fig. 4–7).** Physiologic umbilical hernia at 9 weeks.

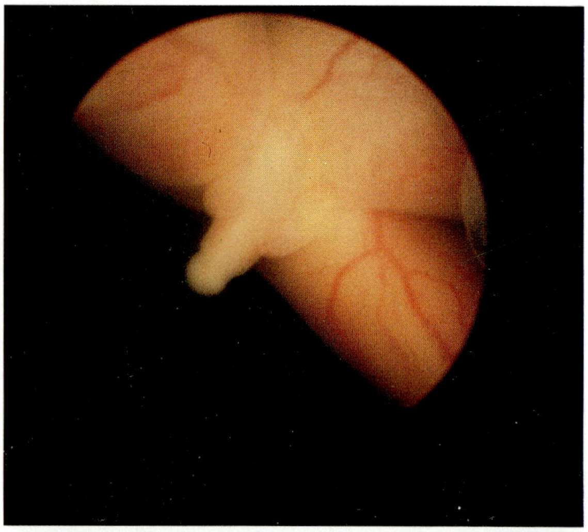

**Color Fig. 6 (Fig. 4–8).** External genitalia at 9 weeks. Ultimate phenotype is not certain at this gestational age.

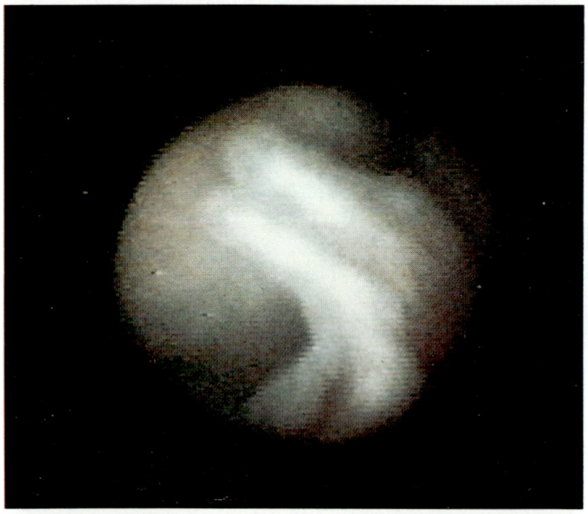

**Color Fig. 7 (Fig. 4–9).** Digital anomalies—syndactyly.

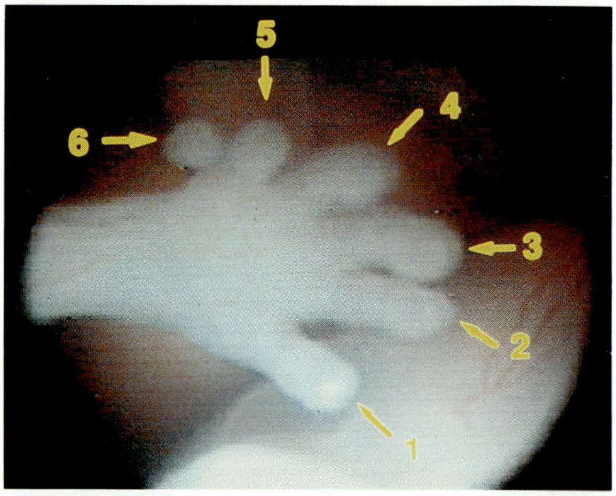


**Color Fig. 8 (Fig. 4–10).** Polydactyly showing 6th digit.

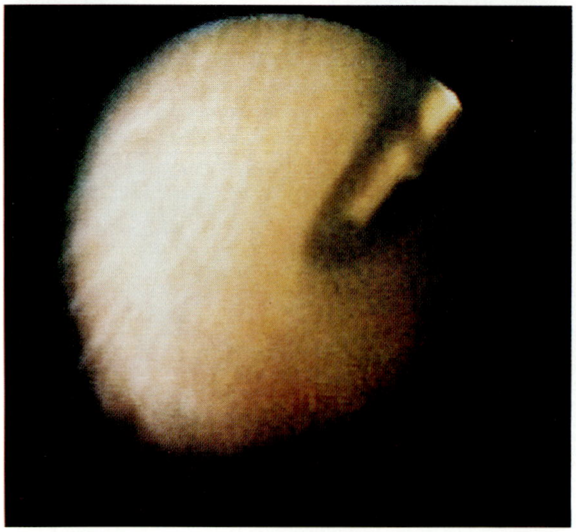

**Color Fig. 9 (Fig. 4–11).** Fetal muscle biopsy gun about to enter fetal skin at 19 weeks gestation.

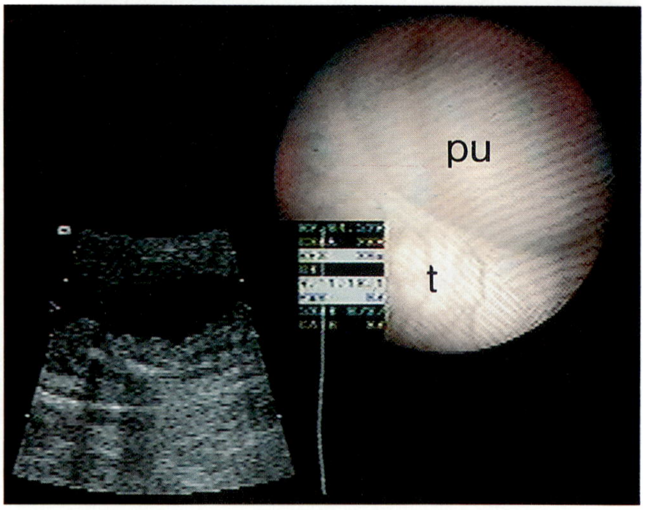


**Color Fig. 10 (Fig. 5–8).** Fetal cytoscopy in a 23-week pregnancy complicated by posterior urethral valves. Note tense dilation of proximal urethra and marked trabeculations of the trigone due to long-standing urethral obstruction. PU = proximal urethra, T = trigone region of posterior bladder.

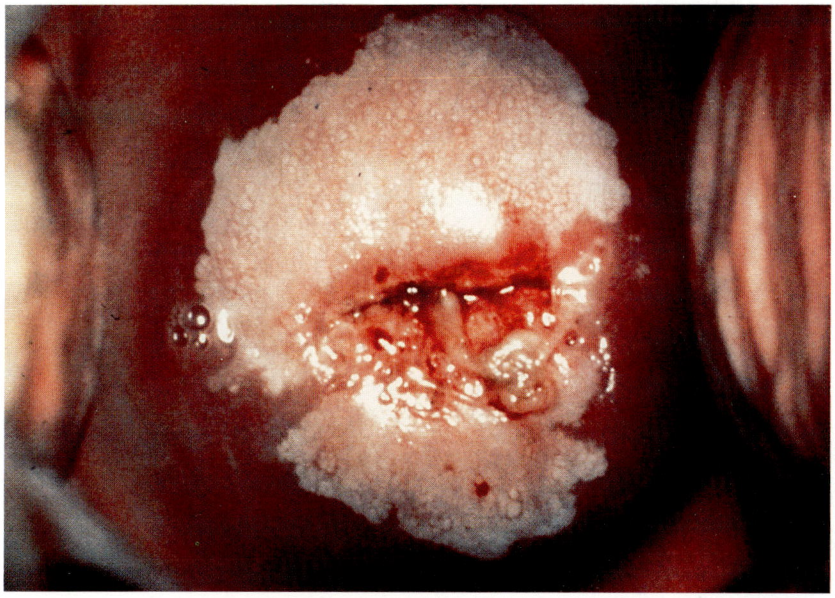

**Color Fig. 11 (Fig. 9–4).** Colpophotograph showing the characteristic yellow staining reaction seen with quarter strength Lugol's iodine.

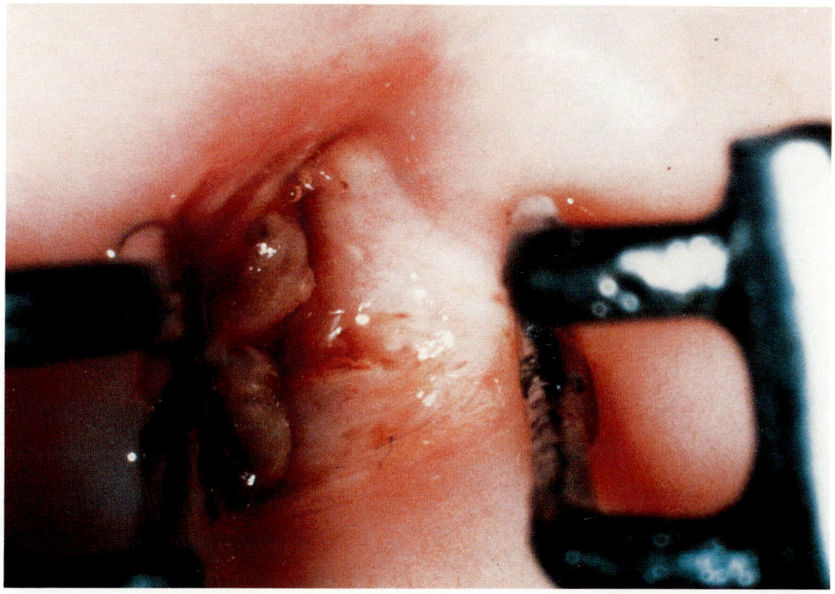

**Color Fig. 12 (Fig. 9–9).** Colpophotograph showing an epithelial lesion extending into the endocervical canal, well out of colposcopic range; an inadequate examination.

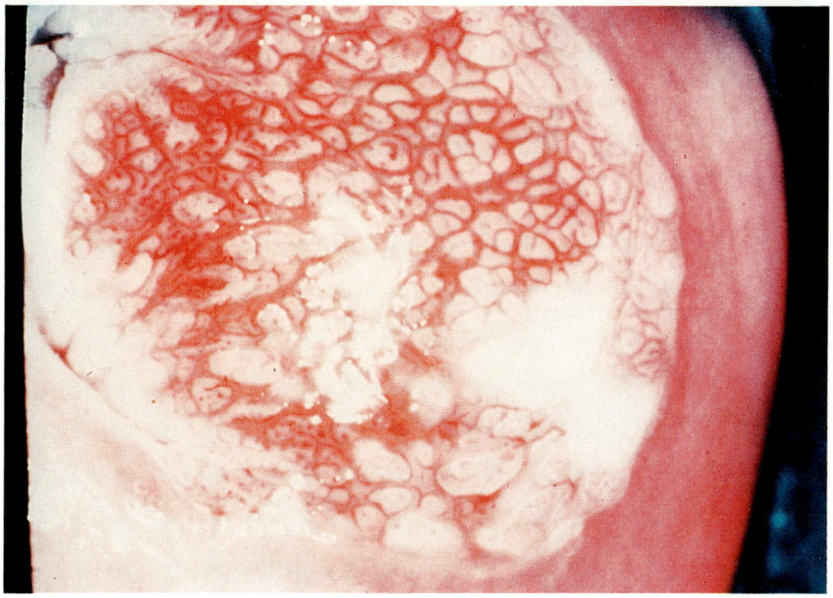

**Color Fig. 13 (Fig. 9–10).** Colpophotograph showing white epithelium and vascular mosaicism.

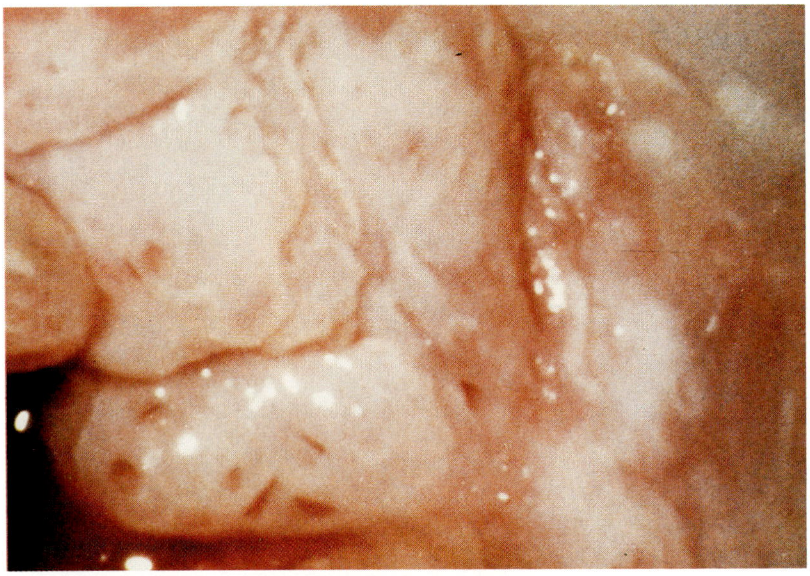

**Color Fig. 14 (Fig. 9–13).** Colpophotograph showing white epithelium encroaching on the endocervical canal.

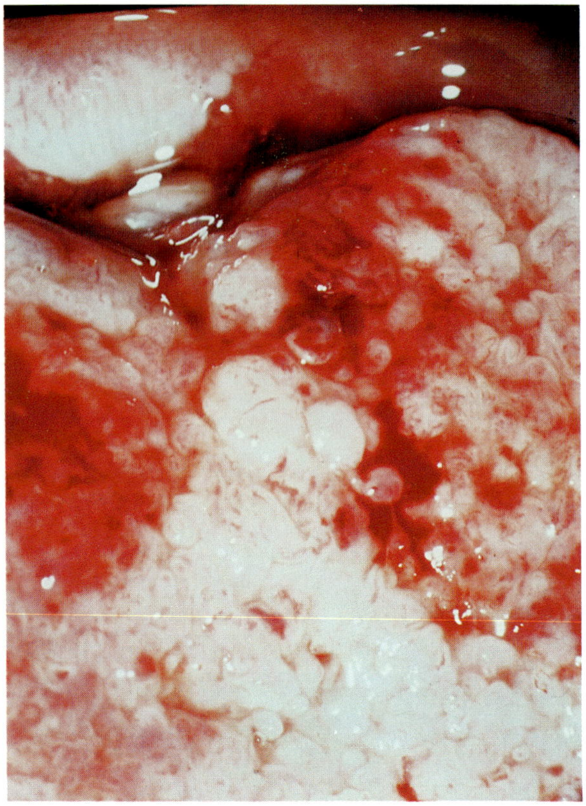

**Color Fig. 15 (Fig. 9–14).** Colpophotograph showing overt carcinoma, recognized by the blunt, exophytic excrescences and horizontally running tumor vessels.

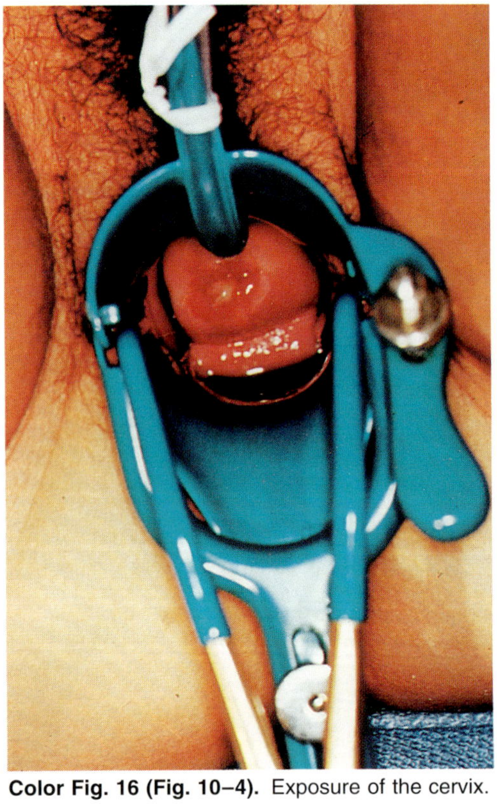

**Color Fig. 16 (Fig. 10–4).** Exposure of the cervix.

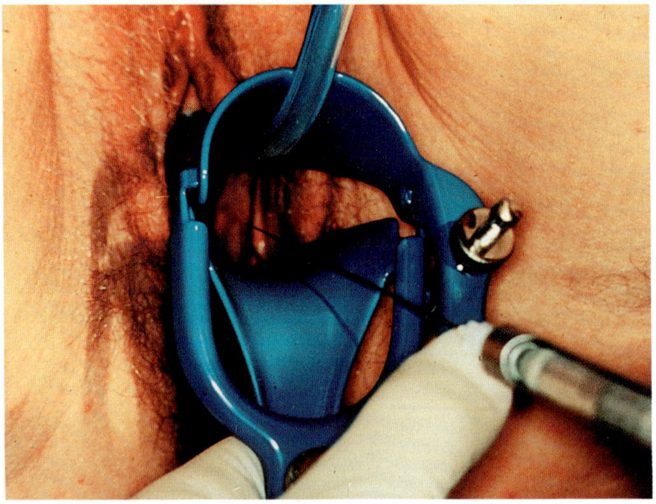

**Color Fig. 17 (Fig. 10–9).** Anesthetic application to the cervix.

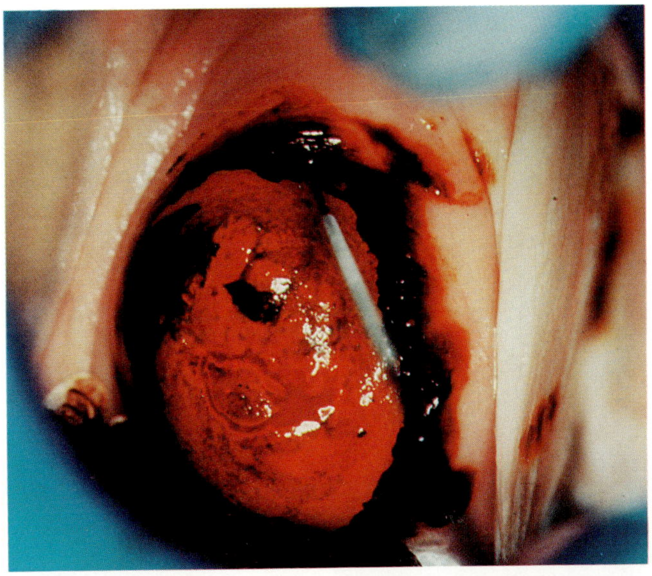

**Color Fig. 18 (Fig. 10–10).** Subepithelial anesthetic application.

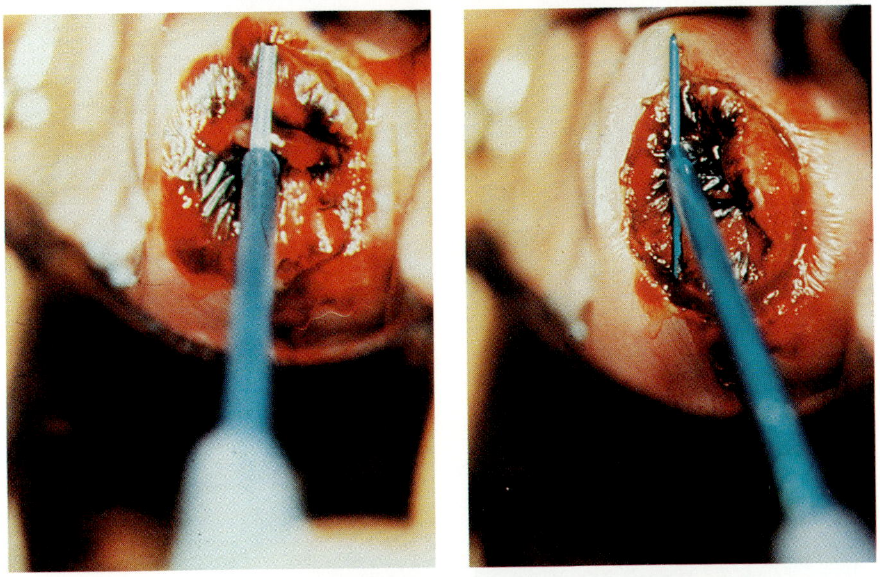

**Color Fig. 19 (Fig. 10–11).** Use of the exo-loop (see text for details).

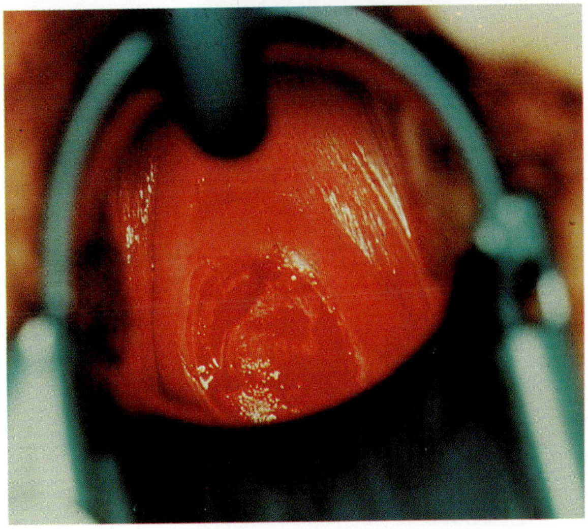

**Color Fig. 20 (Fig. 10–12).** Postexcision colposcopic examination.

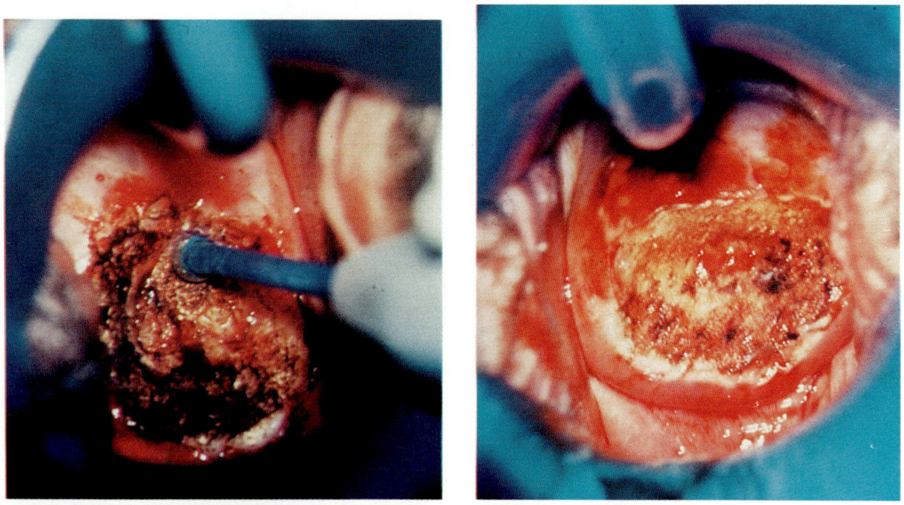

A,B

**Color Fig. 21 (Fig. 10–13).** Use of the ball electrode for electrofulguration.

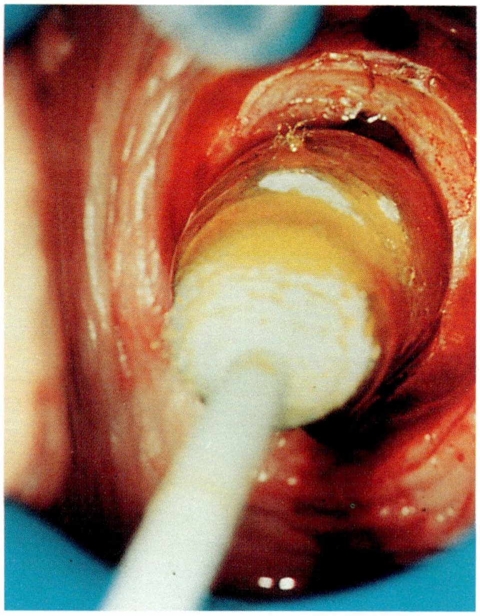

**Color Fig. 22 (Fig. 10–14).** The crater is filled with Monsel's paste.

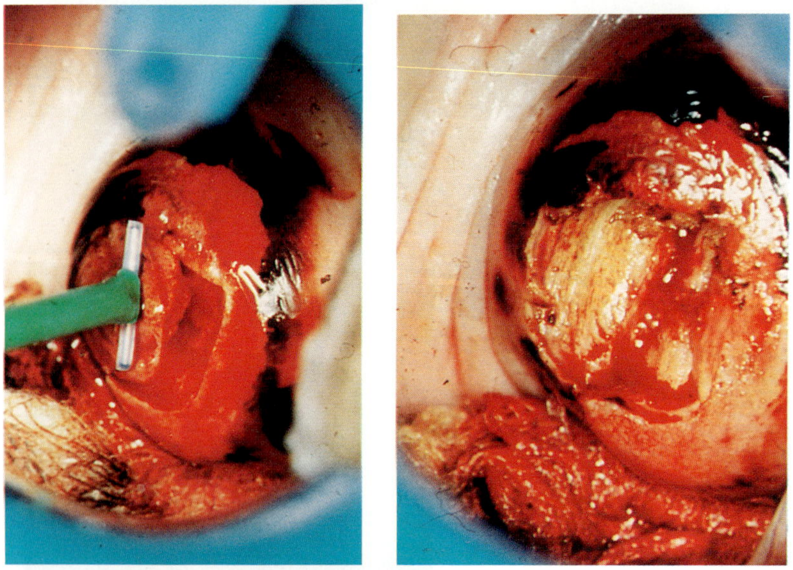

**Color Fig. 23 (Fig. 10–17).** Large exocervical lesion.

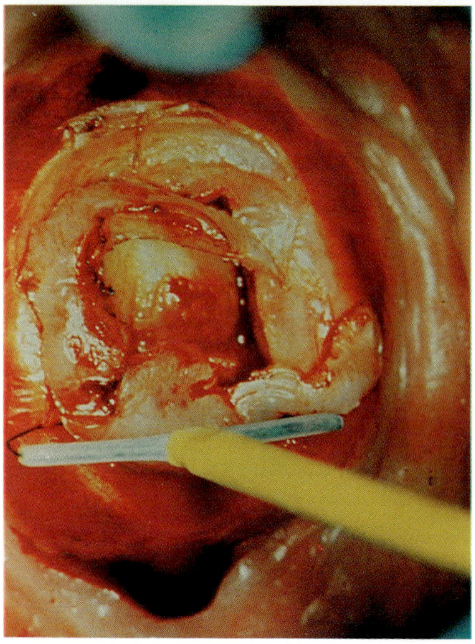

**Color Fig. 24 (Fig. 10–18).** Endoloop excising additional endocervical canal tissue.

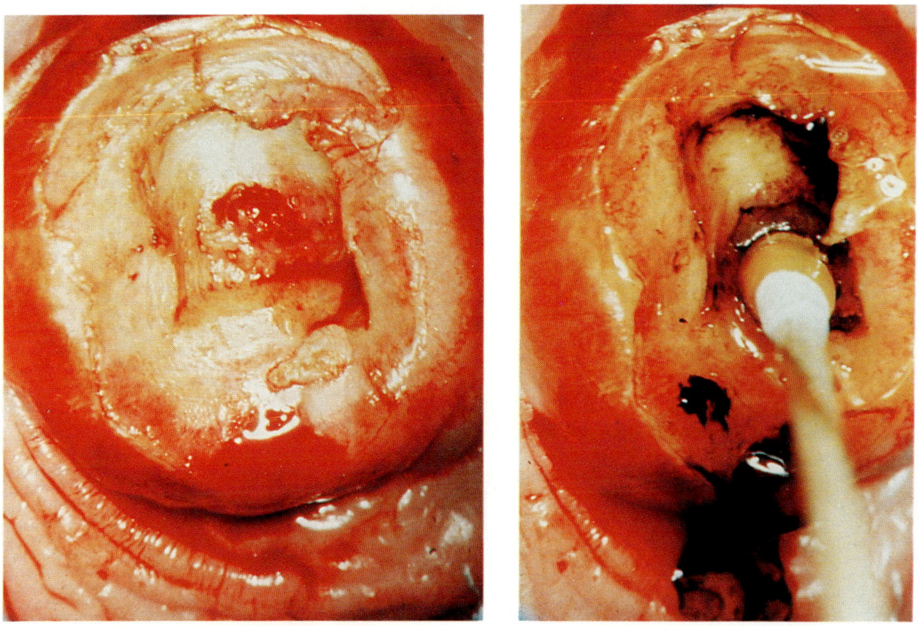

**Color Fig. 25 (Fig. 10–19).** "Cowboy hat" crater (left) and application of Monsel's paste (right).

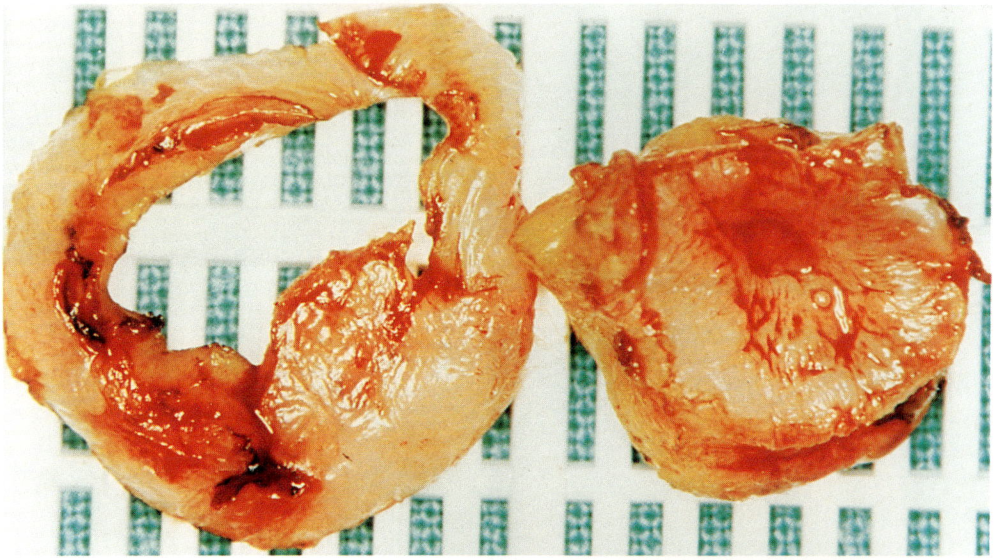

**Color Fig. 26 (Fig. 10–20).** Exo- and endoloop excised tissues prepared for pathologic examination.

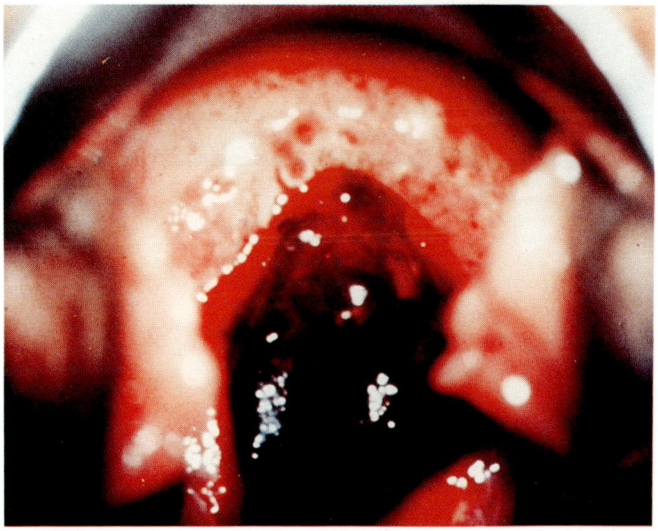

**Color Fig. 27 (Fig. 10–21).** Post LEEP residual bleeding.

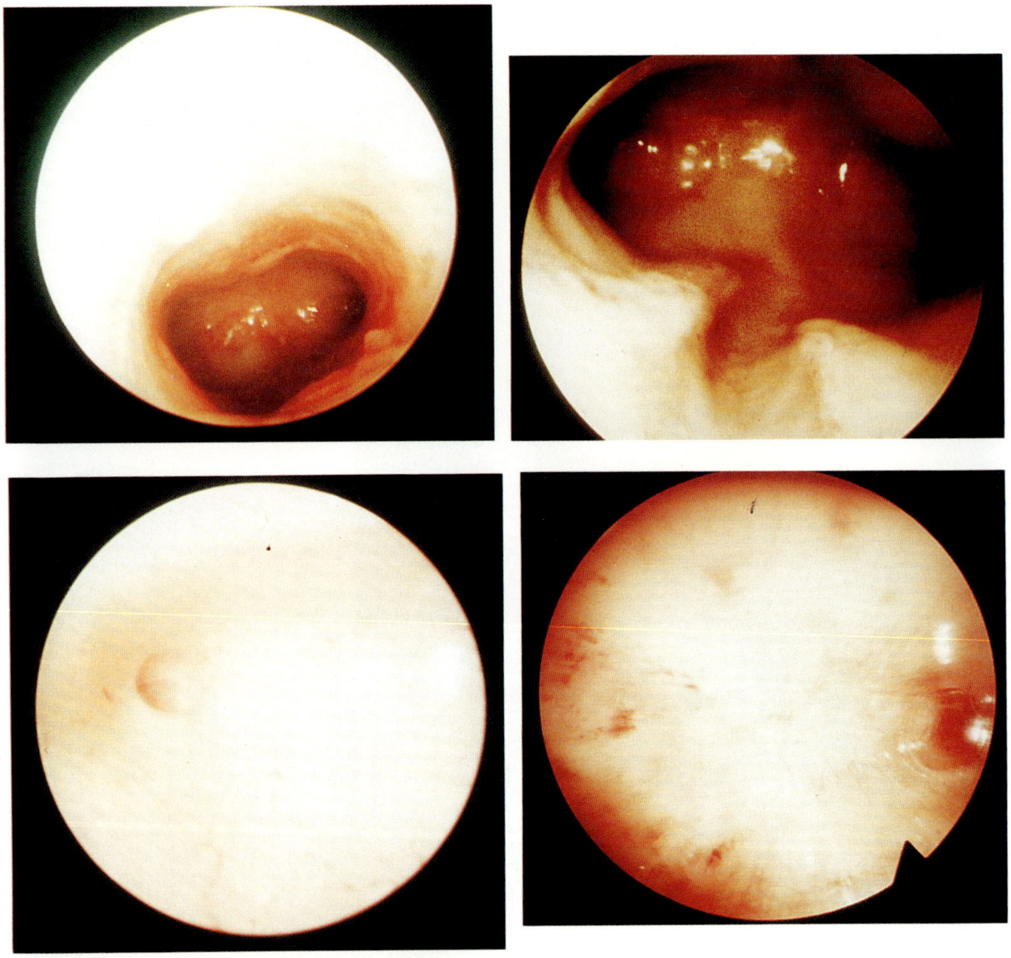

A,B

C,D

**Color Fig. 28 (Fig. 12–2).** (A) Endocervical canal and lower uterine segment are visible with fundus (dark area) in the background. (B) The fundus and both horns come into view. The trough is made to show the depth of the endometrium. Central ridge in fundus in the site of fusion of the 2 Mullerian ducts. (C) Right uterotubal ostium is noted. (D) Left uterotubal ostium has a bubble over it.

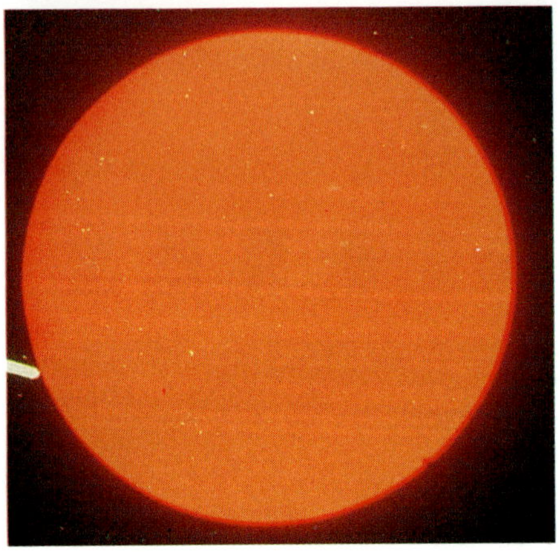

**Color Fig. 29 (Fig. 12–4).** "Red sign" can be caused by blood at the tip of the lens, insufficient uterine distention, or a lens placed against the endometrial surface.

### *VULVAR BIOPSY*

Office vulvar biopsy should be liberally performed because adequate therapy is based on an accurate diagnosis. This very simple office procedure is virtually free of complications and is essentially painless when performed under local anesthesia. Small discrete lesions are best handled by excisional biopsy. For biopsy of large or widespread skin lesions, the Keyes cutaneous punch biopsy instrument can be used (Fig. 11–1). A sharp, disposable cutaneous biopsy instrument is also available and has the advantage of not requiring the periodic sharpening necessary with the Keyes punch. A 4 mm instrument is adequate in most instances. However, occasionally, the 6 mm dermal punch is valuable in totally excising small lesions.

The area from which the biopsy specimen will be obtained is first infiltrated with 1% lidocaine solution using a small-gauge (30 mm) needle (Fig. 11–2). The solution should be infiltrated just beneath the skin or mucosal surface, then inserted into the most superficial subcutaneous tissue for adequate infiltration of the solution. The dermal punch is used like a ''cork borer.'' The sharp edges of the instrument are twisted in a circular fashion into the site to be biopsied (Fig. 11–3). The epithelium and dermis should be cut through. After this has been accomplished, the circular portion of tissue is lifted with a small forceps and the base of the tissue is severed with a small scissors. Utilizing a 4 mm punch, a suture is usually not required to control bleeding. Hemostasis is easily accomplished by the application of Monsel's solution (Fig. 11–4) or cauterized with the tip of a silver nitrate applicator. When the 6 mm dermal punch is utilized it is usually necessary to approximate the skin edges with 3–0 or 4–0 absorbable sutures.

The tissue specimen should be oriented on a small piece of filter paper or paper towel with the epithelial surface on top. This allows for proper orientation of the tissue when the

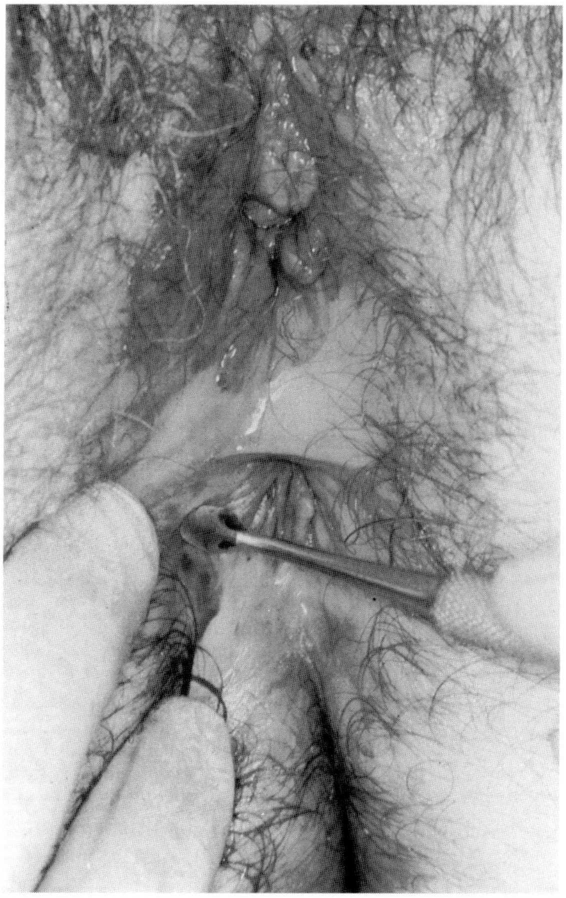

**FIG. 11–3.** Dermal punch is rotated into the site being biopsied.

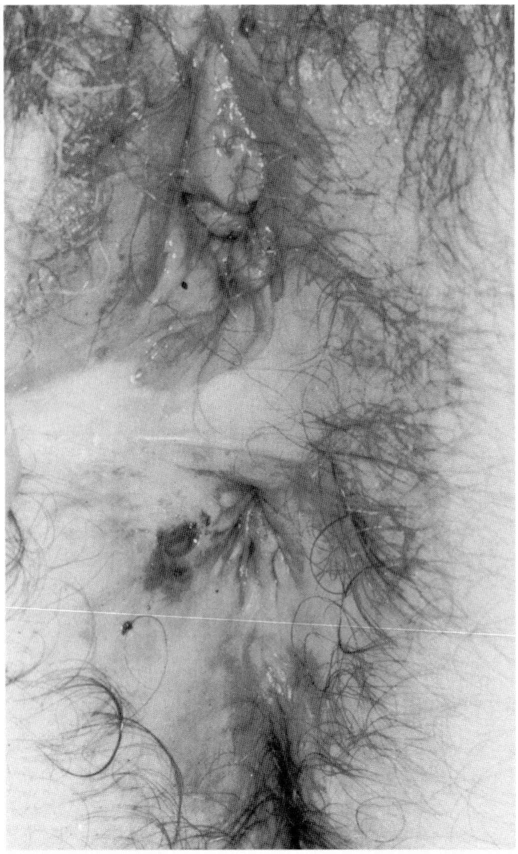

**FIG. 11–4.** The biopsy site has been treated with Monsel's solution. This adequately controls the bleeding.

sections are cut. A poorly oriented tissue specimen may result in tangential cutting that occasionally can lead to an erroneous diagnosis.

Washing the vulva with 3–5% acetic acid will highlight mucosal lesions such as intraepithelial neoplasia, which often turn aceto-white after the application of the solution. These changes are also often seen in the presence of HPV infection. Staining the vulva with 1% toluidine blue is sometimes of help in selecting a biopsy site. The vulva is covered with 1% toluidine blue and, after the stain has dried, the tissues are washed with 1% acetic acid. This should result in the removal of the toluidine blue. Because nuclei retain toluidine blue, lesions such as invasive and intraepithelial carcinoma retain the dye. However, dye is retained on any ulcerated site and, frequently, when a thick keratin layer covers the surface of intraepithelial or invasive carcinoma, the dye will not be retained. Thus, this is not a very sensitive or specific method for accurately selecting a biopsy site.

In the presence of multifocal or diffuse lesions, it is advisable to obtain biopsies from several different locations.

When an erosive or bullous lesion involves the vulva, the differential diagnosis is often confusing. Immunofluorescent staining will often be of value in establishing the correct diagnosis. Direct immunofluorescence testing using the patient's own tissue is most often utilized. This type of study is of value in distinguishing the different chronic ''autoimmune'' vesiculobulous diseases, lupus erythematosus, and leukocytic vasculitis.[1] When this type of study is performed it is important that the biopsy not be taken directly from the eroded area, but rather from the normal appearing tissue adjacent to it. The specimen must be examined in the ''fresh'' state and should be kept in either a special ''holding solution'' or transported in phosphate-buffered normal saline. The location of various immunoglobulins as well as various antigens, such as CEA, S–100 protein, HMB 45, and so on, will often be of extreme value in clarifying the diagnosis.

## CONTRAINDICATIONS

There are literally no contraindications to obtaining a vulvar biopsy. Usually, the biopsy site is so small that, even in the patient receiving anticoagulation therapy, bleeding can be controlled by the use of Monsel's solution followed by pressure on the biopsy site for several minutes or by the placement of one or two interrupted 3–0 or 4–0 absorbable sutures.

## COMPLICATIONS

Rarely will a complication follow a biopsy taken from the vulva; any complication consists primarily of bleeding and infection. Occasionally, oozing from the biopsy site is persistent, in which case it is easily controlled by placing one or two interrupted sutures of absorbable material. On the rare occasion when the biopsy site becomes infected, appropriate cultures should be taken and the patient started on appropriate antibiotic therapy.

## REFERENCES

1. Lever WF, Schaumberg-Lever G. Histopathology of the skin, 7th (ed.). Philadelphia: JB Lippincott, 1989.

*Invasive Outpatient Procedures in Reproductive Medicine*, edited by Mark I. Evans, et al. Lippincott–Raven Publishers, Philadelphia © 1997.

# 12 Hysteroscopy

Alvin M. Siegler

## INDICATIONS

The most common indications for panoramic diagnostic office hysteroscopy are to locate the cause of abnormal uterine bleeding, to evaluate an abnormal hysterogram, to locate occult IUDs, to search for intrauterine adhesions, to explore the lower uterine segment, to locate an endometrial adenocarcinoma, and to evaluate the results of previous therapeutic procedures. No special perioperative care is needed and complications are infrequent. A carefully performed procedure in properly selected patients can eliminate the need for additional interventions or delineate the precise nature of a problem. Hysteroscopy using carbon dioxide as the distending medium is ideal for an office procedure because it is a dry medium, easily instilled with a properly monitored apparatus, and has a long history of safety.[1–4]

Any practicing gynecologist knows that procuring a grossly indentifiable endometrial polyp during a curettage for abnormal uterine bleeding is infrequent. Hysteroscopic examinations after unsuccessful dilation and curettage for abnormal uterine bleeding followed by targeted endometrial sampling have disclosed important abnormalities missed by the curettage.[5,6] The curettage has been used to detect causes of abnormal uterine bleeding but the operation finds the cause in less than 50% of women and is often not therapeutic. Especially in the postmenopausal patient in whom the curettings often yield "tissue insufficient for diagnosis," a look inside of the uterine cavity that shows an atrophic endometrium is reassuring. The future growth and development of this relatively simple, office-based procedure is inevitable.[7]

A brochure describing the procedure, the technique, and expectations should be given to the patient before the examination.

## TECHNIQUE

Office hysteroscopy should include a review of the patient's history and previous hysterosalpingogram to alert the physician to specific concerns, and a pelvic examination to ascertain the uterine position and size. The speculum should be unhinged on one side to enable increased manipulation of the hysteroscope (Fig. 12–1). A tenaculum is placed on the anterior lip of the cervix for traction. The carbon dioxide flow rate (hysteroflator) is adjusted and the fiberoptic light cord is attached to the light post on the hysteroscope. The flow rate of $CO_2$ is set between 40–60 mL/min and remains constant, depending on the resistance at the uterotubal junctions. Occluded tubes cause the pressure to rise to 200 mm Hg as the flow rate falls to zero. The interdependence between flow rate and intrauterine pressure is a very important safety feature. Although some $CO_2$ escapes from the external os, it does not prevent adequate, sustained dilation of the uterine cavity. No cervical cap or occlusive device is required to prevent escape of the gas from the cervix. Leakage from a patulous cervix usually can be prevented by

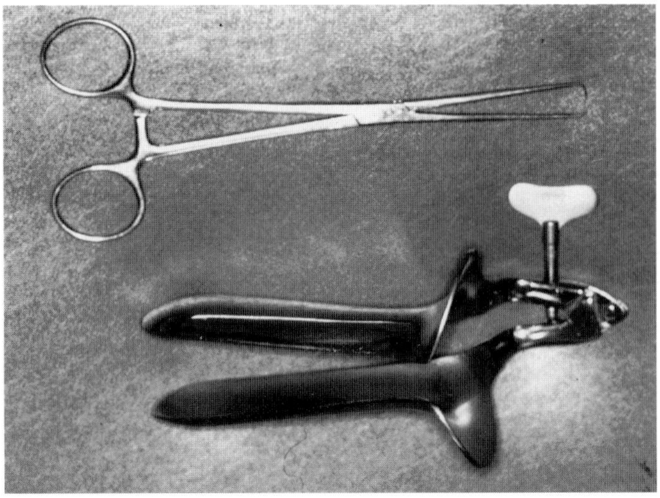

**FIG. 12–1.** Short tenaculum (6 inches in length) and unhinged vaginal speculum.

readjusting the tenaculum to narrow the os. With the carbon dioxide medium, the flow rate rather than the volume of gas used is most important.

For diagnostic purposes, hysteroscopy can be performed in the office using $CO_2$ to distend the uterine cavity.[8] In most patients, a hysteroscope with a 5 mm OD sheath can be introduced into the uterine cavity without the need for either a local block or analgesia. Whenever a local anesthetic is required, it can be administered by injecting about 10 mL of an appropriate agent into the vaginal mucous membrane beneath the cervix to create a wheal or intracervically into 4 sites (3, 6, 9, and 12 o'clock positions). The tip of the hysteroscope and its sheath are inserted gently into the cervical canal, while the surgeon observes through the ocular lens or on a video monitor. As the endocervix fills, the plicae or endocervical glands sometimes can be seen within the canal during its dilation. Slow rotation of the scope using the light post as the guide often facilitates its passage, although some resistance is encountered just before the uterine cavity is entered. Systematic exploration of both horns and ostia, the lateral, anterior and posterior walls of the uterine cavity is begun (Fig. 12–2, Color Fig. 28). As the normal cavity is distended, the endometrium appears pale yellow, tan, or pink, with occasional hemorrhagic spots. The blood vessels can be seen clearly as they traverse through the endometrial tissue.

When learning diagnostic hysteroscopy, the proliferative phase should be selected for easiest interpretations because in this phase the endometrium is thin. The secretory endometrium is thicker and its depth can be estimated after penetrating it with the end of the hysteroscope. The uterotubal junctions can be located by manipulating the instrument until the uterine horn comes into view; the tubal ostia will be at the apex. The amount of manipulation or rotation of the hysteroscope depends on the angle of the lens. Frequently, the cavity, both horns and ostia, can be seen simultaneously. As the hysteroscope is withdrawn, the isthmic and endocervical canals are reinspected. Following their removal, the hysteroscope and its sheath are cleaned and irrigated with a disinfectant solution. Most studies are completed within 5 minutes so that rarely more than 250 mL of $CO_2$ is used.

## POTENTIAL PROBLEMS

***Pain.*** Inject 10 mL of 1% lidocaine (without epinephrine) into the vaginal mucous membrane beneath the cervix to create a wheal. This volume of fluid will intravasate into the region of the uterosacral ligaments and paracervical tissues. Use a 25-gauge needle on a needle extender or a tonsil needle (Fig. 12–3). An alternative method is to inject the anesthetic directly into

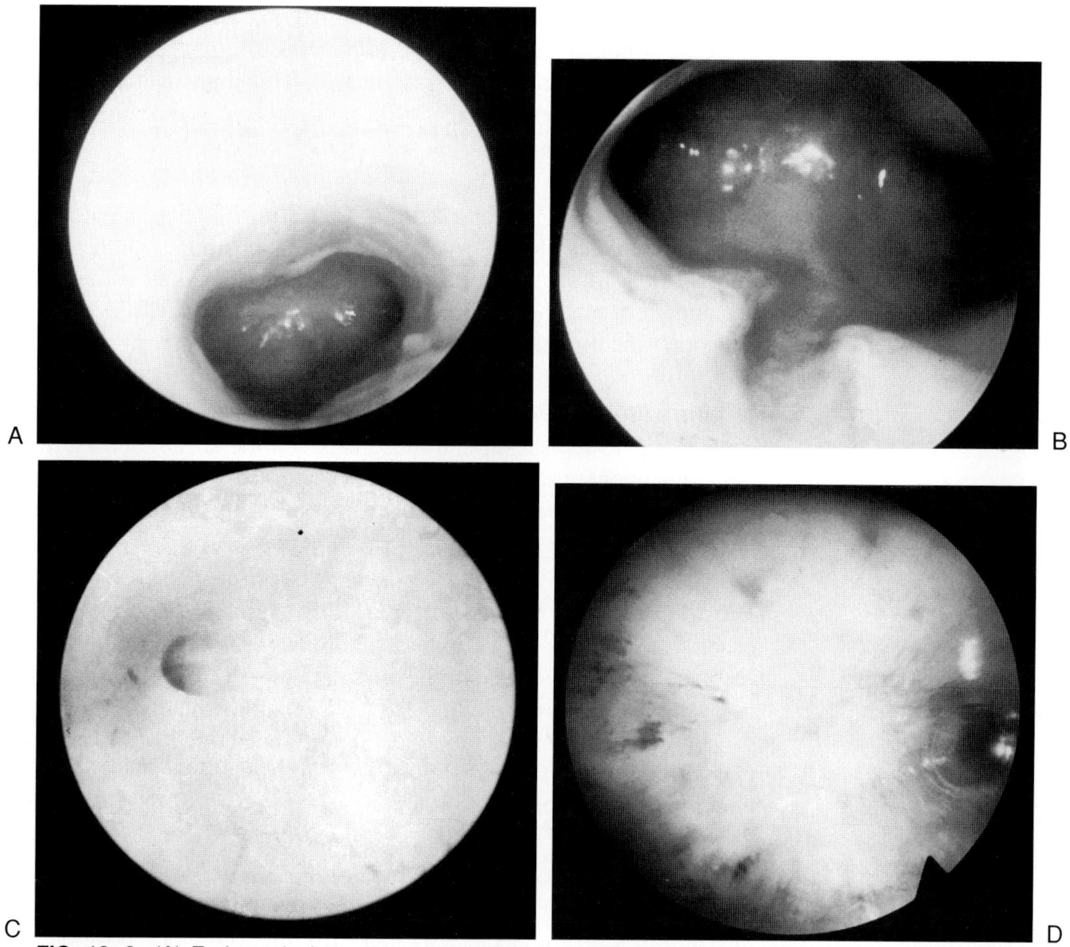

FIG. 12–2. (A) Endocervical canal and lower uterine segment are visible with fundus (dark area) in the background. (B) The fundus and both horns come into view. The trough is made to show the depth of the endometrium. Central ridge in fundus is the site of fusion of the 2 Mullerian ducts. (C) Right uterotubal ostium is noted. (D) Left uterotubal ostium has a bubble over it. See Color Fig. 28.

the cervical tissue into 4 quadrants. In most instances, even in patients not previously pregnant, a hysteroscope with a sheath with an OD that measures slightly over 5 mm can be introduced into the uterine cavity without the need for either a local anesthetic or analgesia. Although there is some discomfort for the patient as the diagnostic hysteroscope passes through the lower uterine segment, no medication is required for relief of pain in over 80% of patients.

***The Cervical Canal is Narrow.*** If the scope and sheath do not pass easily, check the precise course of the uterine cavity with a uterine sound. Gently dilate the canal to 5 mm and then reinsert the instrument. A local anesthetic should be used for this procedure. Avoid exces-

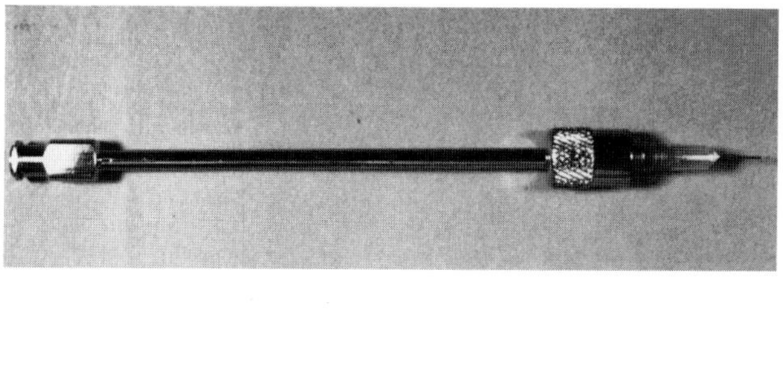

FIG. 12–3. Needle extender has a 25-gauge needle at one end.

sive cervical dilatation—the canal can become too wide and maintaining uterine distention could be a problem. Postmenopausal patients often have a stenotic external os. A tonsil clamp is inserted into the os and slowly opened. This maneuver can overcome the stenosis in most instances. Sometimes premarin is prescribed for 2 weeks and then the hysteroscopic examination can be performed.

***The "Black Area" in the Canal is Not Seen.*** This dark area in the background represents the fundus and should be seen in the 6 o'clock position with the 30° scope. As the gynecologist moves the instrument toward this area, the uterine cavity comes into view. If this dark area is not apparent, manipulate the scope slowly because a 30° angled lens can be misleading in indicating the direction for advancement of the instrument.

***No Intrauterine Pressure is Recorded on the Insufflating Apparatus.*** Check the connections to the sheath and those between the sheath and the hysteroscope to be sure that the connections are fastened securely. The most important dial on the hysteroflator is the measurement of the intrauterine pressure because without an indication of intrauterine pressure the uterine cavity will not appear distended.

***Blood Obscures the Landmarks Within the Cavity.*** Although slight mucosal bleeding occasionally occurs during manipulation, adequate observation should be possible. The intrauterine pressure developed during instillation of the medium helps to reduce bleeding. Endometrial sampling causes minimal bleeding. Even immediately following curettage adequate hysteroscopic observations are possible. Never advance the hysteroscope in a cloudy field or in a cavity that is not distended (Fig. 12–4, Color Fig. 29). Observe the insufflating apparatus and note the flow rate of $CO_2$; the intrauterine pressure should be at least 30 mm Hg.

***The Uterotubal Ostia are Not Seen.*** Slowly rotate the hysteroscope so that angle of vision is directed toward the uterine cornua. Use the light post as a guide and rotate it toward the right or left (9 o'clock, 3 o'clock) from its 6 o'clock position to inspect the entire cavity. The ostia appear in many sizes and shapes and often seem to open and close as the gas passes through a patent tube.

***Patient Complains of Shoulder Pain on Sitting up After Test.*** Arranging the examination table in the Trendelenburg position will quickly relieve the shoulder pain. The discomfort is caused by the $CO_2$ and is not unlike the postoperative pain experienced following a uterotubal insufflation.

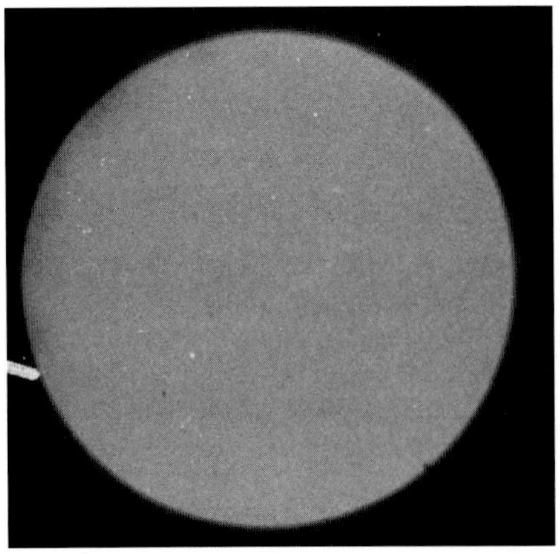

**FIG. 12–4.** "Red sign" can be caused by blood at the tip of the lens, insufficient uterine distention, or a lens placed against the endometrial surface. See Color Fig. 29.

***Loss of $CO_2$ at the Cervical Os.*** To prevent the loss of gas from the cervical os during the procedure, the tenaculum can be adjusted to narrow the canal or a second tenaculum can be applied. Do not over dilate. Laminaria are contraindicated because the cervical dilation resulting from their insertion is unpredictable.

***The Uterus is Displaced (Retroflexion, Retroversion).*** To see a retrodisplaced uterus clearly, it may be necessary for the gynecologist to rotate the scope during its insertion so that the light post is reversed (12 o'clock position). These uteri can be difficult to explore hysteroscopically and such examinations require extreme care.

***Bubbles of Gas Mixed with Blood or Mucus Obscure Vision.*** In most instances, waiting for 1 minute, without additional manipulation of the hysteroscope and sheath, will solve this problem. Alternatively, the sheath can be left in situ, the scope removed, and the lens cleaned with alcohol before reinsertion.

## CONTRAINDICATIONS

### *ABSOLUTE CONTRAINDICATIONS*

***Pelvic Infection.*** Salpingitis is an absolute contraindication to hysteroscopy. Infection in the lower genital tract can spread to the tubes by extension from the vagina or cervix, causing an endomyometritis or salpingitis. Hysteroscopy should be deferred in a woman who gives a history of recent pelvic inflammatory disease or who has adnexal tenderness so as to prevent salpingitis or peritonitis.

***Cervical Carcinoma.*** Patients who have a cervical malignancy should not have hysteroscopy because the findings would not alter therapy. However, suspicion of an endometrial carcinoma is not a contraindication to hysteroscopy. Although curettage has been the most reliable method for the diagnosis of endometrial carcinoma, some localized lesions can be missed. Many small lesions can be detected early; therefore, a prompt diagnosis can lead to suitable treatment with minimal delay. At some medical centers hysterography has been used in the preoperative work-up of patients having endometrial cancer and no increase in metastases has been reported.[9] In about 50% of patients with endometrial carcinoma, tubal patency has been observed, but in others the tubes were not patent because the tumor spreads into the myometrium and blocks the intramural segment. In the latter group distant metastases were evident earlier, even though the surface spread of the carcinoma appeared limited.

The use of hysteroscopy to examine patients with endometrial carcinoma has been questioned because of the risk of perforation, hemorrhage, and dissemination of cancer cells. The presence of displaced endometrial cells has been found in the peritoneal washings of patients who had endometrial adenocarcinoma. Although such a finding may alter the staging of the disease, it may not alter the prognosis.

Sugimoto[10] performed hysteroscopic examinations in 182 women who had endometrial adenocarcinoma and noted no increased risk of dissemination of cancer cells. Although most circumscribed, exophytic growths with polypoid, nodular, or papillary processes were accompanied by necrosis, ulceration, and infection, no instances of endometritis, salpingitis, or fever were caused by hysteroscopy.

### *RELATIVE CONTRAINDICATIONS*

***Uterine Bleeding.*** When $CO_2$ is used as the distending medium, the presence of uterine bleeding generally prevents adequate observations of the uterine cavity. Liquid media can be used in such situations.

Regardless of the distending medium used, hysteroscopy should not be performed if bleeding is excessive. Heavy bleeding should be suppressed so that a proper interpretation of the endometrial cavity can be made and vascular intravasation of the distending media is less likely to occur.

***Pregnancy.*** Hysteroscopy usually is not indicated during pregnancy. However, in selected instances, in a patient who inadvertently becomes pregnant with an IUD in situ, the device can be removed under hysteroscopic control without disturbing the pregnancy.[11] Patients must be made aware of the risks of abortion, infection, and bleeding.

When postabortal bleeding occurs, hysteroscopy is a simple method to search for retained placental tissue. Salat-Baroux and coworkers[12] used the hysteroscope to check the uterine cavity of uncomplicated cases of elective abortion and to detect early sequelae of spontaneous or induced abortions. The first group included 118 patients who had elective abortions before the 10th week of gestation. The second study included 33 women: 13 had complications after spontaneous abortion and 20 after elective abortion. The postoperative appearance of the uterine cavity was practically the same when only aspiration was used or when it was combined with curettage. No untoward effects were noted from a hysteroscopic examination in these patients.

***Cardiovascular or Systemic Diseases.*** Hysteroscopy in patients who have cardiovascular or systemic diseases can be accomplished safely under local anesthesia. Proper precautions include adequate and appropriate medications. Indeed, a successful hysteroscopic examination showing a normal uterine cavity may even enable these women to avoid a curettage or additional uterine operations.

## COMPLICATIONS

### *TRAUMA*

Excessive traction on the tenaculum can cause a cervical laceration. Forceful cervical dilatation can provoke unnecessary bleeding, perforate the lower uterine segment, or create a false passage or tract. If the hysteroscope is advanced without panoramic vision or with undue force, perforation becomes a potential hazard. Unless there is concern about a potential bowel injury, laparotomy is not indicated.

Simultaneous laparoscopy is indicated in women whose uterine landmarks tend to be obscured, as in severe intrauterine adhesions. When the uterine fundus, the cornua, and the uterotubal ostia are not seen or a hysterogram shows vascular intravasation associated with an abnormal uterine shadow, a laparoscopically controlled hysteroscopic study is indicated. If a perforation occurs during a diagnostic examination with a 5 mm sheath, the consequences are minimal. As the endoscope is withdrawn, contractions of the myometrium close the defect. If perforation occurs during a therapeutic procedure, the decision to resort to laparoscopy or laparotomy depends on the energy sources used. The patient should be informed about the complication, although the medical consequences usually are minimal. Uterine perforations occur more frequently following therapeutic procedures than following diagnostic examinations and more often in the fundus than in the lower uterine segment. The displaced uterus (retroflexion, retroversion), the scarred uterine cavity, and the atrophic uterus are conditions predisposing patients to uterine perforation.

Probes inserted into the tubal ostia to overcome proximal tubal obstruction during hysteroscopic tubal cannulation can create a false passage and perforate the intramural segment. This procedure should be monitored by concomitant laparoscopy to enable the physician to evaluate the distal tubal segments.

### *HEMORRHAGE*

Slight uterine bleeding a few days subsequent to hysteroscopy does occur, but hemorrhage is unusual. Postoperative bleeding has been reported after resection of submucous myoma; currently, this operation is not an office procedure.

## INFECTION

Pelvic infections are rare following either diagnostic or therapeutic hysteroscopy. Salat-Baroux and colleagues[13] noted only 7 mild infections in 4,000 hysteroscopic examinations, 90% of which were done in an office setting. These authors took secretions from the cervix and material from the surface of the instruments before and after consecutive use in 6 patients. Cultures of the instruments and disinfectant before use were negative. After the procedure, cultures of material from the tip of the hysteroscope contained the same organisms found in the preoperative cervix. There was no patient-to-patient transmission of bacteria, and no infection occurred in these 6 patients.

## ELECTROSURGICAL INJURIES

Hysteroscopic sterilizations have been performed as an office-based procedure with the use of electrosurgical probes to coagulate the intramural tubal segment. The method fell into disfavor because of serious complications caused by inadvertent thermal injuries to the intestine, caused by uterine perforation, and an unacceptable failure rate.[14]

## COMPLICATIONS FROM MEDIA

The choice of the medium for uterine distention depends on the familiarity of the surgeon with the medium, ease of instillation, clarity, complexity of the equipment for instillation, messiness, and potential side effects.

Carbon dioxide is the only safe gas for distending the uterine cavity. The advantages of this medium include:

1. Excellent image, refractive index 1.00
2. Rapid absorption
3. Volume of gas used unimportant
4. Long history of safety
5. Ideal for office hysteroscopy

The disadvantages of this medium include:

1. Special insufflator essential
2. Gas bubbles annoying
3. Less than ideal for operative hysteroscopy
4. Difficult to use with laser (plume evacuation)

It must be instilled only with a special device that does not permit more than 100 mL/min at a maximal pressure of 100 mm Hg. Early signs of carbon dioxide entering the circulation can be detected by auscultation of a characteristic metallic heart sound during cardiac contractions. Some authors suggest auscultory surveillance during carbon dioxide hysteroscopy in order to avoid serious cardiovascular complications.[15]

Potential complications from liquid media used for uterine distention depend on the type of solution used, the amount absorbed, and the intrauterine pressure. Office-based procedures do not require large amounts of fluid so that cardiovascular overload, resulting in pulmonary edema and significant changes in serum electrolytes, is not a problem encountered during diagnostic office hysteroscopy.

High molecular dextran-70 (Hyskon) has special characteristics and instances of anaphylactoid reactions have been reported.[16] No more than 500 mL of this fluid should be used because each mL of dextran can draw 7 mL of extracellular fluid into the vascular space.

## MORTALITY

The most common cause of death during hysteroscopy has been attributed to media used to distend the uterine cavity during therapeutic hysteroscopic procedures. Large volumes of $CO_2$, rapidly instilled, has resulted in serious morbidity and deaths from pulmonary embolism. Excessive absorbtion of liquid can cause near-fatal consequences including noncarcinogen pulmonary edema and hyponatremia.

## PREVENTION OF COMPLICATIONS

To reduce the occurrence of complications, the physician should obtain a careful history and perform a pelvic examination to identify patients with contraindications or pelvic abnormalities. The hysteroscopic equipment should be disassembled, rinsed, flushed, and disinfected before each examination. The equipment should be rinsed completely because the solution used to disinfect it can irritate the mucous membranes and peritoneum. Gas sterilization of the endoscope is not essential.

Disinfection should be performed according to the manufacturer's instructions. If the manufacturer's recommendations concerning disinfecting solutions are followed, infections will not be caused by contaminated instruments.

Moderate bleeding precludes adequate observation of the cavity and open vessels predispose the patient to vascular intravasation and, possibly, embolism. Observations should begin as the sheath and hysteroscope are inserted into the endocervical canal, without advancing the instrument except in a clear field of vision. A reddened or cloudy view may be caused by juxtapostion of the hysteroscope to the uterine wall, inadequate uterine distention, or a lens with adherent blood or mucus. Additional force may result in uterine perforation and the intestines quickly come into endoscopic view. Simultaneous laparoscopy reduces the consequences of accidental perforation and, therefore, is recommended whenever intrauterine observation is limited or landmarks can not be identified because of intrauterine disease. Usually, hysteroscopy is an endoscopic procedure free of complications. Faulty techniques and selection of inappropriate patients are the most frequent causes of sequelae. Adverse effects as a result of diagnostic hysteroscopy are fewer than those following therapeutic hysteroscopy. Reports of numerous examinations and treatments under hysteroscopic control reveal comparatively few adverse reactions, which are generally not serious.

Remember the main landmarks: the cervical canal, the internal os, the cornua, and uterotubal ostia. Note the angle of the lens. Is it 12° or 30°? Look at similar areas through hysteroscopes with different angled lenses. Using a 30° lens, remember that when the light post is at the 6 o'clock position the viewer is looking toward the anterior uterine wall. Using the light post as the quide the scope is rotated to inspect the entire uterine cavity. Magnification of objects viewed hysteroscopically varies inversely with the distance of the telescope from the object.

When using the video camera, maintain it in one position and rotate the scope. The distinctive feature of the camera for orientation is that its cord is always in the 6 o'clock position. This fact is especially important when performing operative hysteroscopic procedures.

## REFERENCES


1. Rubin IC. Uterine endoscopy, endometroscopy with the aid of uterine insufflation. Am J Obstet Gynecol 1925;10:313.
2. Palmer R. Un novel hysteroscope. Bull Fed Soc Gynecol Obstet Franc 1957;9:300.
3. Lindemann HJ. Eine neue untersuchungsmethode fur die Hysteroskopie. Endoscopy 1971; 4:194.
4. Hamou J. Microhysteroscopy: a new procedure and its original applications in gynecology. J Reprod Med 1981;26:375.
5. Brooks PG, Serden SP. Hysteroscopic findings after unsuccessful dilation and curettage for abnormal uterine bleeding. Am J Obstet Gynecol 1988;158:1354.

6. Loffer FD. Hysteroscopy with selective endometrial sampling compared with dilation and curettage for abnormal uterine bleeding: the value of a negative hysteroscopic view. Obstet Gynecol 1989;73:16.
7. Valle RF. Future growth and development of hysteroscopy. Obstet Gynecol Clin No Am 1988;15:111.
8. Siegler AM, Valle R, Lindemann HJ, Mencaglia L. Therapeutic hysteroscopy: indications and techniques. St. Louis; CV Mosby, 1990.
9. Stock RJ, Gallup DG. Hysterography in patients with suspected uterine cancer: radiographic and histologic correlation and clinical significance. Obstet Gynecol 1987;69:872.
10. Sugimoto O. Diagnostic and therapeutic hysteroscopy. Tokyo; Igaku-Shoin, 1978.
11. Wagner H. Diagnosis and treatment of complications of intrauterine devices. In: van der Pas H, Herendael BJ, Lith DAF, et al (eds). Hysteroscopy. Boston; MTP Press, 1983.
12. Salat-Baroux J, Hamou JE, Uzam S, et al. Postabortal hysteroscopy. In: Siegler AM, Lindemann HJ (eds). Hysteroscopy: principles and practice. Philadelphia: JB Lippincott, 1984.
13. Salat-Baroux J, Hamou JE, Maillard G, et al. Complications from microhysteroscopy. In: Siegler AM, Lindemann HJ (eds). Hysteroscopy: principles and practice. Philadelphia: JB Lippincott, 1984.
14. Darabi KF, Roy K, Richart RM. Collaborative study on hysteroscopic sterilization procedures: final report. In: Sciarra JJ, Zatuchini GI, Speidel JJ (eds). Risks, benefits, and controversies in fertility control. Hagerstown: Harper and Row, 1978.
15. Brundin J, Thomasson K. Cardiac gas embolism during carbon dioxide hysteroscopy: risk and management. Eur J Obstet Gynecol Reprod Biol 1989;33:241.
16. Trimbos-Kemper TCM, Veering BT. Anaphylactic shock from intracavitary 32% Dextran-70 during hysteroscopy. Fertil Steril 1989;51:1053.

*Invasive Outpatient Procedures in Reproductive Medicine,* edited by Mark I. Evans, et al. Lippincott–Raven Publishers, Philadelphia © 1997.

# 13 Hysterosalpingography

Kamran S. Moghissi

## INTRODUCTION

Hysterosalpingography (HSG) is an office procedure designed to diagnose abnormalities of the uterus and fallopian tubes. It provides useful information about the integrity of the uterine cervix, uterine cavity, and endosalpinx, as well as the adnexal region. Precise nature of some anomalies detected by HSG may require confirmation by hysteroscopy and laparoscopy. Thus, HSG, hysteroscopy, and laparoscopy are complimentary procedures rather than mutually exclusive.

The development of hysterosalpingography (HSG) dates to 1909. Various substances were introduced into the uterine cavity to visualize the fallopian tubes by x-ray. Two factors accelerated the development of HSG; the introduction of uterotubal insufflation by Rubin in 1920 and the use of lipiodol as a contrast medium. HSG is now accepted as a standard first step for the evaluation of endometrial cavity abnormalities and to test tubal patency.

### *ANATOMIC CONSIDERATIONS*

The uterus is formed by the fusion of Mullerian ducts. Abnormal or incomplete fusion of these ducts results in various congenital deformities of the uterus that range from the extreme case of a double uterus to an inconspicuous notching of the fundus of the uterine cavity. Acquired pathologic conditions such as leiomyoma of the uterus, uterine synechia, and polyps may distort the uterine cavity and interfere with normal reproductive processes.

The uterus is involved in sperm transport, implantation of conceptus, maintenance of a healthy environment for fetal development, and eventually parturition.

The fallopian tubes are muscular structures derived from the paramesonephric ducts (Müllerian ducts), that are approximately 10–12 cm in length and extend laterally from the fundus of the uterus toward the ovaries. The tube begins at the cornu of the uterine cavity, courses through the myometrium, and emerges from the uterus posterior to the round ligament. Anatomically, three distinct sections of the oviducts are recognized: isthmus (2–3 cm); ampulla (>5 cm), and infundibulum. The diameter of the tubal lumen varies from less than 1 mm at its ostia in the uterine cavity to 2.5 mm in the isthmic portion, widening to 6 mm in the ampulla. The trumpet-shaped infundibulum ends in a number of fringe-like processes called fimbriae. The largest fimbria is in contact with the ovary and is known as fimbria ovarica. The mucosal surface of the oviducts consists of cylindrical epithelium of ciliated and secretory types. The ratio of ciliated to secretory cells varies in different segments of the fallopian tube, being higher in ampullary and fimbriated portions compared to the isthmus. The blood supply of the tubes is derived from the adnexal branch of the uterine artery and tubal branch of the ovarian artery. The lymphatics drain into the mesosalpinx, broad ligament network, and para-aortic nodes.

The fallopian tubes have a number of essential functions in reproduction. These include assisting sperm migration to the site of fertilization, ovum capture from the surface of the

**TABLE 13–1. INDICATIONS FOR HSG**

| Uterus | Fallopian Tubes |
|---|---|
| Demonstration of normal uterine cavity (infertility) | Demonstration of tubal patency |
| Congenital anomalies of the uterus | Partial or total absence of fallopian tubes |
| Myoma of the uterus | Tubal obstruction |
| Uterine polyp | Peritubal adhesions |
| Uterine synechia | |
| Adenomyosis | |
| Incompetent cervical os | |
| Foreign body (IUD) | |
| DES deformity | |

ovary at ovulation, providing a suitable environment for fertilization and embryo development, and transferring fertilized cleaving ovum into the uterine cavity. Inflammatory processes due to gonoccocal, chlamydial, tuberculous, postpartum, or postabortal infections are the major cause of pathologic findings of the fallopian tubes. Other inflammatory conditions, such as endometriosis, intraperitoneal infections, and operative procedures may cause peritubal adhesions.

## INDICATIONS AND PREPARATION

Assessment of uterotubal integrity may be made using three different procedures: HSG, laparoscopy, and tuboscopy. The latter two procedures are invasive and require anesthesia. HSG provides an image of the uterine cavity and endosalpinx and is an excellent screening procedure for detection of uterotubal pathology. Suspected pathological findings revealed by HSG may subsequently be confirmed by hysteroscopy and laparoscopy. Major clinical indications for HSG are shown in Table 13–1. Table 13–2 shows contraindications to HSG.

***Timing.*** The HSG should be performed after cessation of menses but prior to expected time of ovulation. The best timing is before the tenth day of a normal cycle, when the endometrial proliferation has not reached its peak.

***Instruments.*** A sterile instrument tray (Fig. 13–1) should be available for this procedure and include:

- bivalve speculum
- single-toothed tenaculum
- rubber acorn (small and large size)
- HSG cannula (Jarcho)
- 20 mL syringe
- betadine preparation
- sterile sponge and cotton
- contrast medium (warmed)
- drapes

**TABLE 13–2. CONTRAINDICATIONS TO HSG**

| |
|---|
| Acute or simmering pelvic inflammatory disease |
| Sensitivity to contrast media |
| Pregnancy |
| Menstruation or uterine bleeding |

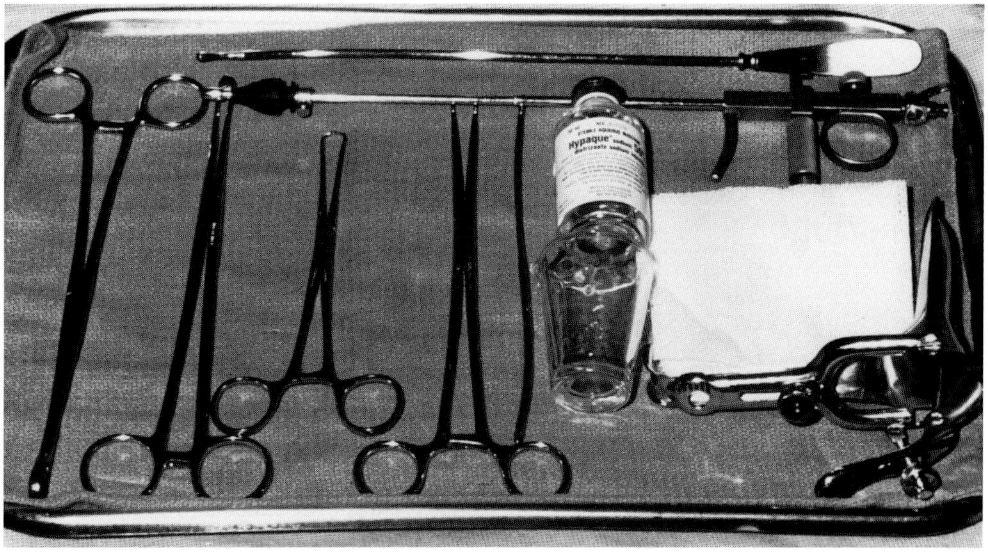

**FIG. 13–1.** Instrument tray for HSG.

A variety of cannula are available for HSG. No single instrument can be successfully used in all patients. Examples of cannula and devices available include vacuum uterine cannula, metal cannula, and balloon catheter.

***Patient Preparation.*** The patient should be informed of the nature of the procedure. It is helpful to administer a nonsteroidal analgesic approximately an hour before the procedure to alleviate discomfort.

***Oily Contrast Medium.*** Introduction of contrast medium into the uterine cavity and fallopian tubes is essential to illustrate these structures by radiography. Two types of contrast media are used for HSG: oil-based medium and water-soluble medium. The oily solutions are very slowly absorbed and, because of their high viscosity, provide a sharp and distinct radiographic image. For diagnostic purposes, these solutions provide excellent pictures during the procedure as well as on delayed films. They are usually well tolerated and produce no pain, but may produce tissue reaction. In occluded fallopian tubes the oily contrast medium may persist for a long time and cause acute flare-up of a chronic infection or granuloma formation. Also, intravasation of oily contrast medium may cause embolization, respiratory distress, and even fatal complications.[1] For these reasons the use of oily contrast medium has been abandoned by most physicians.

***Aqueous Contrast Medium.*** These media (*e.g.*, omnipaque, Sanofi Winthrop Pharmaceuticals, New York) are iodine-containing water soluble preparations that are absorbed rapidly by surrounding tissues when injected in a body cavity. They are well-tolerated but the radiographic image they provide is not as sharp as those seen with oily contrast media. They are less likely to cause granuloma formation, exacerbation of a chronic infection, or embolization when they penetrate the vascular system. Some older studies[2] have reported a higher pregnancy rate following HSG with oil-based medium when compared to water-based medium. A small prospective clinical trial did not confirm these findings.[3] However, a larger randomized prospective study of 398 patients showed a significantly higher pregnancy rate within three months among women after HSG with the use of ''ethiadol poppy seed oil,'' compared to three water-soluble contrast media.[4] Therapeutic effect of oil-soluble contrast media compared with water-soluble contrast media after HSG in infertile couples was also assessed by a meta-analysis of four randomized clinical trials and six nonrandomized controlled reports evaluating pregnancy rates after the procedure. The results indicated that pregnancy rates were significantly higher in the oil-soluble media group. This apparent benefit was greatest for patients with unexplained infertility.[5]

## TECHNIQUE

Hysterosalpingography should be performed by a physician who is familiar with the technique and with the condition of the patient. It is commonly performed by a gynecologist with the assistance of a radiologist. The examination is best performed using image-intensified fluoroscopy to regulate the rate of injection and determine appearance of uterus, tubes, and any pathologic features. Radiographic or spot films are obtained to document various findings and for permanent record. A delayed film is usually taken to demonstrate spillage of the contrast medium from the fimbrial end of the tubes and its spread in the pelvic cavity. The physician should wear a lead apron for protection from radiation. Adequate lighting should be available for instrumentation. The patient should be advised of various steps of the procedure to secure her cooperation.

The patient is placed in lithotomy position and draped. The bivalve speculum is placed in the vagina and the cervix exposed. The vagina and cervix are cleansed with an antiseptic preparation, such as betadine solution, and the cervix is grasped with the tenaculum. Gentle sounding of the uterus may be performed to determine its position. However, in most instances this step is unnecessary and may cause undue discomfort. The cannula is prepared by injecting enough contrast medium into it to evacuate the air within the cannula and prevent air bubble formation in the uterus. The cannula is then inserted gently into the cervical canal under direct vision, allowing the tip to reach the level of internal os, and secured to the tenaculum. The bivalve speculum is then removed and the patient's legs are extended (Fig. 13–2).

Under fluoroscopic control, 2 mL of contrast medium are injected to outline the uterine

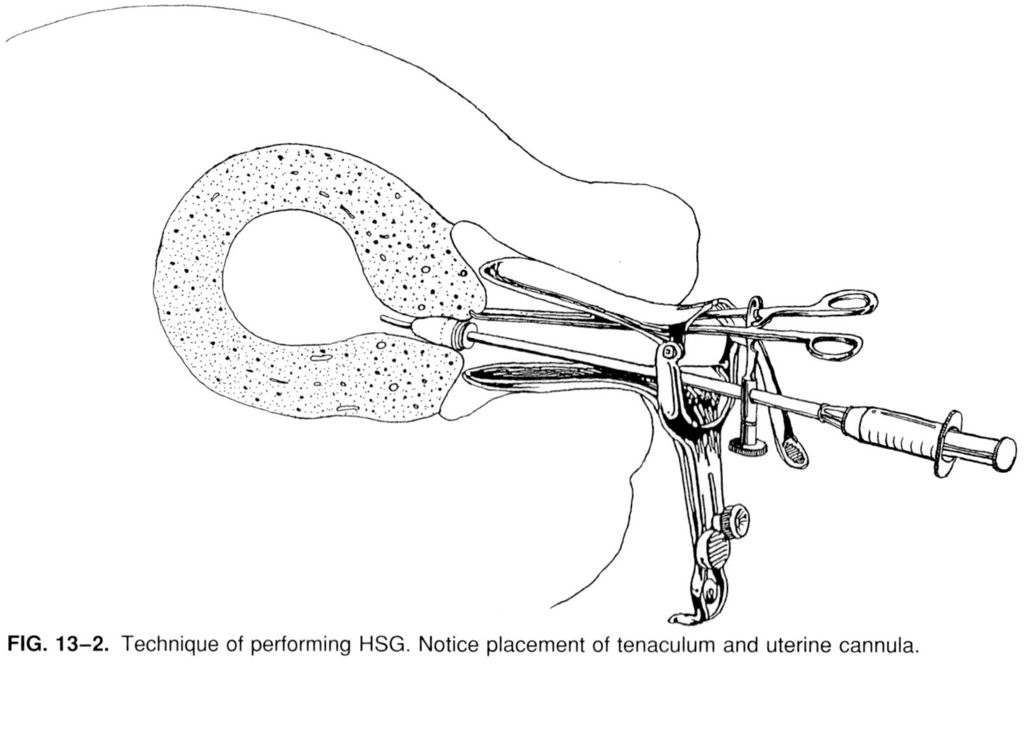

**FIG. 13–2.** Technique of performing HSG. Notice placement of tenaculum and uterine cannula.

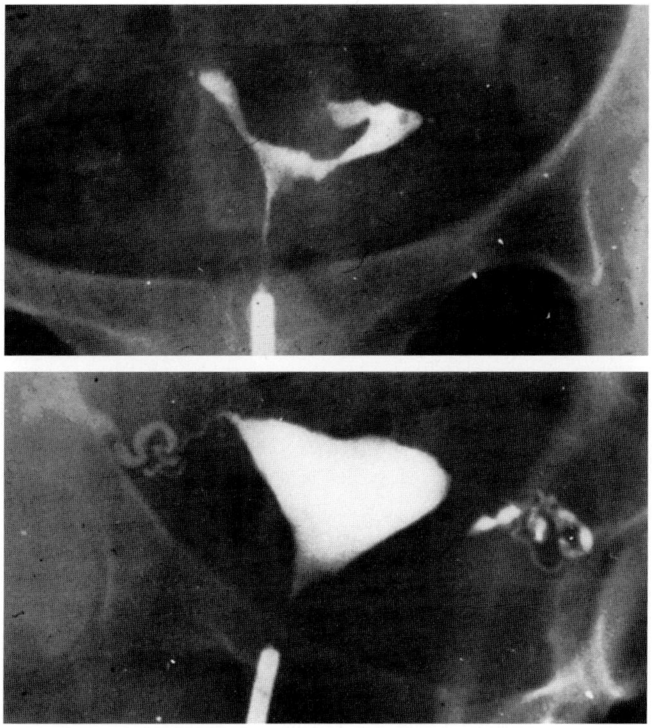
A
B

**FIG. 13–3.** (A) Injection of less than 2 mL of contrast medium results in demonstration of uterine cavity abnormalities (in this case a submucus myoma). (B) Filling the uterine cavity rapidly obscures intrauterine pathology.

cavity (Fig. 13–3). Sufficient amount of contrast medium is then injected gently and slowly to outline the oviducts and confirm intraperitoneal spread. Gentle traction on the tenaculum will allow for visualization of the uterus and fallopian tubes on a single plane and to obtain informative films. Frequently during injection one can observe contractile activity of the tube and pulsatile discharge of the contrast medium from the fimbriae. When using an aqueous contrast medium, a delayed film should be obtained approximately 5–10 minutes later to demonstrate the spread of the medium in the pelvic cavity. With a longer interval the contrast medium may be absorbed. Since the oil-based contrast medium persists for much longer before being absorbed, it is recommended that the delayed film be obtained after 24 hours.

The use of local anesthesia is usually unnecessary; the majority of patients experience only minimal discomfort. It has also been suggested to administer glucagon or a β-mimetic agent to overcome cornual spasm (apparent cornual obstruction). Again, this is rarely done.

The patient is instructed to rest on the examination table (supine position) until her cramps or discomfort subside to avoid occasional instances of dizziness and fainting resulting from a vagal reaction.

## INTERPRETATION OF RESULTS

Hysterosalpingograms should be interpreted by a knowledgeable physician who participated in fluoroscopic procedure. Figure 13–4 shows a normal HSG. The uterine cavity and fallopian tubes are well delineated. The uterine cavity shows no deformity or filling defect and the fallopian tubes appear to be patent. The contrast medium has spilled from the fimbrial end of the fallopian tubes and has spread normally in the pelvic cavity.

## ABNORMALITIES

Incompetent cervix may appear as a widened canal and is readily recognized both during fluoroscopy and on still films. Congenital anomalies of the uterus result from absent or incom-

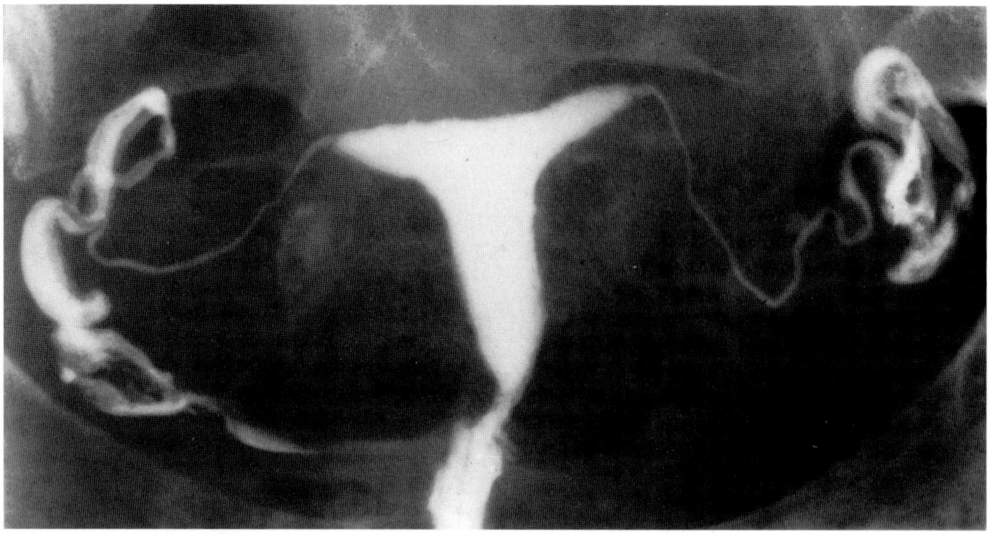

**FIG. 13–4.** Normal HSG.

plete fusion of Mullerian ducts. They include arcuate (Fig. 13–5) and bicornuate (Fig. 13–6) uteri, partial or complete septum, uterine didelphys unicornuate uterus (Fig. 13-7) and T-shaped uterus characteristic of diethylstilbestrol (DES) exposure in utero (Fig. 13–8). These malformations are easily detected by HSG. Experience and familiarity is, however, required to recognize these deformities. Filling defects may be due to polyps or submucous myoma (Fig. 13–9). Care should be taken not to confuse air bubbles with filling defects. Synechia usually appears as irregular or linear interauterine filling defects that are not obliterated by increased amounts of contrast medium (Fig. 13–10).

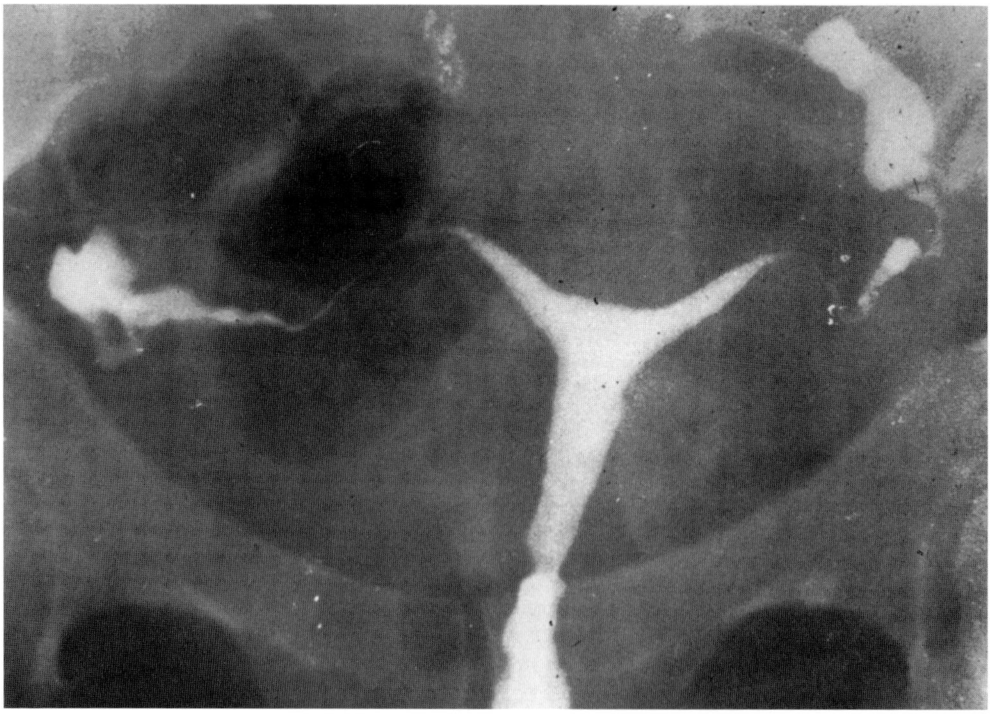

**FIG. 13–5.** Typical arcuate uterus with fimbrial tubal obstruction and moderate hydrosalpinx.

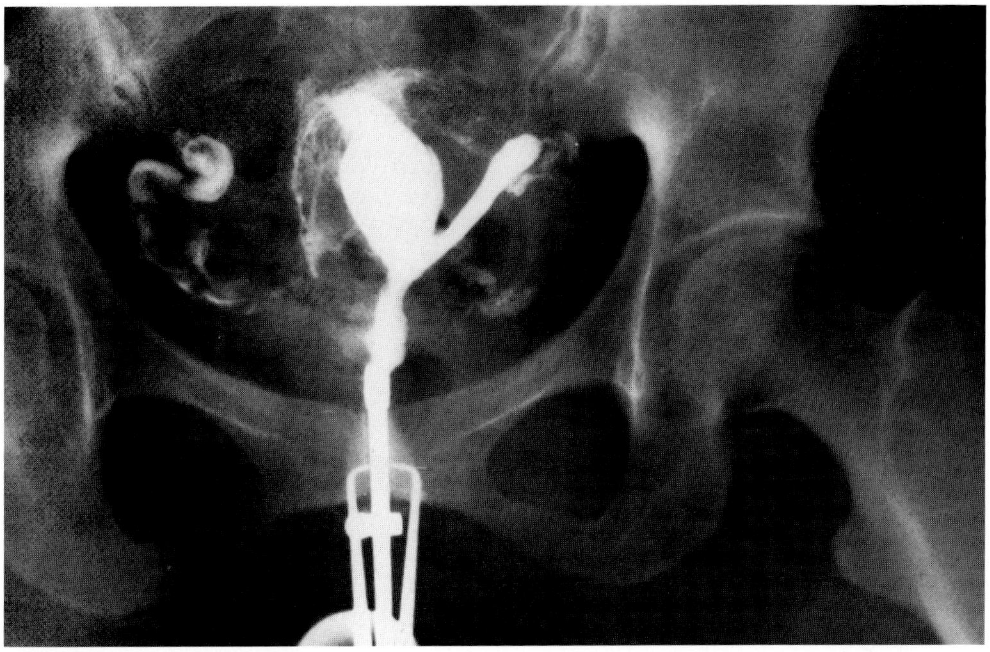

**FIG. 13–6.** Bicornuate uterus.

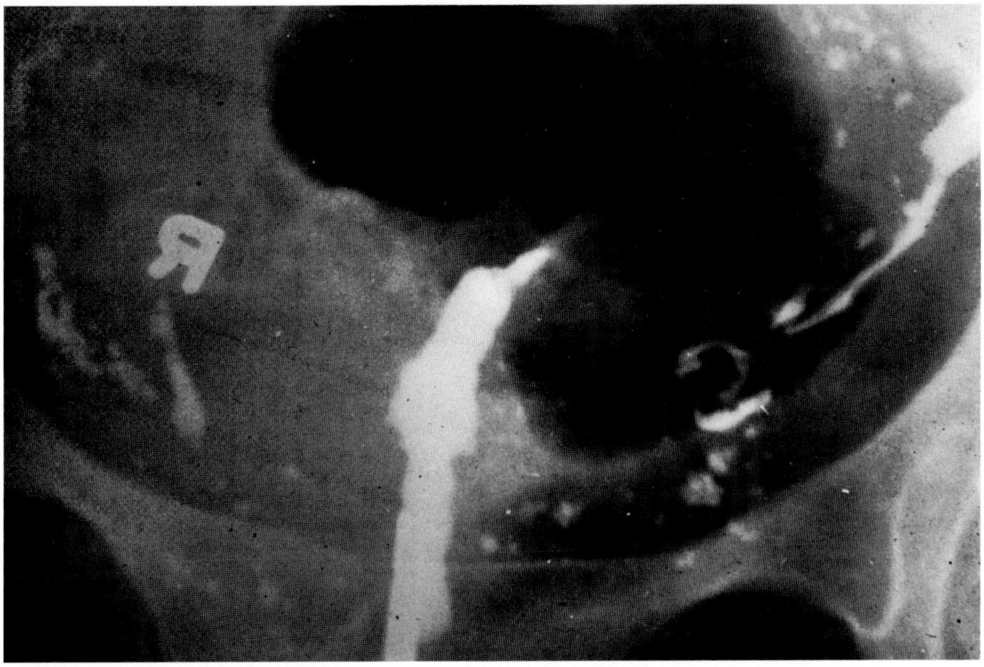

**FIG. 13–7.** Unicornuate uterus.

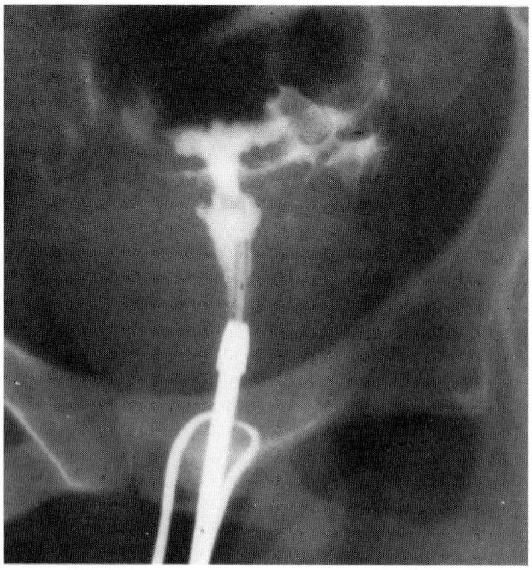

**FIG. 13–8.** Typical DES uterus. Notice severe hypoplastic T-shape and punched out filling defects.

HSG is the best method for the examination of endosalpinx. Tubal obstructions, at cornual portion, result in absent delineation of the tube and may be due to spasm, mucus plug, salpingitis, isthmica nodosa, or endosalpingiosis (Fig. 13–11). Ampulary or fimbrial obstruction is characterized by absence of peritoneal spillage of the contrast medium and various degrees of tubal dilatation (hydro- or pyosalpinx). Peritubal adhesions may be suspected when there is a distortion of fallopian tube, peritubal loculation, or lack of normal spread of contrast medium within the pelvic cavity.

## TECHNICAL PROBLEMS AND COMPLICATIONS

Conditions that limit access to cervical canal or uterine cavity may result in failure to perform the procedure successfully. These include cervical stenosis, severe anteflexion or distortion of the cervix, and, occasionally, a very large uterine cavity. Intravasation of contrast medium into the vascular or lymphatic system may occur when excessive pressure is used, in cases of cornual occlusion of fallopian tubes, or when the procedure is performed during menses. Even though the use of water-soluble contrast media has minimized complications such as dyspnea, respiratory distress, and embolization, the procedure should be stopped whenever intravasation occurs.

Other complications consist of hypersensitivity to iodine, uterine perforation, and pelvic infection. To prevent exacerbation of an existing chronic infection, it is recommended to use a broad spectrum antibiotic for 2–3 days, when unsuspected pelvic inflammatory disease is detected in the course of the procedure.

## ACCURACY

The accuracy of HSG for the diagnosis of tubal uterine pathology has been compared to those of ultrasound, hysteroscopy, and laparoscopy. Taylor[6] questioned the validity of HSG as an initial screening procedure to detect uterotubal anomalies and suggested that a combination of hysteroscopy and laparoscopy offers a more rapid and accurate initial approach to infertile women. False-positive rates of approximately 15–19% have been reported in the diagnosis of tubal obstruction by HSG.[6–8] Peritubal adhesion is the pathologic process most commonly missed by HSG but subsequently diagnosed by laparoscopy. HSG may also falsely diagnose

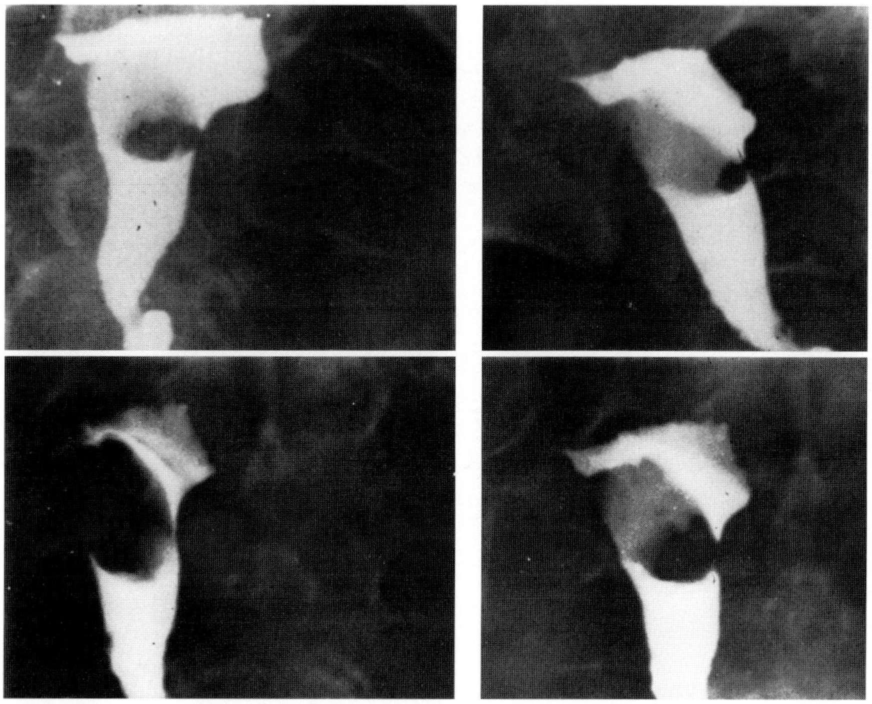

**FIG. 13–9.** Large submucus myoma of the uterus.

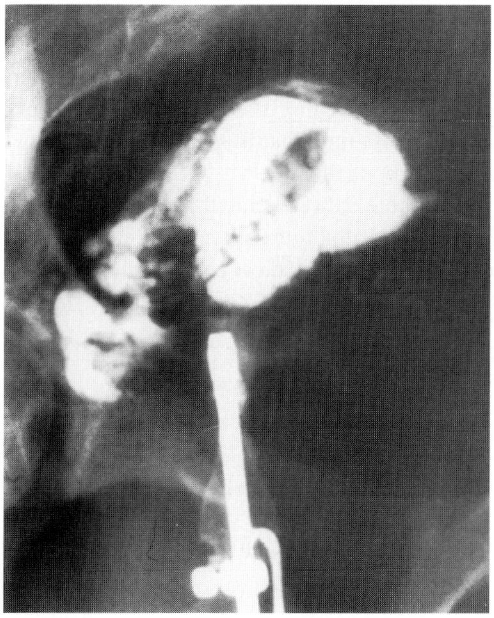

**FIG. 13–10.** Severe intrauterine adhesions (synechia) obstructing almost entirely the uterine cavity.

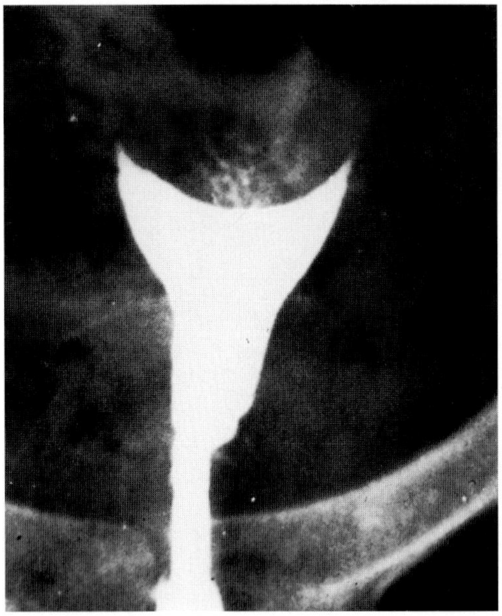

**FIG. 13–11.** Bilateral cornual obstruction of the fallopian tubes.

tubal cornual obstruction resulting from spasm. On the other hand, an occasional cornual obstruction diagnosed by laparoscopy is found to be false by a subsequent HSG.

To assess usefulness of real-time ultrasonography (US) as an alternative to HSG in the evaluation of uterine abnormalities and tubal patency, Randolph et al[9] used ultrasound with instillation of saline into the uterus to provide contrast immediately before hysteroscopy or laparoscopy. Their results indicated that this procedure was as accurate as HSG in demonstrating uterine pathology and provided a more complete assessment of abnormalities. US was also as accurate as HSG in demonstrating the presence of tubal patency, but less accurate in establishing which tubes were patent. A more recent report has confirmed these findings.[10]

Other studies have documented that hysteroscopy does not offer greater diagnostic accuracy as an initial screening procedure.[11]

Collectively, the available data indicate that HSG is an important, relatively inexpensive, informative, and safe procedure for initial screening of uterotubal abnormalities.[11] Hysteroscopy and laparoscopy should be reserved only for the confirmation and treatment of pathologic entities discovered by HSG.

## CONCLUSIONS

HSG should be the initial procedure for evaluation of utero-tubal anomalies. Because of its safety, an aqueous contrast medium is usually utilized by most physicians. Abnormalities detected by HSG may require further confirmation by hysteroscopy and laparoscopy.

## References

1. Levinson JM. Pulmonary oil embolism following hysterosalpingography. Fertil Steril 1963;14:21.
2. DeCherney AH, Kort H, Barney JB, et al. Increased pregnancy rate with oil soluble hysterosalpingography dye. Fertil Steril 1980;33:407.

3. Alper MM, Garner PR, Spence JEH, Quarrington AM. Pregnancy rates after hysterosalpingography with oil and water soluble contrast media. Obstet Gynecol 1986;68:6–9.
4. Rasmussen F, Lindequist S, Larsen C, Jurstensen P. Therapeutic effect of hysterosalpingography: oil- versus water-soluble contrast media—a randomized prospective study. J Radiology 1991;179:75–78.
5. Watson A, Vandekerckhove P, Lilford R, et al. A meta-analysis of the therapeutic role of oil-soluble contrast media at hysterosalpingography: a surprising result. Fertil Steril 1994; 61:470–477.
6. Taylor PJ. The case against HSG as a first line procedure. Contemporary OB/GYN 1985; 25:49–71.
7. Snowden EU, Jarrett JC, Dawood MY. Comparison of diagnostic accuracy of laparoscopy, hysteroscopy and hysterosalpingography in evaluation of female infertility. Fertil Steril 1984;41:709–713.
8. Moghissi KS, Sim GS. Correlation between hysterosalpingography and pelvic endoscopy for the evaluation of tubal factor. Fertil Steril 1975;26:1178–1181.
9. Randolph J, Ying YK, Maier DB, Schmidt CL, Riddick DH. Comparison of real-time ultrasonography, hysterosalpingography and laparoscopy/hysteroscopy in the evaluation of uterine abnormalities and tubal patency. Fertil Steril 1986;46:828–832.
10. Schlief R, Deichert U. Hysterosalpingography—contrast sonography of the uterus and fallopian tubes: results of a clinical trial of a new contrast medium in 120 patients. Radiology 1991;178:213–215.
11. Fayez JA, Mutri G, Schneider PJ. The diagnostic value of hysterosalpingography and hysteroscopy in infertility investigation. Am J Obstet Gynecol 1987;156:558–560.

*Invasive Outpatient Procedures in Reproductive Medicine,* edited by Mark I. Evans, et al. Lippincott–Raven Publishers, Philadelphia © 1997.

# 14 Endometrial Biopsy

Richard E. Leach, Nilsa C. Ramirez

## INTRODUCTION

The endometrial biopsy (EB) dates to the precommon Greek era as a means of therapy for abnormal uterine bleeding.[1] In the early 1950s, the morphological characteristics of the normal cycling endometrium were established, which led to the application of endometrial dating to diagnose luteal phase defects. Today it remains an important office procedure for the collection of endometrial tissue for histological evaluation. This chapter covers the indications, interpretation, technique, and complications of the endometrial biopsy.

## INDICATIONS AND CONTRAINDICATIONS

The most common indications for collecting endometrial tissue are evaluation of the luteal phase (LP), diagnosis of atypical histological changes in abnormal uterine bleeding, and monitoring the effect of HRT on endometrium.

Contraindications for endometrial biopsy include pregnancy, pelvic inflammatory disease, and uterine anomalies that would prevent adequate sampling of the cavity.

### *LUTEAL PHASE DEFECT*

Jones first developed the concept of luteal phase defect (LPD) due to insufficient progesterone secretion from the corpus luteum with resulting inadequate secretory transformation of the endometrium.[2] The prevalence of LPD ranges from 3–30% for infertility patients and 25–60% in women with habitual abortion.[3–5] Deficient progesterone secretion has been shown to prevent adequate endometrial development, which may preclude embryo implantation.[6] This dysynchrony may arise from inadequate progesterone secretion from the corpus luteum or inherent abnormalities of the endometrial lining in face of normal progesterone levels (Table 14–1).[7]

The first four entities are diagnosed by uterine cavity evaluation with endometrial biopsy, hysterosalpingography, or hysteroscopy. Progesterone receptor defect has been described in only a few cases and, therefore, is not a clinically important entity. However, its description would suggest the importance of repeating the biopsy after treatment to ensure correction.[8–10]

Traditionally, the diagnosis of LPD is made by finding two EB equal or greater than 2 days out of phase, as determined retrospectively by establishing the time of ovulation (LH surge), the onset of the next menses as day 28, counting back to the day of the EB, and comparing to the histological date provided. The diagnosis has been characterized more precisely in the research setting but remains controversial in the clinical setting.

The EB could be collected late in the LP to reflect the total accumulative progesterone

**TABLE 14–1. CAUSES OF LUTEAL PHASE DEFECT IN FACE OF NORMAL PROGESTERONE LEVELS**

| |
|---|
| Septate uterus |
| Asherman's Syndrome |
| Endometritis |
| Submucous myomas |
| Cycle after danazol |
| Progesterone receptor defect |

secretion from the corpus luteum, as abnormal progesterone secretion may not manifest in an altered secretory histology in a biopsy collected too soon.[11] The fundal region of the uterus has been shown to be the most advanced area by histological dating in a study sampling posthysterectomy specimens. Therefore, the most histologically advanced portion of the specimen is taken to represent the dates of the EB and account for this regional variability.[3]

## TECHNIQUE

Common instruments used in performing office endometrial biopsy are the vaginal speculum, tenaculum, aseptic solution (betadine), cotton swab and sponges, ring forceps, uterine sound, and pipelle (or similar biopsy device).

The patient is placed in the dorsal lithotomy position. A prebiopsy bimanual exam should identify the orientation of the uterus to more easily guide the insertion of the cannula. Once complete visualization of the cervix is achieved the cervix is swabbed with betadine and the excess removed to prevent contamination. With a normal-sized external os a tenaculum is generally not required with the pipelle and is used only about 15% of the time.[3] Manually curving the tip of the cannula in the sterile package to accommodate the natural curve of the endocervical canal allows for easier insertion. In an anteverted, anteflexed uterus the curved tip is gently guided along the anterior surface of the endocervical canal until the intrauterine cavity is reached. In a retroverted uterus the reverse of the above description would be followed. Without manually curving the cannula, the straight tip is embedded into the posterior or anterior wall of the canal, increasing the pain and difficulty associated with this approach. With instances of increased resistance, the plastic pipelle will bend in that region found outside the cervix, usually midway between the plunger handle and the tip. Placing a pipelle with a curved tip in the freezer until needed will generally keep it rigid enough to overcome this problem. With the increased rigidity, uterine perforation should be considered and avoided.

Once the pipelle is in the uterine cavity it should be slowly and gently advanced until the fundus is reached. This is determined by increasing resistance and by a feeling of uterine cramping by the patient (Fig. 14–1). Stabilization of the cannula with the left hand with controlled and complete withdrawal of the plunger with the right hand generally results in an

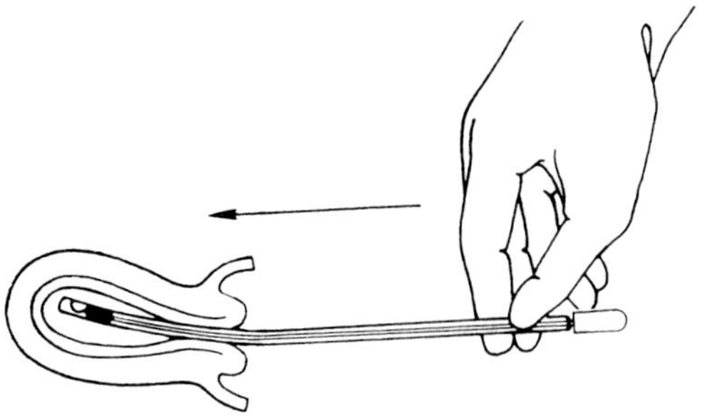

**FIG. 14–1.** With piston fully advanced within sheath, insert pipelle through cervical canal into uterine cavity until resistance is felt. Prior determination of uterine depth and direction with a uterine sound is recommended.

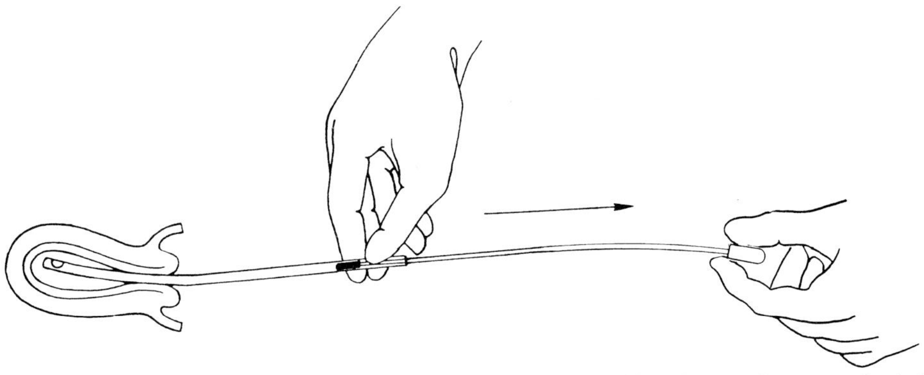

**FIG. 14–2.** While holding sheath, pull piston back completely and without interruption to proximal piston stop, thus creating maximum negative pressure within sheath. Leave piston fully retracted.

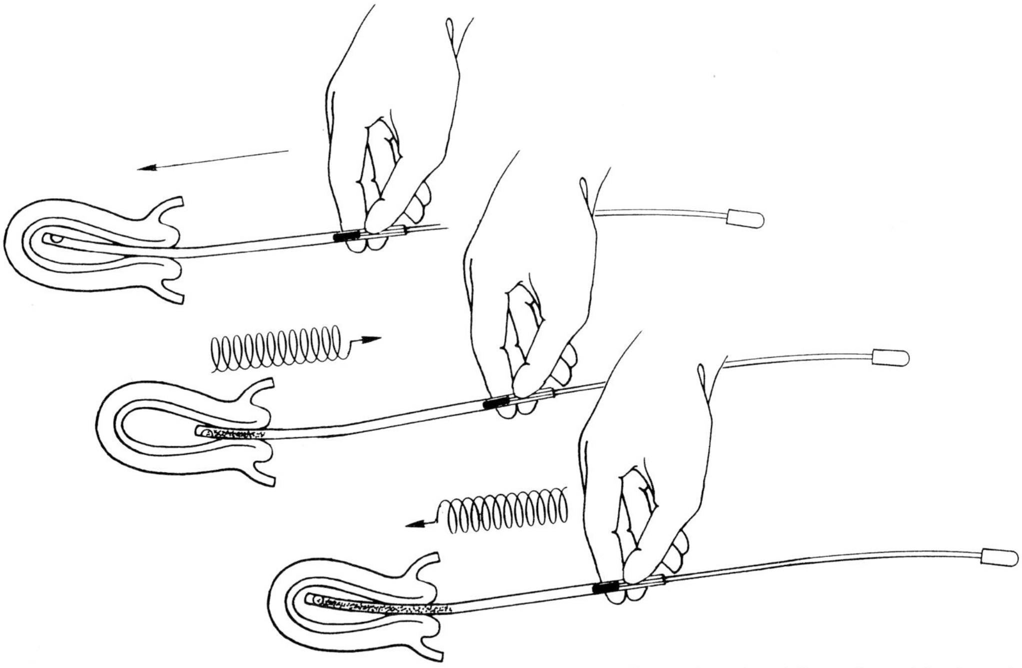

**FIG. 14–3.** Simultaneously roll (twirl) sheath between fingers while moving sheath laterally and back and forth (in and out) between the fundus and internal os 3 or 4 times to obtain sample.

adequate negative pressure (Fig. 14–2). The pipelle is rotated between the thumb and index finger as it is gently advanced and withdrawn between the fundus and internal os three or four times, generally yielding an adequate sample (Fig. 14–3). When using a Vabra aspirator, a single withdrawal is usually sufficient. If a sufficient sample is not retrieved, which is not uncommon in postmenopausal patients, the steps mentioned above should be repeated. Once an adequate specimen is obtained, the cannula is removed and the contents directly introduced into fixative (Figs. 14–4 and 14–5). The patient is then allowed to rest until any discomfort is relieved and is observed for vasovagal response.

## INTERPRETATION OF RESULTS

### *DATING*

The full thickness of the endometrial mucosa is divided into two zones: the functionalis and the basalis. The functionalis corresponds approximately to the upper two-thirds of the mucosa

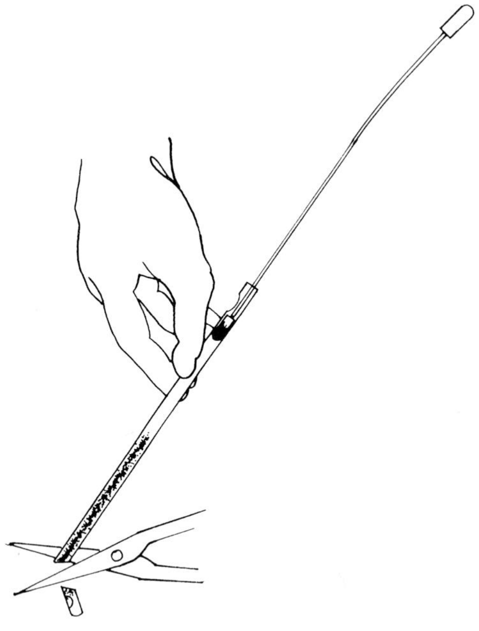

**FIG. 14–4.** Remove pipelle from uterus and cut off distal tip just proximal to curette opening.

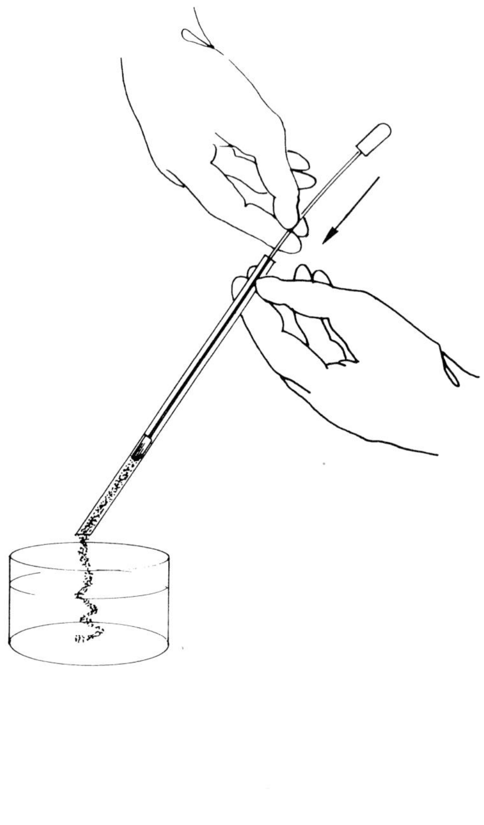

**FIG. 14–5.** Grasp piston rod close to sheath and advance it to expel sample into transport medium.

in which the cyclic hormonal influences induce glandular and stromal changes. During the proliferative phase of the cycle (corresponding to the follicular ovarian phase) the functionalis exhibits histological changes that result primarily from the influence of estrogen. With ovulation comes the ovarian luteal phase, accompanied by rising levels of estrogen and progesterone responsible for inducing histological changes in the endometrium, known as the secretory phase. Due to the decline of serum estrogen and progesterone levels at the end of the secretory phase, the functionalis undergoes degeneration and necrosis and sheds during menstruation.

The lower third of the endometrial mucosa corresponds to the basalis. This area exhibits essentially the same histological features throughout the menstrual cycle, reflecting a different sensitivity to cyclic hormonal stimulation than that of the functionalis. The integrity of the basalis is needed in order to accomplish the regeneration of the functionalis after menstruation occurs.[12] This area is characterized by straight glands lined by columnar cells with nuclear pseudostratification and rare mitotic figures. The stroma is spindled and lacks mitotic activity. The arteries of the basalis exhibit a subendothelial elastica similar to that seen in the myometrial arteries. This histologic feature is not present in the arteries of the functionalis.[13] The presence of arterial elastic membranes contributes to vasoconstriction during menstruation and ultimately controls bleeding.[12] The basalis interdigitates with the myometrium at the endomyometrial junction, which is usually a very irregular zone (Fig. 14–6). Another area that lacks synchrony with the functionalis is the mucosa of the lower uterine segment, or isthmus, of the uterus. This feature becomes more evident during the secretory phase of the cycle. The isthmic mucosa, together with the basalis and the endometrium of the peritubal ostium, participate in the regeneration of the functionalis.[14,15]

The classic work of Noyes et al[16] describes histological features seen in the endometrium associated with the hormonal changes that occur during the menstrual cycle. A system of dating was based on the determination of ovulation by basal body temperature charting and compared to the corresponding endometrial histological characteristics. The preovulatory or

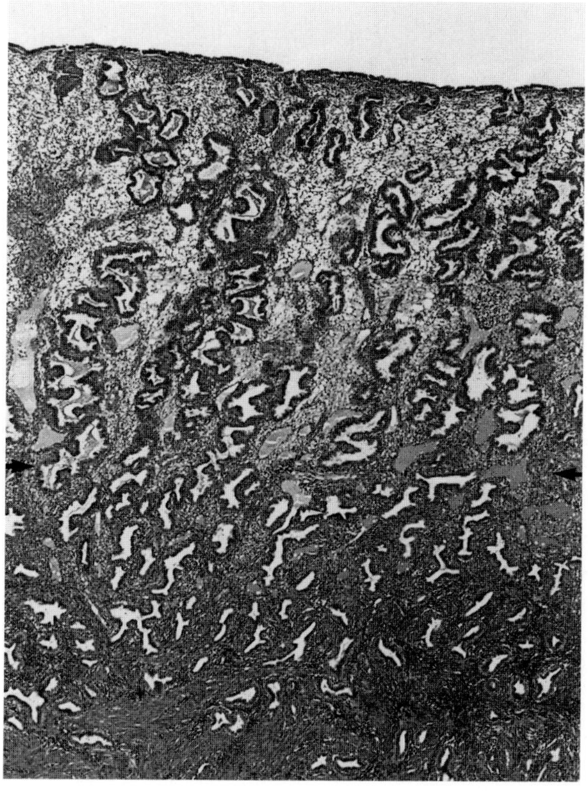

**FIG. 14–6.** The area above the arrows represents the functionalis. Glandular and stromal secretory changes are evident and exhibit the response to the changing levels of $E_2$ and progesterone that occur during the luteal phase. The area below the arrows represents the basalis. Note the lack of synchrony with the secretory type changes seen in the functionalis.

follicular phase is characterized by the changes induced by estrogen in the glands and stroma. The fact that these changes are not dramatically different from day to day precludes dating. However, certain features permit the identification of early, mid, and late events in this proliferative phase, the purpose of which is to prepare the endometrium for the changes induced by ovulation.

The first day of menstruation is considered the first day of the menstrual cycle, the evaluation of which is based on an "ideal" 28-day cycle, with ovulation occurring on the 14th day. Ideally, by day 5 of the cycle, the surface of the functionalis has been completely reepithelialized.[15] It is believed that the repair that takes place in the endometrium immediately following menstruation is not due to estrogen exposure since the circulating levels, as well as the receptors for estrogen and progesterone, are not different from premenstrual levels, despite increased DNA synthesis.[17] However, the proliferative phase shows evidence of estrogen influence during days 7–12, in which an increase in DNA synthesis and a proliferation of all components of the mucosa are seen (Fig. 14–7).[17] These changes are possible because of the increase in estrogen receptors seen in epithelial and stromal cells.[18,19] During the early proliferative phase the endometrium is thin with edematous-spindled stroma and thin-walled noncoiled spiral arteries. The glands are tubular and lined by columnar cells with increased nuclear to cytoplasmic ratio, coarse nuclear chromatin, and numerous mitotic figures. Ciliated epithelial cells begin to appear.[20] The mid proliferative phase is characterized by glands showing a degree of coiling with pseudostratification of the nuclei and numerous mitotic figures. The spindled stroma is edematous with numerous mitosis. The vessels also show coiling and, together with the glands, appear to be growing at a faster rate than that of the stroma.[20] It is during days 8–10 of the cycle that the concentration of plasma estrogen peaks, coinciding with increased mitotic activity and estrogen receptors concentration.[19] The late proliferative phase shows

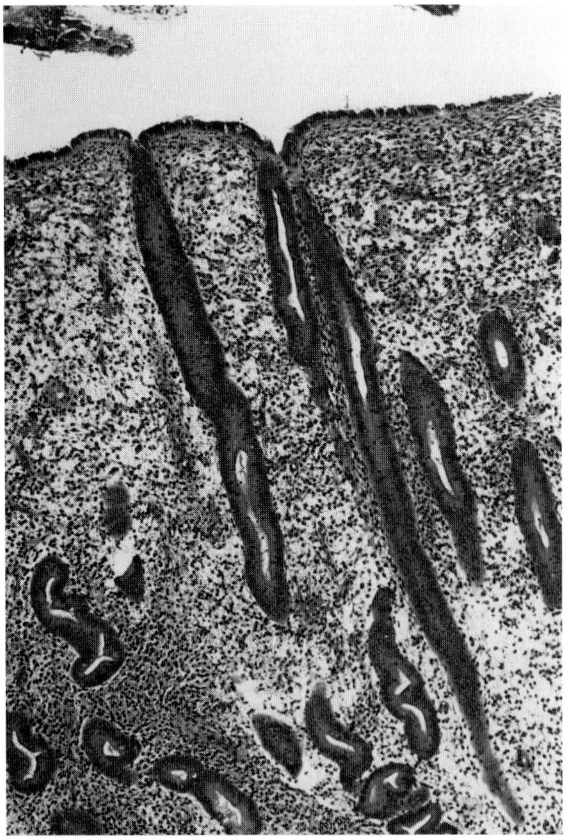

**FIG. 14–7.** Mid-proliferative endometrium. Note the straight glands perpendicular to the surface and the presence of stromal edema.

coiled glands that still exhibit marked nuclear pseudostratification as well as mitosis. The stroma, however, is not as edematous as the early or mid proliferative endometrium.[20] During ovulation the effect of the rising progesterone levels on the estrogen-primed endometrium are not immediately apparent. In fact, day 14 and day 15 (POD 1) endometrium show features similar to those of late proliferative endometrium. Scattered, small subnuclear vacuoles appear on day 16 (POD 2), but they are poorly formed and seen in less than 50% of the glands.[20] A similar histological picture can be seen in association with anovulatory cycles. Some authors refer to this histological picture as ''interval'' endometrium.[20] In order to assess ovulation based on the endometrial biopsy, more than 50% of the glands have to show well-developed subnuclear vacuoles in the glandular epithelium as well as palisading of the nuclei of those cells.[20] The glycogen vacuoles are the earliest histological manifestation of ovulation and are evident as early as 36 hours following that event.[20] On cycle day 17 (POD 3) the majority of the glands show subnuclear vacuoles, palisading of the nuclei, and few mitoses. This histological picture is reminiscent of the keys of a piano (Fig. 14–8). The presence of supranuclear vacuoles is characteristic of day 18 (POD 4); mitotic figures are uncommon. The contents of the supranuclear vacuoles are secreted into the lumen between days 19 and 20 (POD 5 and 6); the secretion is apocrine in nature and consists of glycoproteins, mucopolysaccharides, and plasma transudate.[21,22] The maximum concentration of glandular luminal secretions (that coincides with implantation of the blastocyst) is seen on day 21 (POD 7), when stromal edema is also evident; the latter reaches its peak during the luteal phase on day 22 (POD 8). Mitotic figures become more prevalent in the perivascular stroma, the glands are dilated with secretions and lined by low columnar epithelium. On day 22-23 (POD 8-9) predecidualization starts in the perivascular stromal cells. Vascular endothelial proliferation is also seen and it results in coiling of the arterioles. Prostaglandins have been shown to mediate stromal edema and

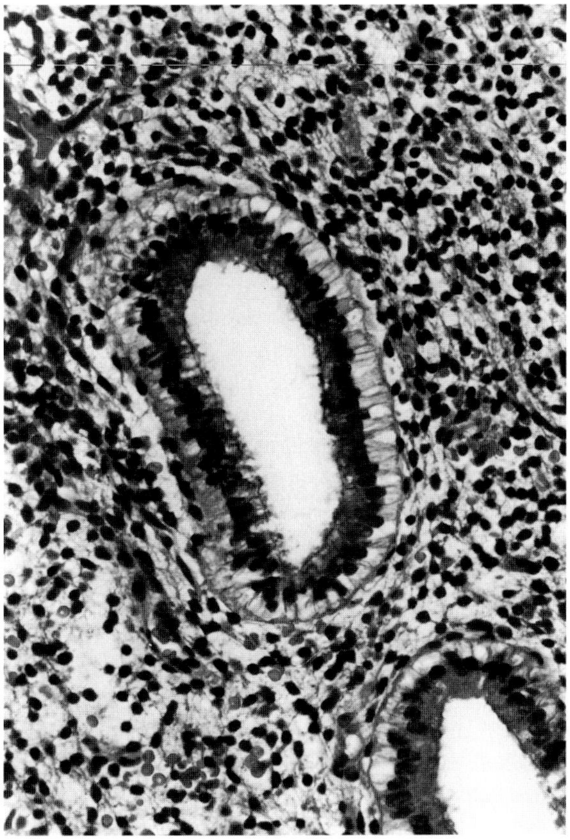

**FIG. 14–8.** Secretory phase endometrium, day 17. Note the presence of subnuclear vacuoles in the glandular epithelium ("keys of a piano").

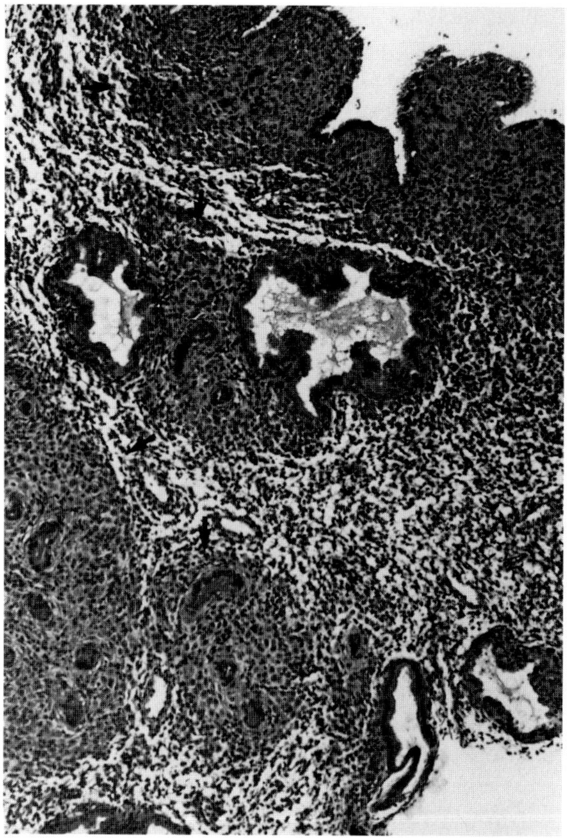

**FIG. 14–9.** Secretory phase endometrium, day 25. Note the stromal predecidual reaction around blood vessels and also beneath the surface epithelium (arrows).

predecidualization as well as coiling of the arterioles.[23] Prostaglandin production is augmented in midluteal phase under the stimulatory influence of estrogen on cyclooxygenase.[24] Also, on day 23 (POD 9) the glands show the formation of intraluminal epithelial projections, also known as "ferning."[12] By day 24 (POD 10), the predecidual reaction is more prominent. The stromal fibroblasts that undergo predecidual reaction become eosinophilic with increased cytoplasm and enlarged nuclei. These cells are the precursors of the decidual cells that develop if implantation occurs.[12] Predecidual cells have phagocytic properties and it is felt that they, among other things, may contribute to the breakdown of endometrial stroma during menstruation.[20,21] By day 25 (POD 11), the transformation of the stroma into predecidual cells extends into the area under the surface epithelium and the compacta layer is created (Fig. 14–9). By days 26 and 27 (POD 12 and 13), there is glandular exhaustion and the upper two-thirds of the endometrial stroma show a predecidual reaction and permeation by extravasated polymorphonuclear leukocytes (POD 13), as well as metrial cells or granulocytes. The latter exhibit a granular eosinophilic cytoplasm and a single kidney-shaped nucleus; they are members of the large granular lymphocyte series.[12] Metrial granulocytes are also seen during days 20 to 22, which coincides with the time of implantation of the blastocyst.[12] They, also, have been shown to contain relaxin, a polypeptide hormone also produced by the decidua and responsible during labor for the activation of the collagenolytic system.[22] If implantation does not occur, the degeneration of the functionalis with eventual necrosis and shedding of the tissue ensues. Glandular cells from the lower functionalis and basalis can be seen phagocytizing the cellular debris on day 28, as well as on days 1 and 2 of the cycle.[12] The menstrual period is estimated to last approximately 4 days. The degenerating tissue consists of exhausted secretory glands mixed with predecidual cells, lymphocytes, and acute inflammatory cells; the aggregates of degenerating stromal cells are referred to as "stromal balls." Lysosomal autodigestion mediates the tissue degeneration.[12] Prostaglandins also contribute to the vasomotor, as well as to expulsive mechanisms involved in menstruation.[21] Vasoconstriction of the basal (endometrial) arteries, as well as the radial and arcuate myometrial arteries control the bleeding.[14] The first 2 days of the cycle are when shedding is more prominent. Days 3 and 4 are characterized by proliferation of the basalis and subsequent development of the previously described features seen in the proliferative phase. Two factors are important to recognize when evaluating an endometrial biopsy for the purpose of dating. First, fragments should contain surface endometrium in order to be sure that the tissue being evaluated corresponds to the functionalis. Second, the date assigned to the endometrium is that of the more advanced area, and the time interval between that area and the less developed one in the biopsy should not exceed 48 hours.[18]

When LPD occurs, the endometrial tissue can show a secretory pattern with a lag of greater than 2 days from the expected date, or an abnormal secretory pattern in which there is glandular–stromal dissociation (dyssynchronous endometrium) (Fig. 14–10).[18] There is some variability in dates found by pathologists and even by one pathologist reviewing the same slide.[25]

The method of chronologically dating the day of EB requires determining the day of ovulation. One study looked at both prospective methods including basal body temperature charting (BBT), transvaginal ultrasonography (TVUS), and serum LH determination, or retrospectively by counting back from the first day of the next menses (NMP).[26] Prospective dating was shown to be a more effective means to document ovulation, with identification of follicular collapse by TVUS being the most accurate method.[26] The observed error in documenting ovulation by subtracting 14 days from the next menses is based on three factors.[27] First, the luteal phase has been shown to last 14 days in only 26% of 327 regularly cycling women.[28] Second, the late luteal phase biopsy is often followed by spotting, making it difficult to determine reliably the first day of the next menstrual cycle.[27] Third, the EB itself may shorten the luteal phase by one day.[28] Taking into account the above factors, a prospectively timed EB, either by LH surge testing or TVUS, collected from the fundal region of the uterus, would yield the best results.

A properly obtained EB evaluated by an experienced pathologist should be considered out of phase if the histological dating and chronological dating are different by 3 or more days. The endometrial biopsy remains the best current method for the diagnosis of LPD when standard guidelines for its use are followed. The EB remains an important tool in the evaluation of the endometrium in women being treated for LPD.

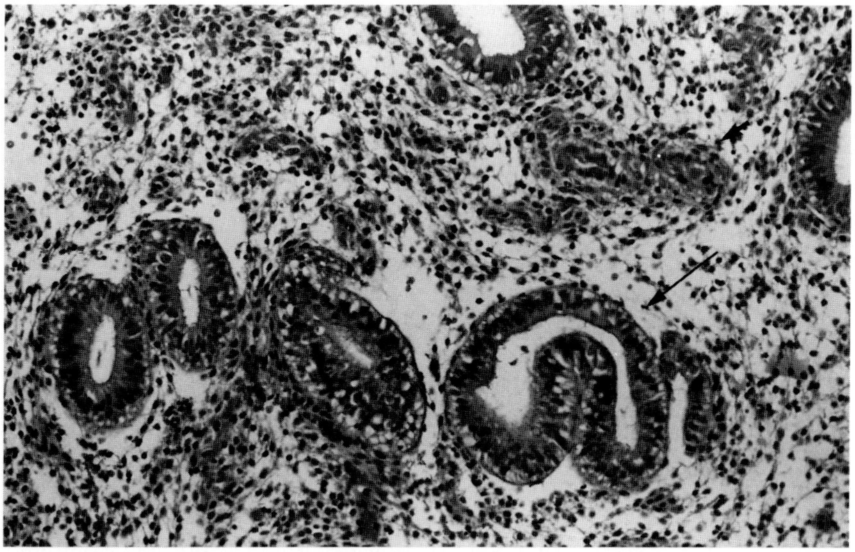

**FIG. 14–10.** Dyssynchronous secretory endometrium can result from a luteal phase defect. Note the early (days 17–18) secretory gland type changes (long arrow) and the stroma exhibiting edema and a perivascular predecidual reaction (short arrow), the last feature usually seen as early as day 22-23 of the cycle.

### *ABNORMAL UTERINE BLEEDING*

The EB is an important procedure for screening women at risk for endometrial hyperplasia and neoplasia. Dilation and curettage (D&C) was previously the gold standard for obtaining endometrial tissue for histological diagnosis. Today, several sampling devices are available that can be used safely in the office setting, without the cost and associated risks of D&C.

In 1970, the Vabra aspirator was introduced and has proven to be an efficacious means of sampling the endometrium when compared to D&C. The Vabra aspirator is a thin stainless steel cannula 23 cm long and 3 mm in diameter, with a serrated end containing a 3 mm opening. Connected to the opposite end is a plastic tissue trap. The trap is in turn connected to a vacuum pump, which applies negative pressure to collect the endometrial contents. There was initial concern as to the ability to achieve adequate sampling with this device. In Jensen's original report, only 5 of 350 patients sampled were found to have insufficient tissue, with none having endometrial cancer.[29] Grimes documented that the Vabra aspirator was less expensive, incurred less complication, and was more convenient. The diagnostic accuracy of 96% was comparable to that of D&C. The disadvantage of this approach is the associated pain in performing the biopsy. However, the Vabra aspirator is an accepted alternative to D&C in the investigation of abnormal bleeding.[30]

The pipelle endometrial suction curette was introduced in 1986 for sampling the endometrium. The pipelle is a flexible polypropylene cannula, 23.5 cm in length and 3 mm in diameter, with a distal side port through which the tissue is aspirated. Within the cannula is a piston, which, when withdrawn within the uterus, creates negative pressure, drawing endometrial tissue into the lumen. One study found that in 56 women biopsied with both the Vabra and the pipelle, those sampled with the pipelle provided more tissue and suffered considerably less pain.[31] Because the tip of the pipelle is smooth and flexible it can be envisioned to be less traumatic as it passes through the endocervical canal. In another study, pipelle biopsies were performed in 40 women with known endometrial cancer before hysterectomy.[32] In only 1 of 40 specimens was the correct histological diagnosis not confirmed. The histological similarity between specimens collected by D&C, pipelle, and hysterectomy confirmed that in no case was the pipelle specimen less informative and in no cases would therapy have been altered.

### *HISTOLOGICAL CHANGES ASSOCIATED WITH ESTROGEN EXPOSURE*

Unopposed exposure to estrogen can induce specific histological changes in the endometrium. These changes are a function of the duration of the exposure as well as of the level of hormone present. Estrogen induces the proliferation of endometrial glands during the follicular phase of the menstrual cycle. When ovulation fails to occur the architecture of the glands, the epithelial lining, the vasculature, the stroma, and the volume of the endometrial tissue are affected. When the levels of estrogen diminish, breakdown of this estrogen-primed endometrium occurs. The histological pattern of changes seen in anovulatory cycles is similar to that found in the endometrium exposed to replacement therapy with estrogen alone. When bleeding associated with anovulatory cycles occurs, a biopsy will reveal a pattern of estrogen withdrawal endometrial breakdown. This pattern results from the sudden decrease in estrogen levels (due to the regression of the ovarian follicle or follicles) affecting a proliferative-type endometrium. It is characterized by fragmented proliferative glands, sometimes artifactually crowded, mixed with necrotic stroma. Glandular cells can be seen with phagocytized nuclear debris.[33] Do not confuse this pattern with menstrual endometrium. In the latter, exhausted secretory glands, as well as predecidualized degenerated stroma are evident. Another change seen in the estrogen withdrawal endometrium is fibrin thrombi in ectatic thin-walled vessels. Increased numbers of thin-walled vessels and inhibition of spiral arterioles are changes associated with excess estrogen exposure.[34]

Numerous endometrial patterns (including endometrial hyperplasias) are also associated with unopposed estrogen exposure. In disordered proliferative endometrium, the glandular architectural features vary from one area to another; it consists of glands showing noncomplex budding and mild cystic dilation alternating with areas exhibiting proliferative-type glands.

The epithelial lining of the glands lack atypical features. There is a moderate increase in endometrial volume.[20]

The endometrial hyperplasias are classified according to the International Society of Gynecological Pathologists and the World Health Organization as follows:

1. simple hyperplasia.
2. complex hyperplasia (adenomatous hyperplasia without atypia).
3. simple atypical hyperplasia.
4. complex atypical hyperplasia (adenomatous hyperplasia with atypia).

A characteristic feature of simple hyperplasia without atypia, also known as cystic or mild hyperplasia, is that the glands are of various sizes, many of which show cystic dilation, and the stroma is abundant (Fig. 14–11). The epithelium lining the glands resembles the proliferative type, with no atypical changes; mitotic figures are frequent and sometimes luminal secretions are seen.[20] The complex hyperplasias exhibit a greater degree of glandular architectural anomalies consisting of complex budding and branching, as well as crowding of the glands. The lining epithelium shows stratification, although sometimes this feature may be absent. The degrees of epithelial mitotic activity may also be extremely variable. In the atypical hyperplasias the glandular epithelium exhibits atypical features consisting of loss of polarity, enlarged nuclei (with increased nucleus-to-cytoplasmic ratio), pleomorphic coarse nuclear chromatin, and prominent nucleoli. The nuclei become round, different from the typical oval nuclei seen in the nontypical hyperplasias. The degree of epithelial mitotic activity is also variable. The architecture of the glands can be simple (cystically dilated) with abundant intervening stroma and, in this case, will be classified as simple atypical hyperplasia. Alternatively, the glands can exhibit marked complexity and crowding with very little intervening stroma, in which case they are classified as complex atypical hyperplasia. The higher the degree of atypia, cellular stratification, and mitotic activity seen in the endometrial biopsy, the higher the association with an endometrial carcinoma.[35] Endometrial hyperplasia can progress to carcinoma in a certain percentage of patients, with the percentages varying with the type of hyperplasia. The type of carcinoma, however, is usually of a low grade and lacks myometrial

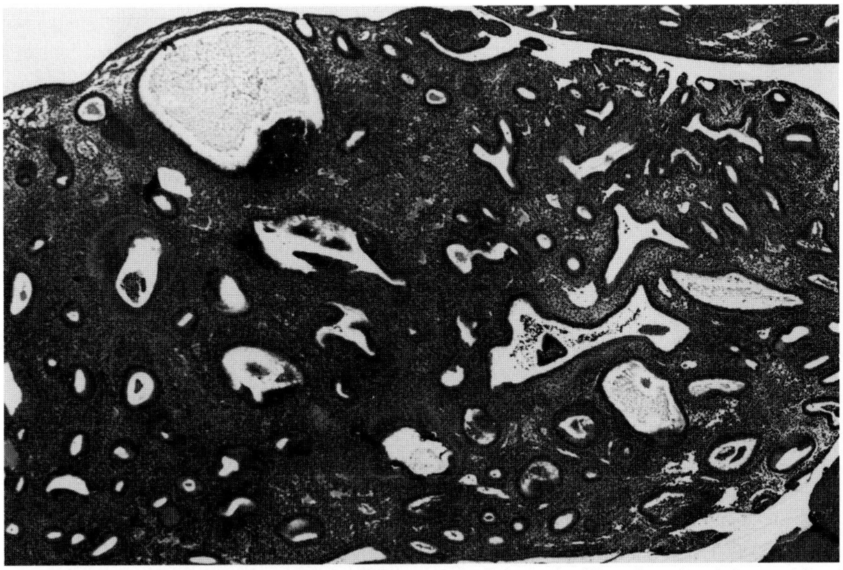

**FIG. 14–11.** Simple endometrial hyperplasia without epithelial atypia. Note the glandular architecture, with the cystically dilated glands, and the abundant stroma.

invasion, contrary to the more aggressive types of endometrial carcinoma arising in association with atrophic endometrium.[36] A well-differentiated endometrial adenocarcinoma exhibits complex glands that have invaded the intervening stroma and have merged to form a cribiform pattern. This pattern can be confused with a tangentially cut complex gland present in a complex atypical hyperplasia. Other changes associated with endometrial hyperplasia include the different forms of metaplasias that can be associated with hyperestrogenic states. The metaplasias (defined as the presence of mature cells of a type that is not normal for that tissue) can be seen in other conditions such as polyps, endometritis, trauma, and carcinoma.[33] The metaplasias include squamous, mucinous, ciliated-cell (tubal), eosinophilic, clear-cell, hobnail, and papillary syncytial. Remember that the terms ''simple'' and ''complex'' are used to define the architecture of the glands. Atrophic endometrium can have cystic dilation of glands but they are typically lined by a flattened single layer of cuboidal epithelium.

## COMPLICATIONS

Endometrial biopsy is associated with little risk. Reported complications include cramping, vasovagal reaction, perforation, postbiopsy endometritis, and pelvic inflammatory disease. In one series of endometrial biopsies collected over a 10-year period 28 complications out of 774 biopsies occurred (Table 14–2).[37]

In postmenopausal women the external os is often stenotic, making an office biopsy difficult. A lacrimal duct probe may be utilized to determine the true course of the endocervical canal and to avoid burrowing a false passage. Often in this situation the use of a tenaculum is required to stabilize the cervix and facilitate passage of the cannula.

The cervix should be observed for signs of cervicitis or purulent discharge and, if present, the cervix should be cultured, gram stain obtained, and the biopsy abandoned.

Women with a cardiac disease should receive prebiopsy antibiotic prophylaxis to prevent endocarditis.[38]

Uterine cramping and pain is decreased with prebiopsy ingestion of a nonsteroidal anti-inflammatory medication. Local paracervical block is rarely required.

The patient should be allowed to lie in the supine position for at least 5 minutes after the biopsy with supervision to monitor for vasovagal response, which typically presents as nausea, vomiting, bradycardia, hypotension, and fainting.

Fundal uterine perforation is generally without serious sequelae and requires only expectant observation.

The incidence of conception in the cycle of biopsy ranges from 1.4 to 4%.[1,39] The risk of pregnancy interruption due to endometrial biopsy is on the order of 1/1500 biopsies total and 1/500 in conception biopsies. Subsequent spontaneous abortion rate is 20%, similar to the infertility population in general, with no evidence of increased congenital anomalies or preterm

**TABLE 14–2. COMPLICATIONS ASSOCIATED WITH ENDOMETRIAL BIOPSY[37]**

| Complication | Rate |
|---|---|
| Cervical stenosis | 12/28 |
| Excessive bleeding | 5/28 |
| Fever | 4/28 |
| Excessive pain | 2/28 |
| Vasovagal reaction | 2/28 |
| Uterine perforation | 2/28 |
| Interrupted pregnancy | 1/28 |

delivery. The couple should be counseled to abstain from intercourse or use barrier contraception to avoid the small chance of disturbing an early pregnancy. A sensitive serum hCG test the morning of the biopsy may help avoid this occurrence.

## CONCLUSION

The endometrial biopsy is an important and commonly performed office procedure. Understanding the indications and its accuracy will provide the physician with a useful tool in the care of women. When applied to the patient with abnormal uterine bleeding, the endometrial biopsy will enable the objective recommendation for hormone therapy or the management of the diagnosed malignancy. Although the endometrial biopsy has not been validated for the recognition of luteal phase defect, when performed using standard guidelines is considered the best clinical method for its diagnosis.

## REFERENCES


1. Karrow W, Gentry W, Skeels R, Payne S. Endometrial biopsy in the luteal phase of the cycle of conception. Fertil Steril 1971;22:482–495.
2. Jones GES. Some newer aspects of management of infertility. JAMA 1949;141: 1123–1129.
3. Brodie B, Wentz AC. An update on the clinical relevance of luteal phase inadequacy. Sem Reprod Endo 1989;7:138–154.
4. Rosenbergh SM, Luciano AA, Riddick DH. The luteal phase defect: the relative frequency of and encouraging response to treatment with vaginal progesterone. Fertil Steril 1980; 34:17–20.
5. Tho PT, Byrd JR, McDonough PG. Etiologies and subsequent reproductive performance of 100 couples with recurrent abortion. Fertil Steril 1979;32:389–395.
6. Caspo AI. The luteo-placental shift, the guardian of prenatal life. Postgrad Med J 1969; 45:57–64.
7. Wentz A. Luteal phase inadequacy. In: Behrman SK, Kistner RW, Patton G. Progress in infertility. Boston: Little, Brown 1988:435.
8. Rosenfeld DL, Chudow S, Bronsen RA. Diagnosis of luteal phase inadequacy. Obstet Gynecol 1980;56:1193–1196.
9. Witten BI, Martin SA. The endometrial biopsy as a guide to the management of luteal phase defect. Fertil Steril 1985;44:461–465.
10. Shangold M, Berkeley A, Gray J. Both midluteal serum progesterone levels and late luteal endometrial histology should be assessed in all infertile women. Fertil Steril 1983;40: 627–630.
11. McNeely M, Soules M. The diagnosis of luteal phase deficiency: a critical review. Fertil Steril 1988;50:1–15.
12. Ferenczy A. Anatomy and histology of the uterine corpus. In: Kurman RJ (ed). Blaustein's pathology of the female genital tract. (4th ed). New York: Springer-Verlag, 1987:257–291.
13. Orcel L, Smadjt A, Roland J, Minh HN. Nouvelle hypothese sur le mechanisme intime de la menstruation. Rev Fr Gynecol 1973;68:477.
14. Ferenczy A. Studies on the cytodynamics of human endometrial regeneration: scanning electron microscopy. Am J Obstet Gynecol 1976;124:64.
15. Ferenczy A. Studies on the cytodynamics of human endometrial regeneration: transmission electron microscopy and histochemistry. Am J Obstet Gynecol 1967;124:582.
16. Noyes RW, Hertig AT, Rock J. Dating the endometrial biopsy. Fertil Steril 1950;1:3.
17. Ferenczy A. Regeneration of the human endometrium. In: Fenoglio CM, Wolff M (eds). Progress in surgical pathology. (vol 1). New York: Masson Publishing, 1980;157–173.
18. Ferenczy A. The endometrial cycle. In: Sciarra JJ (ed). Gynecology and obstetrics. (vol 5). New York: Harper and Row, 1981;1–14.

19. Ferenczy A, Bertrand G, Gelfand MM. Proliferation kinetics of human endometrium during the normal menstrual cycle. Am J Obstet Gynecol 1979;133:859.
20. Hendrickson MR, Kempson RL. Surgical pathology of the uterine corpus. In: Bennington JL (ed.). Major problems in pathology. (vol 12). Philadelphia: WB Saunders, 1980.
21. Ferenczy A, Guralnick M. Endometrial microstructure: structure–function relationships throughout the menstrual cycle. Semin Reprod Endocrinol 1983;1:205.
22. Ferenczy A, Richart RM. Female reproductive system: dynamics of scan and transmission electron microscopy. New York: John Wiley and Sons, 1974.
23. Levitt MJ, Tobon H, Josimovich JB. Prostaglandin content of human endometrium. Fertil Steril 1975;26:296.
24. Abel MH, Baird DT. The effect of 17 β-estradiol and progesterone on prostaglandin production by human endometrium maintained in organ culture. Endocrinology 1980;106: 1599.
25. Join ES, Cummings DC, Honore LH, Scott JZ, Williams KP. The luteal phase in infertile women: comparison of simultaneous endometrial biopsy and progesterone levels. Fertil Steril 1985;43:715–719.
26. Shoupe D, Mishell D, Lacarra M, Lobo R, Horenstein J, d'Ablaing, Moyer D. Correlation of endometrial maturation with four methods of estimating day of ovulation. Obstet Gynecol 1989;73:88–92.
27. Li TC, Rogers AD, Lenton EA, Dockery P, Cooke I. A comparison between two methods of chronological dating of human endometrial biopsies during the luteal phase, and their correlation with histological dating. Fertil Steril 1987;48:928–932.
28. Lenton EA, Landgren BM, Sexton L. Normal variation in the length of the luteal phase of the menstrual cycle: identification of the short luteal phase. Br J Obstet Gynaecol 1984; 91:685.
29. Jensen JG. Vacuum curettage: out-patient curettage without anesthesia: a report of 350 cases. Dsn Med Bull 1970;17:192–202.
30. Grimes DA. Diagnostic dilatation and curettage: a reappraisal. Am J Obstet Gynecol 1982; 142:1–6.
31. Kaunitz A, Masciello A, Ostrodwski M, Rovira E. Comparison of endometrial biopsy with the endometrial Pipelle and Vabra aspirator. J Reprod Med 1988;33:427–431.
32. Stovall T, Photopulus G, Poston W, Long F, Sandles L. Pipelle endometrial sampling in patients with known endometrial carcinoma. Obstet Gynecol 1991;77:954–956.
33. Kurman RJ, Mazur MT. Benign diseases of the endometrium. In: Kurman RJ (ed). Blaustein's pathology of the female genital tract. (4th ed). New York: Springer-Verlag, 1994;367–410.
34. Kurman RJ, Norris HJ. Endometrial hyperplasia and related cellular changes. In: Kurman RJ (ed). Blaustein's pathology of the female genital tract. (3rd ed). New York: Springer-Verlag, 1994;411–438.
35. Kurman RJ, Norris HJ. Evaluation of criteria for distinguished atypical endometrial hyperplasia from well differentiated carcinoma. Cancer 1982;49:25–45.
36. Beckner ME, Mori T, Silverberg SG. Endometrial carcinoma: nontumor factors in prognosis. Int J Gynecol Path 1985;4:131–145.
37. Davidson B, Thrasher T, Seraj I. An analysis of endometrial biopsies performed for infertility. Fertil Steril 1987;48:770–774.
38. McCurdy C, Noln T. Endocarditis: reviews and update on the prophylaxis in the obstetric and gynecology patients. Female Patient 1993;18:16–28.
39. Wentz AC, Herbert C, Maxson W, Hill G, Pittaway D. Cycle of conception endometrial biopsy. Fertil Steril 1986;46:196–199.

*Invasive Outpatient Procedures in Reproductive Medicine,* edited by Mark I. Evans, et al. Lippincott–Raven Publishers, Philadelphia © 1997.

# 15 Oocyte Retrieval and Embryo or Gamete Transfer

Charla M. Blacker, Kenneth A. Ginsburg

## INTRODUCTION

Since the birth of Louise Brown in 1978[A1], the techniques involved in assisted reproductive technology (ART) have evolved by seemingly opposing forces, becoming increasingly sophisticated and yet more oriented toward patient acceptance and low cost. Thus hospital laparoscopy for oocyte retrieval under general anesthesia has now been replaced by outpatient or office transvaginal ultrasound-guided oocyte retrieval under intravenous sedation. Alternative regimens have also been proposed or reported for oocyte stimulation and monitoring, gamete or embryo transfer, and as alternatives to the traditional laboratory for embryo culture. These modifications have increased the accessibility to these techniques by making the procedures less intrusive and invasive, while controlling costs.

This chapter will review the in vitro fertilization (IVF) procedure in detail, focusing on modifications that allow it and related ARTs to be successfully transported to the office setting.

## INDICATIONS, PATIENT SELECTION AND CONTRAINDICATIONS

While IVF was first used in patients with irreparable tubal disease, with time the indications for its use have extended to a variety of disorders including endometriosis, male factor, immunologic infertility, and unexplained infertility. The general criteria for selecting patients for IVF do not differ from those employed for other infertility therapies (Table 15–1).

Importantly, however, contraindications and exclusion criteria for IVF have become considerably less absolute. Thus, ultrasound-guided follicle aspiration has made IVF available to women with severe pelvic adhesions and ovaries inaccessible by laparoscopy. Donor oocytes may be used successfully in women unable to produce oocytes because of ovarian failure or oophorectomy. Briefly, the donor undergoes controlled ovarian stimulation, and oocytes are retrieved by transvaginal ultrasound-guided follicle aspiration. These are then inseminated with the male partner's sperm, and resulting pre-embryos are transferred into the infertile woman's uterus, the endometrium having been prepared by exogenous oral or transdermal estrogen followed by progesterone.[1,2] Pregnancy rates of 40–60% per retrieval have been reported utilizing this technique. Similarly, women with an abnormal or absent uterus may undergo oocyte retrieval, and a surrogate can carry the pregnancy.[3]

## TECHNIQUE

In vitro fertilization can be thought of in six discrete steps: recruitment of healthy, mature oocytes; follicle aspiration; preparation of spermatozoa; insemination and culture of oocytes

**TABLE 15–1. PREREQUISITES FOR IN VITRO FERTILIZATION: PATIENT SELECTION**

| |
|---|
| No medical contraindication to pregnancy |
| At least one functioning ovary that is accessible for oocyte retrieval |
| Functioning, accessible endrometrial cavity in which embryos can be replaced |
| Inability to conceive or maintain a pregnancy through other (less costly, invasive, aggressive) therapy |

and embryos; embryo transfer; and luteal phase support. Careful attention to detail at each step is critical to the success of the IVF process.

## OOCYTE RECRUITMENT AND STIMULATION

After Steptoe and Edwards[A1] published their account of the first IVF pregnancy using oocytes obtained during the spontaneous menstrual cycle, a number of groups tried natural cycle IVF with poor results. Subsequently, the natural cycle was abandoned in favor of controlled ovarian stimulation. Stimulation regimens have used clomiphene citrate alone, clomiphene with human menopausal gonadotropin (hMG; Pergonal, Serono Laboratories, Norwell, MA), hMG alone, or hMG combined with follicle-stimulating hormone (pFSH; Metrodin, Serono Laboratories). More recently, gonadotropin-releasing hormone agonists (GnRHa) have been added before gonadotropin stimulation.

Seventy three percent of clinics surveyed by the Society of Assisted Reproductive Technology in 1990 used GnRHa.[4] Through suppression of endogenous gonadotropin production and release, GnRHa qualitatively improve folliculogenesis and prevent spontaneous luteinizing hormone (LH) surges before oocyte retrieval. First used in women with a history of poor response to gonadotropin stimulation, trials utilizing these drugs in patients with no history of inadequate follicular development have reported favorable results.[5] Hughes et al reported a meta-analysis of randomized controlled trials that found increased numbers of oocytes retrieved (6.76 versus 5.25: overall difference 1.5 oocytes per cycle, 95% confidence interval [Cl] 1.18 to 1.87), improved clinical pregnancy rates both per cycle (odds ratio [OR] 1.80, 95% Cl 1.33 to 2.44) and per transfer (OR 1.40, 95% Cl 1.01 to 1.95), and decreased cancellation rates (OR 0.33, 95% Cl 0.25 to 0.44) in cycles that employed GnRHa. Such findings support the routine use of GnRHa for IVF despite the need for significantly more gonadotropin compared to other protocols without GnRHa (31.1 versus 19.0 ampules; overall difference 12.1 ampules per cycle, 95% Cl 11.0 to 14.0). No difference could be demonstrated between GnRHa suppression and flare-up regimens in cancellation rates or clinical pregnancy rates.[6] Our program has had success using a long GnRHa suppression regimen developed by Meldrum et al[7] and shown in Table 15–2.

## NATURAL CYCLE OOCYTE RETRIEVAL

As mentioned above, early attempts at natural cycle IVF yielded disappointing results. Factors contributing to this failure included inaccurate assays for luteinizing hormone (LH), less availability of ultrasound imaging of the ovaries and poor image quality, resulting in low oocyte recovery (46–66%), and premature insemination of immature oocytes resulting in poor fertilization (41–71%) and birth rates (0–12.5%).[8]

Recent improvements in laboratory techniques and follicle aspiration have renewed interest in natural cycle IVF. A typical protocol for monitoring such cycles consists of transvaginal ultrasound, serum estradiol, and urinary LH assays.[9] Serial transvaginal ultrasounds are performed during the first 3 days of the cycle (baseline) and then daily beginning 18 days before anticipated menses. Serum estradiol measurements are obtained daily once follicle diameter reaches 15 mm, and hCG 10,000 IU is administered intramuscularly when follicle maturity criteria are satisfied (Table 15–3). Urine is collected for LH assay every 3 hours, and the cycle is canceled and subsequent hCG timing modified if a spontaneous LH surge is detected. Follicles larger than 10 mm are aspirated under transvaginal ultrasound guidance 36 hours after

**TABLE 15–2. GnRHa-hMG STIMULATION PROTOCOL**

| Protocol Phase | Details |
|---|---|
| GnRHa start | Midluteal phase |
| Initial leuprolide acetate (LA) dose | 1 mg subcutaneously daily dose |
| Start hMG | After 10 days of GnRHa when estradiol <50 pg/mL and follicles <10 mm |
| Initial hMG dose | If weight <70 kg: 225 IU daily × 3 days, then 150 IU daily × 2 days<br>If weight >70 kg: 225 IU daily × 5 days<br>In either case, decrease daily LA to 0.5 mg when starting hMG |
| Adjusted hMG dose | Increase/decrease dose after 5 days of stimulation, based on follicular scan |
| Completion of stimulation | hCG 10,000 IU at follicle maturity |
| Follicle maturity criteria | If progesterone <0.4 ng/mL: 2 follicles with mean diameter = 18 mm<br>If progesterone >0.4 but <0.7 ng/mL: 2 follicles with mean diameter = 16 mm<br>If progesterone >0.7 ng/mL, 2 follicles = 14 mm<br>Estradiol should be approximately 200 pg/mL/codominant follicle |

hCG administration. Similar protocols have been reported by English[8] and French[10] investigators, though some groups advocate timing oocyte retrieval following detection of the spontaneous LH surge instead of cancelling the process. Follicle aspiration has usually been performed using transvaginal ultrasound; although most programs utilize intravenous sedation with narcotics, successful single-follicle aspirations without analgesia have been reported.[11]

Results of natural cycle IVF are generally favorable. In small series, ongoing pregnancy rates of 7–16% are reported, lower than those for cycles employing controlled ovarian stimulation, although per embryo implantation rates are actually higher than those achieved in stimulated cycles (13, versus 9%) (Table 15–4).[12] Importantly, avoiding controlled ovarian hyperstimulation results in medication and monitoring-related cost savings for the patient. Thus, natural cycle IVF gives a reasonable chance of success in patients who are normally ovulatory and are otherwise candidates for IVF at a substantially reduced cost.

## *FOLLICLE ASPIRATION*

Oocyte recovery is typically scheduled 35–36 hours after hCG administration. Relatively few cases are done using laparoscopy, and transvaginal ultrasound-guided IVF follicle aspiration is performed on an outpatient basis under general or spinal anesthesia or by intravenous propofol sedation. The latter is appropriate for office oocyte retrieval. Local anesthetics are not used because of potential toxicity to oocytes and embryos.[13]

The vaginal ultrasound probe (Fig. 15–1) is draped using a sterile cover and a needle guide is affixed to the probe. Sterile coupling gel is used to improve image quality. We have found it convenient to cover the control panel of our ultrasound machine with a sterile plastic drape, which allows the surgeon to adjust the ultrasound controls to optimize the image while

**TABLE 15–3. FOLLICLE MATURITY CRITERIA IN UNSTIMULATED IVF CYCLES**

| Follicle Size (mm) | Serum Estradiol (pg/mL) |
|---|---|
| >20 | >200 |
| >18 | >250 |
| >15 | >300 |

**TABLE 15–4. NATURAL CYCLE IN VITRO FERTILIZATION RESULTS, 1989–1992**

| | Sheffield 1987[8] | Paris 1989[10] | Stockholm 1991[27] | Los Angeles 1992[12] |
|---|---|---|---|---|
| Cycles initiated | 42 | 80 | 51 | 101 |
| Egg collection attempts | 31 | 68 | 32 | 78 |
| Oocytes obtained | 23 | 63 | 31 | 127 |
| Oocytes inseminated | 20 | 62 | 31 | 127 |
| Embryos transferred | 13 | 53 | 20 | 82 |
| Clinical pregnancies | 4 | 18 | 6 | 6 |
| Live births | 3 | 14 | 6 | 9 |
| Cancellation rate (%) | 26.2 | 15.0 | 37.2 | 22.7 |
| Oocyte recovery rate (%) | 74.2 | 92.6 | 96.8 | nk* |
| Embryo transfer rate (%) | 65.0 | 85.5 | 64.5 | 80.7 |
| Pregnancy rate per embryo (%) | 30.8 | 34.0 | 30.0 | 13.4 |
| Live births per cycle (%) | 7.1 | 18 | 12 | 8.9 |
| Percent over 40 years | 8 | 0 | nk | 0 |
| Percent tubal infertility | 100 | 80 | 100 | 89 |
| Percent male infertility | 14 | 0 | 30 | nk |

* nk = not known

gloved. The computed needle track is shown on the ultrasound monitor screen to facilitate follicle puncture.

Once the follicles are identified, a 17-gauge Pivet-Cook double-lumen needle (Cook Ob/Gyn, Indianapolis, IN) is inserted through the vaginal mucosa and into the follicle. Attempt is made to identify a track that allows aspiration of several follicles without repositioning the probe or needle. It is important to gain a three-dimensional perspective of the follicles to avoid trauma to the hypogastric vessels, which are adjacent to the ovary and clearly visualized in most cases. Once the needle tip is positioned within the follicle, an assistant aspirates the follicle contents into a sterile tube held in a 37°C heating block (Fig. 15–2). The follicle is gently curetted by rotating the needle between thumb and forefinger, then flushed twice through

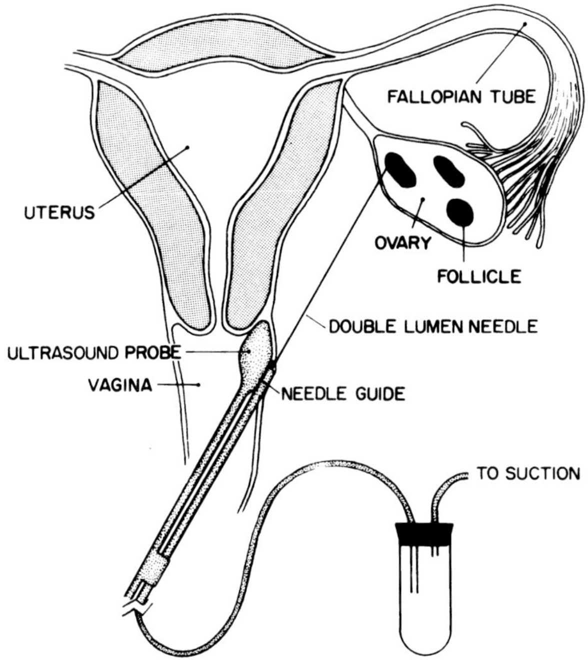


**FIG. 15–1.** Diagrammatic representation of transvaginal oocyte retrieval showing ultrasound probe in lateral vaginal fornix with attached needle guide and double-lumen needle entering a follicle.

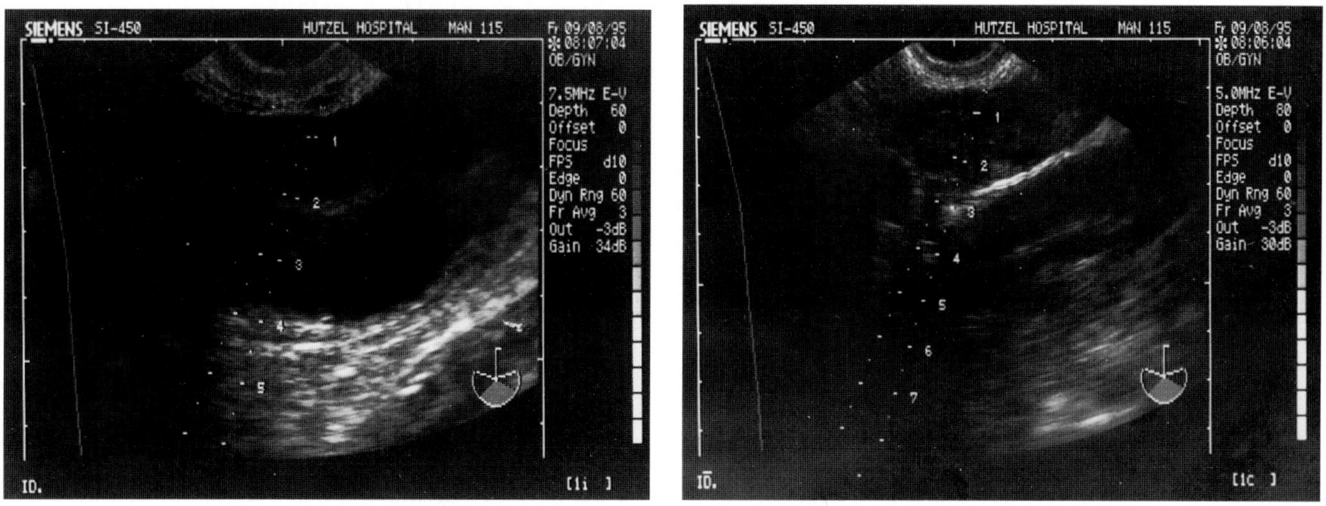


A B

**FIG. 15–2.** (A) Transvaginal sonogram of the ovary demonstrating multiple preovulatory follicles immediately prior to follicular aspiration. Lines delineate the path of the aspiration needle when placed through the needle guide. (B) Transvaginal sonogram of the ovary after follicular aspiration demonstrates collapse of follicular cysts.

the second channel with approximately 1–2 cc of Ham's F-10 media (Gibco Laboratories, Grand Island, NY) (Fig. 15-3).

Aspirates are transported to the embryologist for identification, isolation, and grading of the oocyte. The laboratory requires a laminar flow hood with a dissecting microscope and heated stage. Alternatively, a microscope located within a temperature-controlled neonatal incubator under 5% $CO_2$ suitably maintains temperature and pH. Identified oocytes are rinsed and transferred by pipette into organ culture dishes with 2 cc Ham's F-10 culture media supplemented with 7.5% fetal cord serum, penicillin G 75 mg/L (Sigma, St. Louis, MO), streptomycin 75 mg/L (Sigma, St. Louis MO), calcium lactate (Mallinckrodt, Detroit, MI), and $NaHCO_3$ (Sigma, St. Louis, MO), and incubated until insemination approximately 6 hours later.

Novel approaches have been proposed that challenge our concept of the traditional IVF laboratory and facilitate the transformation of this procedure to the office setting. Taymore and Ranoux recently reported intravaginal oocyte culture within a sealed capsule containing culture media, sperm, and oocyte. Fertilization was achieved in 84% of oocytes and resulted in pregnancy in 10–17% of retrievals.[14,15] Steinkampf et al reported a simplified approach to IVF utilizing clomiphene citrate for stimulation, ultrasound alone for monitoring, in-office egg retrieval, and transport of follicular aspirates to the laboratory in an insulated container with bags of saline prewarmed to 37°C.[16]

## SPERM PREPARATION

Semen is obtained after 48-hour sexual abstinence on the day of follicle aspiration. The sperm preparation protocol is individualized for each couple as determined by results of trial washes during preliminary evaluation. The goal of sperm preparation includes atraumatic isolation of large numbers of highly motile spermatozoa, and capacitation of those sperm by removal of

**TABLE 15–5. SWIM-UP PROTOCOL FOR IVF**

1. Pipet 2 ml of semen specimen into tube and add 2 mL warm equilibrated insemination media (Ham's F-10 with 7.5% patient serum). Mix gently with sterile 1 mL plastic pipet.
2. Centrifuge sample at 1100 rpm for 7 minutes.
3. Gently remove supernatant with sterile 1 mL plastic pipet. Do not disturb sperm pellet when removing supernatant.
4. Add 2 mL warm insemination media to sperm pellet and mix gently with sterile 1 mL plastic pipet.
5. Centrifuge again at 1100 rpm for 7 minutes.
6. Remove supernatant with sterile 1 mL plastic pipet.
7. Add 0.5–3.0 mL insemination media to the tube labeled "swim-up." The amount of media used depends on the size of the pellet and the number of sperm in the original sample.
8. Carefully layer the resuspended pellet underneath the insemination media in the swim-up tube.
9. Place the tube with the cap loosened in an angled test tube rack in a 5% $CO_2$ incubator. Allow 30 minutes to 2 hours for motile sperm to "swim-up." Length of swim-up time is dependent on the quality of the motility in original sample. The poorer the motility, the longer the swim-up time.
10. Following the designated swim-up time, carefully remove tube from the incubator. Using sterile 1 mL plastic pipet, remove top layer of media, leaving settled debris. Place in tube labeled "final sample."
11. Remove aliquot for assessment of sperm motility and count. Maintain final sample in 5% $CO_2$ incubator until used for oocyte insemination.

seminal plasma and exposure to protein-containing buffers. The swim-up procedure shown in Table 15–5 is suitable for the majority of cases. Approximately 6 hours after retrieval, a total of 200,000 motile sperm are added to each oocyte. After overnight incubation, fertilization is confirmed by visualization of two pronuclei and a second polar body. If no fertilization is noted, oocytes are reinseminated with a freshly prepared semen sample.

### *EMBRYO TRANSFER*

Pronuclear embryos identified on the day following retrieval are transferred to growth media (Ham's F-10 supplemented with 15% fetal cord serum) and incubated for an additional 24

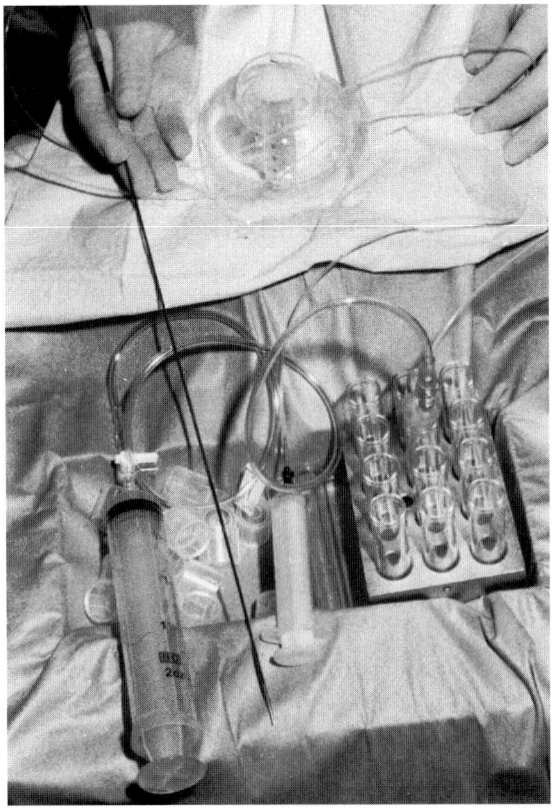

**FIG. 15–3.** Mayo tray for IVF. Double-lumen needle, aspiration traps, syringe, and connecting plastic tubing used for aspiration. Note that traps and media for flushing of follicles are maintained at 37°C within a heating block.

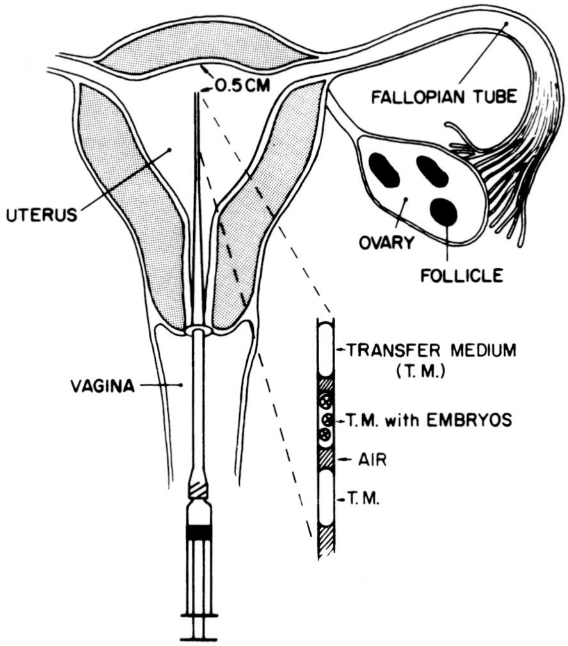


**FIG. 15–4.** Diagrammatic view of embryo transfer catheter inside uterine cavity. Note placement of embryos high in uterine fundus, approximately 0.5 cm from roof of cavity. Embryos are loaded into catheter in transfer medium surrounded by air cushions and additional small volumes of transfer media.

hours. By the morning of the second day after retrieval, cleaved embryos are typically between 2 and 8 cells. To prepare for embryo transfer, the depth of the uterine cavity had previously been measured during a menstrual cycle to allow atraumatic placement of embryos 0.5 cm from the uterine fundus (Fig. 15–4). Embryo transfer is performed in dorsal lithotomy position utilizing a Tefcat catheter (Cook Ob/Gyn, Indianapolis, IN) containing embryos in a small volume (30–35 μl) of transfer medium (Ham's F-10 supplemented with 50% maternal or fetal cord serum). The patient is kept recumbent in the mild Trendelenburg position for 3 hours to allow transfer fluid to absorb.

**TABLE 15–6. LUTEAL PHASE SUPPORT PROTOCOL**

| Serum Estradiol Level (on day of hCG) | Progesterone Dose |
|---|---|
| $<$2500 pg/mL | 12.5 mg IM $\times$ 2 days beginning on day of retrieval, then 50 mg IM daily, and hCG 2,500 IU IM 4 days after transfer |
| 2500–3000 pg/mL | 25 mg IM $\times$ 2 days beginning on day of retrieval, then 50 mg IM daily, and hCG 2,500 IU IM 4 days after transfer |
| $>$3000 pg/mL | 50 mg daily beginning on day after hcG |

### *LUTEAL PHASE SUPPORT*

The least understood part of IVF is the interval after embryo transfer. It has been suggested that high serum estradiol levels in the follicular phase, or decreased luteal progesterone production because of aspiration of large numbers of granulosa cells, act to alter endometrial receptivity, resulting in decreased embryo implantation rates. Support for this position comes from oocyte donation programs, cryopreserved embryo transfer and natural cycle IVF, in which spontaneous or hormonally normal cycles are associated with improved pregnancy rates in some centers. In addition, GnRH agonists cause a shorter luteal phase due to LH suppression, and luteal phase support is especially necessary in regimens containing these agents. In an effort to improve endometrial receptivity, progesterone and hCG are administered intramuscularly (Table 15–6).

## INTERPRETATION OF RESULTS

There is currently no requirement for mandatory reporting of IVF results. Despite this, ART outcome reports are published yearly by the Society of Assisted Reproductive Technology and The American Society for Reproductive Medicine through voluntary participation of 215 Canadian and US programs. In 1991 of the 27,443 cycles of IVF initiated, approximately 86% led to a retrieval. Over 87% (24,410) led to embryo transfer, resulting in 6,321 clinical pregnancies. The overall success (in terms of clinical pregnancies) was 23.0% per retrieval and 25.9% per transfer. A total of 5,103 deliveries were reported (81% of clinical pregnancies), or 18.6% deliveries per retrieval. Overall, 65.9% of deliveries were singletons and 34% were multiple gestation, primarily twins. Twenty percent of the clinical pregnancies were lost, primarily as spontaneous first-trimester abortions. About 1% of IVF transfers resulted in ectopic pregnancies.[17]

Pregnancy rates reported for IVF are affected by a number of factors including expertise of the reporting clinic, patient age, and male factor. Decreasing pregnancy rates have been reported in women over the age of 40. In the 1993 American Society for Reproductive Medicine Registry, women under 40 years of age had a delivery rate of 32% per retrieval. The corresponding rate in women aged 40 years or older was 12%.[17] For this reason, many programs have limited the use of IVF to women 40 years of age or younger. Ovarian age as measured by follicular follicle stimulating hormone (FSH) levels has been reported to be a better predictor of pregnancy rate than age alone.[18] Women with FSH levels above 25 mIU had a pregnancy rate of only 3.6% compared to 17.0% in women with normal FSH levels.

## COMPLICATIONS

Theoretical complications of IVF, whether in the hospital or office setting, include ovarian hyperstimulation syndrome (OHSS); infection from organisms introduced by transvaginal puncture, or inadvertent bowel injury with pelvic inflammatory disease or abscess formation; trauma of the ovary, fallopian tube, or uterus; and vascular injury. Interestingly, when transvaginal oocyte retrieval is followed by laparoscopy for gamete intrafallopian transfer, considerable (100–200 cc) hemorrhage from the ovaries or a retroperitoneal hematoma may be present yet not appreciated by ultrasound. Adnexal adhesions rarely develop after transvaginal retrieval. Mild degrees of OHSS appear to be relatively common, although severe OHSS is rare.

## OTHER ASSISTED REPRODUCTIVE TECHNOLOGIES IN THE OFFICE SETTING

Assisted reproductive technology includes, in addition to IVF, gamete intrafallopian transfer (GIFT); zygote intrafallopian transfer (ZIFT), also known as tubal embryo transfer (TET); and superovulation with gonadotropins followed by intrauterine insemination (IUI). Superovulation with IUI is and always has been an office procedure; transcervical uterine cannulation is a straightforward procedure that requires no anesthesia or complicated instrumentation. The administration of gonadotropins for superovulation requires monitoring capabilities similar to those employed for in vitro fertilization. Spermatozoa for IUI are prepared by washing them from seminal plasma and initiating capacitation; the actual insemination is performed in the office with the patient in dorsal lithotomy position, using one of a variety of commercially available catheters.

Follicle stimulation and oocyte retrieval in GIFT and ZIFT are identical to comparable phases of IVF. However, in the former two procedures a mixture of capacitated spermatozoa and oocytes (GIFT) or embryos (ZIFT) are re-introduced into the fallopian tube. GIFT and ZIFT (TET) have traditionally required laparoscopy to approach the distal end of the fallopian tube through which gametes or embryos were replaced. The development of sonographically guided tubal cannulation, first described by Jansen and Anderson in 1987,[19] has allowed reexamination of our approach toward GIFT and ZIFT, and has also allowed development of direct intratubal insemination procedures.

The tubal cannulation set (Fig. 15–5) includes an obturator to guide the outer cannula past the cervix into the uterus, an outer curved cannula that lodges at the uterotubal junction, and a soft 2-French inner catheter that enters the tube from the uterotubal junction. Several reports have appeared in the literature studying ultrasound-guided transcervical GIFT and ZIFT,[20–23] with a mean intrauterine pregnancy rate of 18%. Tubal cannulation was successful in over 90% of women. A revealing study is the prospective series by Hazout, in which the sonographic cannulation pregnancy rate was 6% compared to 47% for laparoscopic GIFT.[22] Based on preliminary results, ultrasound-guided ZIFT (TET) may be preferred to GIFT; pregnancy rates appear to be slightly higher with zygote transfer. At this point, however, the world experience of both is preliminary, and transcervical GIFT and ZIFT are best viewed as experimental procedures.

Two other techniques for introducing sperm and oocytes, or sperm alone, into the female reproductive track deserve mention because they can be performed in the office. Transvaginal peritoneal oocyte and sperm transfer has been reported by Tan et al[24]; a clinical pregnancy rate of 25% was reported in their small study. Intrafallopian insemination has been reported in two series,[25,26] in one of which donor semen was used in women who had previously failed

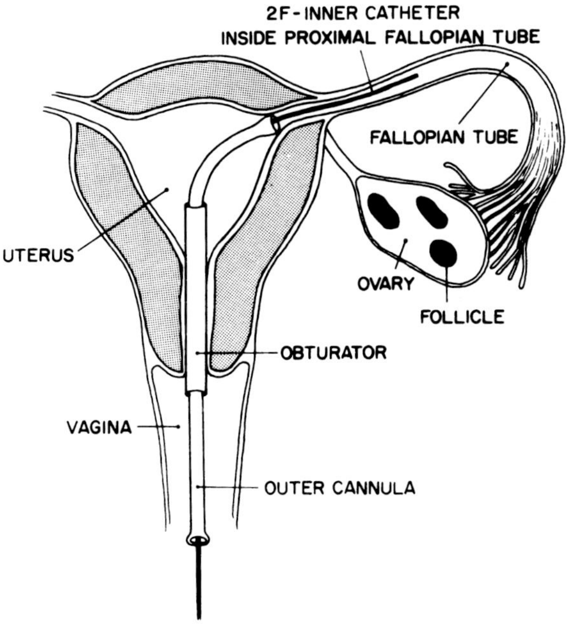


**FIG. 15–5.** Diagram of Jansen-Anderson transcervical catheter inside uterus. Note obturator, outer catheter lodged at uterotubal junction, and 2 F inner catheter inside isthmic portion of fallopian tube.

intracervical insemination. The fecundity and efficacy of intrafallopian insemination were shown to be approximately that of intrauterine insemination with controlled ovarian hyperstimulation. Additional prospective studies are needed to further evaluate these promising techniques.

## REFERENCES


A1. Steptoe PC, Edwards RG. Birth after reimplantation of human embryo. Lancet 1978;2: 336.

1. Doesch K, Navot D, Scott R, Kreiner D, Liu HC, Rosenwaks Z. Transdermal estrogen replacement in ovarian failure for ovum donation. Fertil Steril 1988;50:931–934.
2. Rosenwaks Z, Navot D, Veeck L, Liu HC, Steingold K, Kreiner D, Droesch K, Stumpf P, Muasher SJ. Oocyte donation: the Norfolk program. Ann NY Acad Sci 1988;541: 728–741.
3. Meldrum DR, Wisot A, Hamilton F, Gutlay-Yeo AL, Marr R, Huynh D. Artificial agonadism and hormone replacement for oocyte donation. Fertil Steril 1989;52:509–511.
4. Medical Research International, Society for Assisted Reproductive Technology (SART), The American Fertility Society (AFS). In vitro fertilization-embryo transfer (IVF-ET) in the United States: 1990 results from the IVF-ET registry. Fertil Steril 1992;57:14–24.
5. Meldrum DR, Wisot A, Hamilton F, Gutlay AL, Kempton W, Huynh D. Routine pituitary suppression with leuprolide before ovarian stimulation for oocyte retrieval. Fertil Steril 1989;51:455–459.
6. Hughes EG, Fedorkow DM, Daya S, Sagle MA, Van de Koppel P, Collins JA. The routine use of gonadotropin-releasing hormone agonists prior to in vitro fertilization and gamete intrafallopian transfer: a meta-analysis of randomized trials. Fertil Steril 1992;58:888–896.
7. Meldrum DR. Ovulation induction for in vitro fertilization procedures. Semin Reprod Endocrinol 1990;8:213–218.
8. Lenton EA, Cooke ID, Hooper M, King H, Kumar A, Monks N, Turner K, Verma S. In vitro fertilization in the natural cycle. Bailliere's Clin Obstet Gynecol 1992;6:229–245.
9. Paulson RJ, Sauer MV, Francis MM, Macaso TM, Lobo RA. In vitro fertilization in unstimulated cycles: a clinical trial using hCG for timing of follicle aspiration. Obstet Gynecol 1990;76:788–791.
10. Foulot H, Ranoux C, Dubuisson JB, Rambaud D, Aubriot FX, Poirot C. In vitro fertilization without ovarian stimulation: a simplified protocol applied in 80 cycles. Fertil Steril 1989; 52:617–621.
11. Ramsewak SS, Kumar A, Welsby R, Mowforth A, Lenton EA, Cooke ID. Is analgesia required for transvaginal single-follicle aspiration in in vitro fertilization? A double-blind study. J Vitro Fert Embryo Transfer 1990;7:103–106.
12. Paulson RJ, Sauer MV, Francis MM, Macaso TM, Lobo RA. In vitro fertilization in unstimulated cycles: the University of Southern California experience. Fertil Steril 1992; 57:290–293.
13. Schnell VL, Sacco AG, Savoy-Moore RT, Ataya KM, Moghissi KS. Effects of oocyte exposure to local anesthestics on in vitro fertilization and embryo development in the mouse. Reprod Toxicol 1992;6:323–327.
14. Taymore ML, Ranoux CJ, Gross GL. Natural oocyte retrieval with intravaginal fertilization: a simplified approach to in vitro fertilization. Obstet Gynecol 1992;80:888–891.
15. Ranoux CJ, Aubriot FX, Duboisson JB, Cardone V, Foulot H, Poirot C, Chevallier O. A new in vitro fertilization technique: intravaginal culture. Fertil Steril 1988;49:654–657.
16. Steinkampf MP, Kretzer PA, McElroy E, Conway-Myers BA. A simplified approach to in vitro fertilization. J Repro Med 1992;37:199–204.
17. Society for Assisted Reproductive Technology, American Society for Reproductive Medicine. Assisted reproductive technology in the United States and Canada: 1993 results from the Society for Assisted Reproductive Technology. Fertil Steril 1995;64:13–21.
18. Scott RT, Toner JP, Muasher SJ, Oehninger S, Robinson S, Rosenwaks Z. Follicle-stimulating hormone levels on cycle day 3 are predictive of in vitro fertilization outcome. Fertil Steril 1989;51:651–654.

19. Jansen RP, Anderson JC. Catheterisation of the fallopian tubes from the vagina. Lancet 1987;August 8:309–310.
20. Scholtes MCW, Roosenberg BJ, Alberda AT, Zeilmaker GH. Transcervical intrafallopian transfer of gametes. Fertil Steril 1990;54:283–286.
21. Bustillo M, Munabi AK, Bender S, Dorfmann A, Schulman JD. Transcervical ultrasound-guided intrafallopian placement of gametes, zygotes and embryos (abstract). Presented at the Sixth World Congress on In Vitro Fertilization and Alternate Assisted Reproduction, Jerusalem, Israel, April 2–7, 1989.
22. Hazout A, Glissant A, Frydman R. Transvaginal ultrasound guided gamete intrafallopian transfer (GIFT) (abstract). Presented at the Sixth World Congress on In Vitro Fertilization and Alternate Assisted Reproduction, Jerusalem, Israel, April 2–7, 1989.
23. Anderson JC, Jansen RPS. Ultrasound guided catheterization of the fallopian tube for the nonoperative transfer of gametes and embryos (abstract). Presented at the Sixth World Congress on In Vitro Fertilization and Alternate Assisted Reproduction, Jerusalem, Israel, April 2–7, 1989.
24. Tan SL, Pampiglione J, Steer C, Balen A, Mills C, Campbell S. Transvaginal peritoneal oocyte and sperm transfer for the treatment of non tubal infertility. Fertil Steril 1992;57: 850–853.
25. Jansen RPS, Anderson JC, Radonic I, Smit J, Sutherland PD. Pregnancies after ultrasound-guided fallopian insemination with cryostored donor semen. Fertil Steril 1988;49:920–922.
26. Lucena E, Ruiz JA, Mendoza JC, Ortiz JA, Lucena C, Gomez M, Arango A. Vaginal intratubal insemination (VITI) and vaginal GIFT, endosonographic technique: early experience. Human Reprod 1989;4(6):658–662.

*Invasive Outpatient Procedures in Reproductive Medicine,* edited by Mark I. Evans, et al. Lippincott–Raven Publishers, Philadelphia © 1997.

# 16 IUD Insertion

Howard J. Tatum, Elizabeth B. Connell, Kamran S. Moghissi

## INTRODUCTION

Intrauterine contraceptive devices have been used for centuries. The modern IUDs were developed and tested in the 1960s and 1970s. Many varieties of IUDs of different shapes and sizes have been fabricated and clinically used worldwide. They may be classified to two major categories: inert and medicated. In the United States, IUDs were used extensively prior to 1975. An inert IUD, the Dalkon Shield, introduced in 1970, was found to cause a high incidence of pelvic infection due to defective construction.[1] Dalkon Shield was withdrawn from the market in 1975. However, complications resulting from the use of Dalkon Shield led to a gradual decline in the use of IUDs. Currently in the United States two types of medicated IUD are available: Copper IUD (TCU-380A, ParaGard) and Progestasert.

The TCU-380A is a T-shaped device with a polyethylene frame holding 380 $mm^2$ of exposed area of copper. The pure electrolytic copper wound around the stem weighs 176 mg, and copper sleeves on the horizontal area weigh 66.5 mg. The IUD frame contains barium, making it radiopaque. TCU-380A provides effective contraception for 10 years with a pregnancy rate of 0.5–0.8%, an expulsion rate of 5%, and a removal rate of 14%. This device is a highly effective, safe, and well-tolerated contraceptive.

Progestasert is a T-shaped IUD made of ethylene/vinyl acetate copolymer containing titanium dioxide. The vertical stem contains a reservoir of 38 mg progesterone together with barium sulfate dispersed in silicone fluid. Progestasert releases 65 mcg progesterone per day and duration of its use is limited to 1 year. Another T-shaped hormone-releasing IUD available in Europe releases 20 μg of levonorgestrel (LNG-20) and is effective for 7 years.

The contraceptive action of all IUDs is dependent on the production of an intrauterine environment that is spermicidal. Ovulation is not affected and the IUD is not abortifacient. Contrary to some early suggestion, IUDs do not increase the risk of ectopic pregnancy and may in fact offer some protection against it.[2]

## INDICATIONS

The IUD is well-suited for parous women in a stable, mutually monogamous relationship who wish to prevent future pregnancy but preserve their reproductive function. In selecting appropriate candidates for IUD use, the risk of sexually transmitted disease (STD) should be carefully evaluated.

## CONTRAINDICATIONS

The use of IUD is contraindicated in:

- known or suspected pregnancy
- known or suspected pelvic inflammatory disease (PID) or pelvic malignancy

- undiagnosed vaginal bleeding
- patients at high risk of PID
- uterine size or shape incompatible with IUD use
- Wilson's disease (for Copper device only)
- other medical conditions: valvular heart disease, immune suppression resulting in increased risk of infection

## TECHNIQUE AND TIMING FOR INSERTION OF AN IUD

There are two general methods for IUD insertion. The withdrawal technique consists of the release of the enclosed IUD from the inserter tube by withdrawing the stationary plunger. This results in minimal chance of uterine wall perforation.

The second technique is the push-out process. This results in an upward motion of the IUD and a corresponding increased chance of uterine wall perforation. The withdrawal technique is the safer of the two.

The technique of IUD insertion depends to a certain extent on the phase of the menstrual cycle, parity, and the time relationship to termination of the last pregnancy. The use-effectiveness and the acceptability of the IUD are modified to some extent by the above factors. In general, an IUD may be inserted at any time during the menstrual cycle, provided a pregnancy has been excluded.

Immediate post-placental insertion, although not specifically approved by the US Food and Drug Administration (FDA) is easily accomplished because the cervical canal is dilated and high fundal placement is readily achieved. Spontaneous expulsion is less likely to occur than when insertion is carried out 1–7 days after delivery.[3]

Recent studies have shown that IUD insertion immediately following a curettage for the treatment of an incomplete abortion or therapeutic termination of an early pregnancy is safe and effective.[3,4]

Postcoital IUD insertion (not specifically approved by the FDA) has also been shown to be effective when performed 5–7 days after unprotected intercourse. In a study of 341 women, no pregnancies occurred.[5] Statistically, at least 25 pregnancies would have been expected had no IUDs been used.[6]

The techniques for the actual insertion depend to certain extent on the phase of the menstrual cycle. A comprehensive gynecological examination must precede the insertion. This should include vaginal and cervical cultures for gonorrhea (GC) and chlamydia and a Papanicoloau smear. Cervical erosions and infections should be excluded.

### *INSERTION PROCEDURES*

1. Perform bimanual examination to determine uterine position and size.
2. Administer an analgesic or nonsteroidal anti-inflammatory drug.
3. Place a vaginal speculum to expose the cervix. The vagina and external cervix should be cleansed with an antiseptic solution.
4. Stabilize the cervix by grasping its anterior lip with a single-toothed tenaculum or Allis clamp. Gentle traction on the tenaculum will reduce the angle between the endocervical canal and the endometrial cavity.
5. Sound the uterus with a malleable uterine sound, bent to conform to the position of cervicoendometrial canal. The sound is inserted while gentle traction is applied on the cervical tenaculum. The sound is directed upward until it comes in contact with the top of the endometrial cavity.
6. Measure the distance between the external cervical os and the fundus of the endometrial cavity. A general recommendation is that if the uterus is found to be less than 6 cm or greater than 9 cm, IUD insertion is contraindicated (8.5 cm for Copper IUD and up to 10 cm for Progestasert).

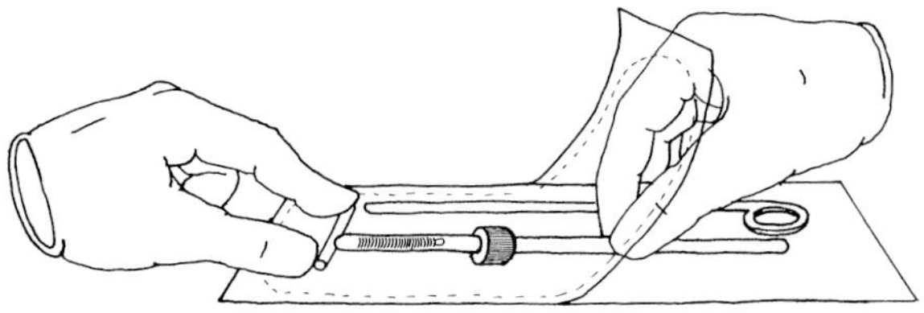

FIG. 16–1. Grasp the arms of the device within the package.

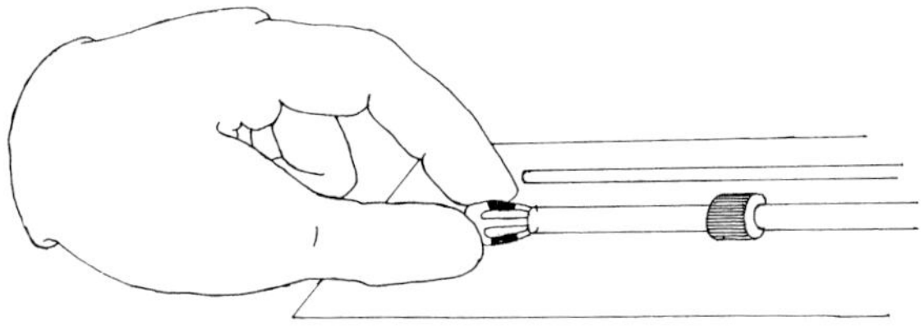

FIG. 16–2. IUD retracted into loading device.

7. Leave the sound in place until the IUD is loaded into the inserter tube.
8. Grasp the arms of the device within the package (Fig. 16–1).
9. Push the arms in the inserter (Fig. 16–2).
10. Remove the sound and gently insert the IUD, using the recommended inserter and until resistance of the fundal top is met (Fig. 16–3).
11. Retract the insertion tube approximately 1.5 cm while the solid rod is not moved. This frees the IUD into the top of the uterine cavity with the transverse arms extended (Fig. 16–4). Move inserter upward gently until resistance of fundus is felt.
12. Remove the inserter tube, leaving the IUD in contact with the fundal wall (Fig. 16–5).
13. Cut the tails to about 4 cm beyond cervical opening. These may need shortening at a later date if found to be too long.
14. Remove the tenaculum and vaginal speculum.
15. Stop if insertion is difficult.
16. Teach the patient how to feel the strings (Fig. 16–6).
17. An antibiotic (Doxycycline 200 mg) administered orally 1 hour prior to insertion may provide protection against insertion-associated pelvic infection.

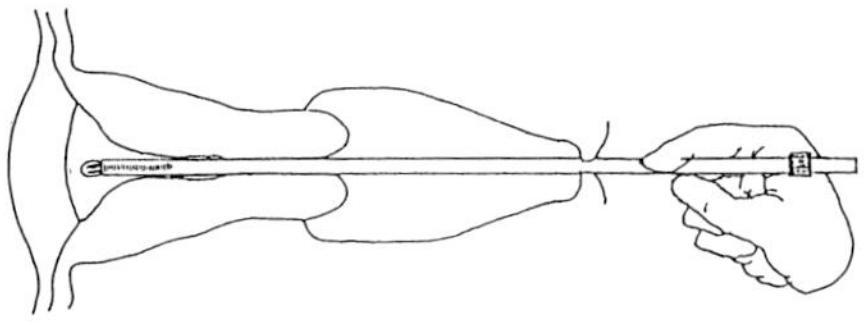

FIG. 16–3. Insertion of the IUD.

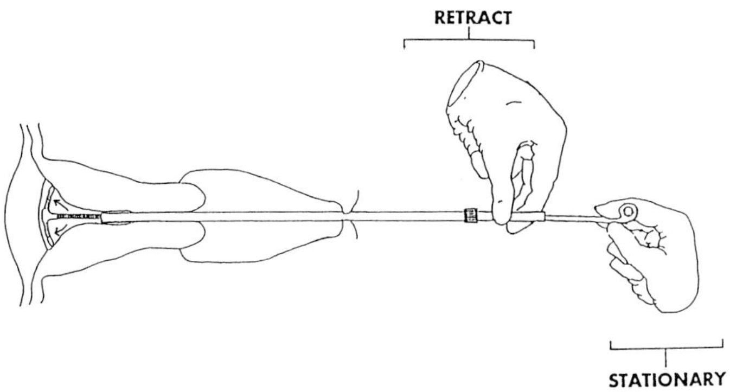


FIG. 16–4. Freeing the IUD with transverse arms extended.

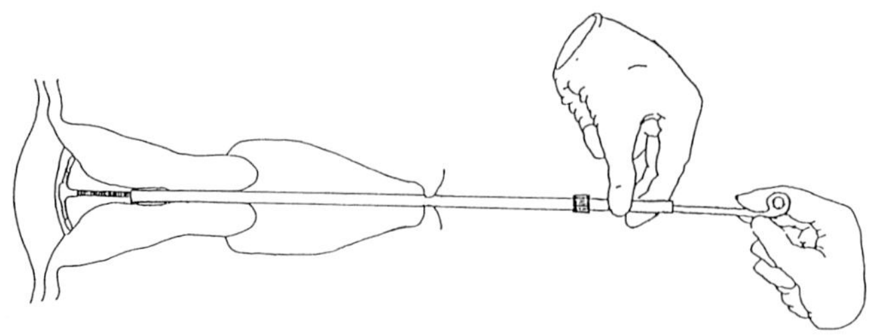


**FIG. 16–5.** Removal of the inserter tube, leaving the IUD in contact with the fundal wall.

**18.** Strings should be palpated at least monthly, usually after menstruation.

Each type of IUD will be found to have slightly different characteristics and recommended procedures for insertion. These directions will be described in the package insert as received from the manufacturer.

### *POSTINSERTION COUNSELING*

The patient should be instructed to report the following symptoms and signs to the physicians or clinic:

- vaginal discharge or lower abdominal pain
- change in length of strings
- heavy bleeding or cramping, which may signal complete or partial expulsion
- missed menstrual period
- signs and symptoms of pregnancy

Patient is asked to return for a check-up after the next menses and subsequently report any episode of amenorrhea.

## COMPLICATIONS

Partial or complete perforation of uterine wall occurs in approximately 1 of 1,000–2,000 insertions[7] and is almost always associated with the insertion procedure.[8] Factors affecting the risk of uterine perforation include the type of IUD, status and configuration of the uterus, the

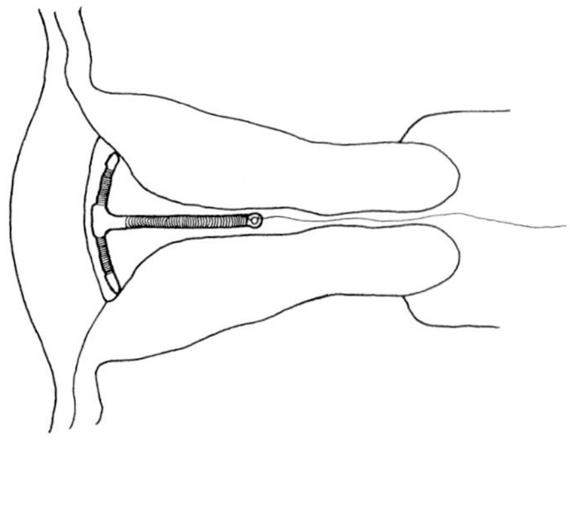

**FIG. 16–6.** IUD in place with string extending out of cervix.

technique of insertion (perforation is less likely to occur when withdrawal technique is used), and the skill and experience of the clinician. Women who are lactating at the time of insertion are more likely to have a uterine perforation.

### *MANAGEMENT OF COMPLICATIONS*

Increased cramping and heavier menstrual flow can occur in some women. In such cases, the possibilities of partial expulsion or infection should be considered and excluded. Oral iron therapy and nonsteroidal anti-inflammatory agents (NSAID) are used to alleviate these problems.

Infection of the lower genital tract (vaginitis) in association with IUD may be managed without the removal of IUD. However, in the presence of endometritis or salpingitis, the IUD may have to be removed and appropriate antibiotic therapy instituted.

If a woman becomes pregnant while wearing an IUD there is a 2–3% chance that the pregnancy will be ectopic.[9] Therefore, the diagnosis of ectopic pregnancy should be considered and ruled out. If intrauterine pregnancy is confirmed, the IUD should be removed as soon as possible. If the IUD cannot be removed, therapeutic abortion should be offered to the patient. However, there is no increased risk of congenital anomalies if the IUD is left in situ.

## CONCLUSION

The modern IUDs are extremely effective, long-acting, and safe. They are grossly underutilized, owing to negative media coverage of some poorly designed IUDs in the past.

## REFERENCES

1. Tatum JH, Schmidt FH, Philips DM, McCarty M, O'Leary WM. Dalkon Shield controversy, structural and bacteriologic studies of IUD tails. JAMA 1975;231:711.
2. Sivin I. IUDs are contraceptives, not abortifacient: a comment on research and belief. Stud Fam Plann 1989;20:355.
3. Tatum HJ. Intrauterine Contraception. Am J Obstet Gynecol 1972;112(7):1000–1023.
4. Tatum HJ. Intrauterine devices: demise of some myths. Obstetrics/Gynecology Report 1992; 2(1):47–53.
5. Lippes J, Tatum JH, Maulik D, Zielezny M. Postcoital copper IUDs: advances in planned parenthood. Excerpta Medica 1979;14(3):87–94.
6. Tietze C. Probability of pregnancy resulting from a single unprotected coitus. Fertil Steril 1960;11:485.
7. ACOG. The Intrauterine Device. Technical Bulletin 164, February 1992, Washington DC.
8. WHO. Mechanism of action and efficacy of intrauterine devices. Technical Report Series, 753, Geneva; 1987;1:91.
9. The Intrauterine Device. In: Speroff L, Darney P (eds). A clinical guide for contraception. Baltimore: Williams & Wilkins, 1992;157–182.

*Invasive Outpatient Procedures in Reproductive Medicine,* edited by Mark I. Evans, et al. Lippincott–Raven Publishers, Philadelphia © 1997.

# 17 Norplant

Kamran S. Moghissi, David F. Archer

## INTRODUCTION

Norplant contraceptive system is an implant contraception method that consists of six flexible capsules each 34 mm in length and 2.4 mm in diameter (about the size of a book of matches). The set contains a total of 2.6 mg of crystallized levonorgestrel, a progestogen used extensively in oral contraceptives. One-third of the drug load is released in 5 years, the currently approved lifetime of the implant. Silicone rubber provides the encapsulating, rate-measuring membrane through which levonorgestrel diffuses into the body.

Levonorgestrel is detectable within 2 hours after insertion, concentrations of 250–600 pg/mL are observed after 3–6 months of use. At 5 years, levonorgestrel levels average 170–350 pg/mL, depending on body weight.

Norplant implants, like progestogen alone oral contraceptives (minipills), exert their contraceptive effect in several ways. The drug has a marked effect on cervical mucus and sperm cervical mucus interaction. Under the influence of circulating, levonorgestrel cervical mucus becomes scanty, viscous, and impenetrable by spermatozoa.[1] The progestin also suppresses the ovulation in approximately fifty percent of women.[2] If ovulation occurs, corpus luteum function is altered and low levels of progesterone consistent with luteal phase deficiency render the women infertile. Additionally, out of phase endometrium potentially interferes with implantation.[1]

## INDICATIONS

Norplant contraceptive system is a highly effective method of contraception suitable for most women of reproductive age. It is particularly indicated for:

- women who desire long-acting protection
- birth control when a reversible method is required
- women who desire a method alternative to sterilization

## INSERTION TECHNIQUE

### *EQUIPMENT*

1. Sterile package of 6 implants and a trocar for insertion
2. A comfortable table for patient to lie on with support for the patient's arm
3. Sterile surgical drapes
4. Sterile tray for the instruments
5. Sterile gloves, soap, and antiseptic solution
6. Local anesthetic, needle, and syringe
7. Scalpel with a #11 blade, pick-up forceps, and hemostats
8. Sterile gauze, butterfly bandage, and bandage

### *PROCEDURE*

Implants may be inserted at any site on the body, but preferably on the inner aspect of the upper arm, which is a convenient site and is a less likely location for fat deposition.[3] Furthermore, the capsules can be readily identified and removed from this site. The patient is usually asked to lie flat on a table, and the appropriate arm is then extended from the body at a right angle and rotated.

The site for insertion is selected between the biceps and the triceps muscle in the midline, approximately 10 cm above the medial condyle of the humerus. The insertion site can be outlined with the use of a template and marker with ink and then painted with a betadine solution. The site is draped with a fenestrated eye drape or appropriate drape to wall off the surrounding area.

The area for insertion is anesthetized, using $\leq$ 5 mL of a 1% xylocaine solution or its equivalent. Do not use a local anesthetic with epinephrine, since epinephrine can cause vasoconstriction and can result in a skin slough. The anesthetic is placed in a wheal in the area where the incision will be made, and then in a spoke-like fashion along the delineated areas for the 6 Norplant capsules to be inserted (Fig. 17–1).

An incision for the insertion of the needle can be performed using a #11 knife blade, or the #10 gauge-needle, with the obturator (plunger) in place and the bevel down, can be inserted through the skin without making an incision (Fig. 17–2). The needle is then rotated so that the bevel is up. The skin is tented with the needle in place by placing the forefinger of the inserting hand underneath the shaft of the needle. This elevates the skin and countertraction is placed with the opposite hand (Fig. 17–3). The needle is advanced to the second notch on the needle, which is 4.5 cm from the tip (Fig. 17–4).

At this time, the obturator is removed (Fig. 17–5) and the Norplant is inserted (Fig. 17–6). It is recommended that thumb forceps be used to pick up and insert the Norplant in order to reduce the transfer of powder from the gloves onto the Norplant capsule. Each capsule

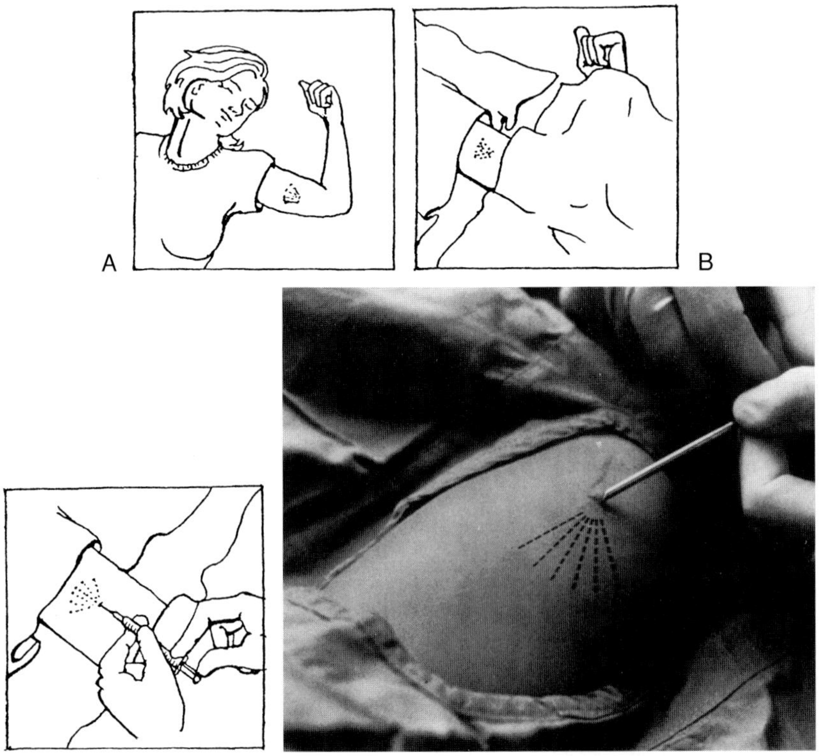

A B C D

**FIG. 17–1.** (A) Patient is positioned, (B) prepped and draped, (C, D) and anesthetic administered.

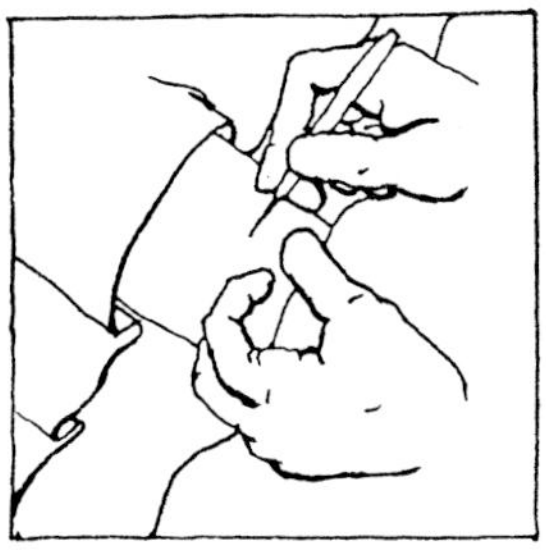

FIG. 17–2. Scalpel incision.

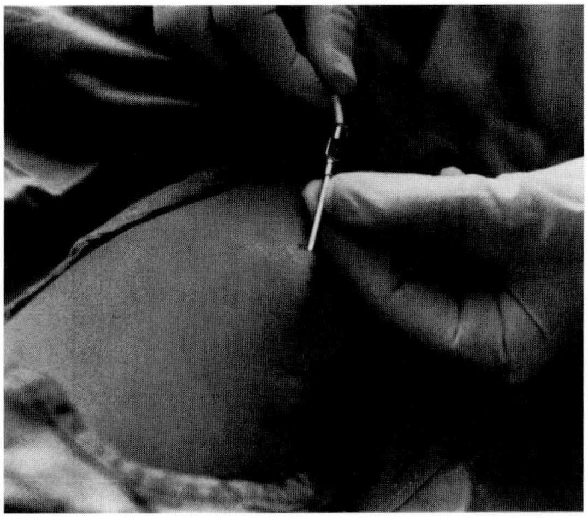

FIG. 17–3. Skin tenting.

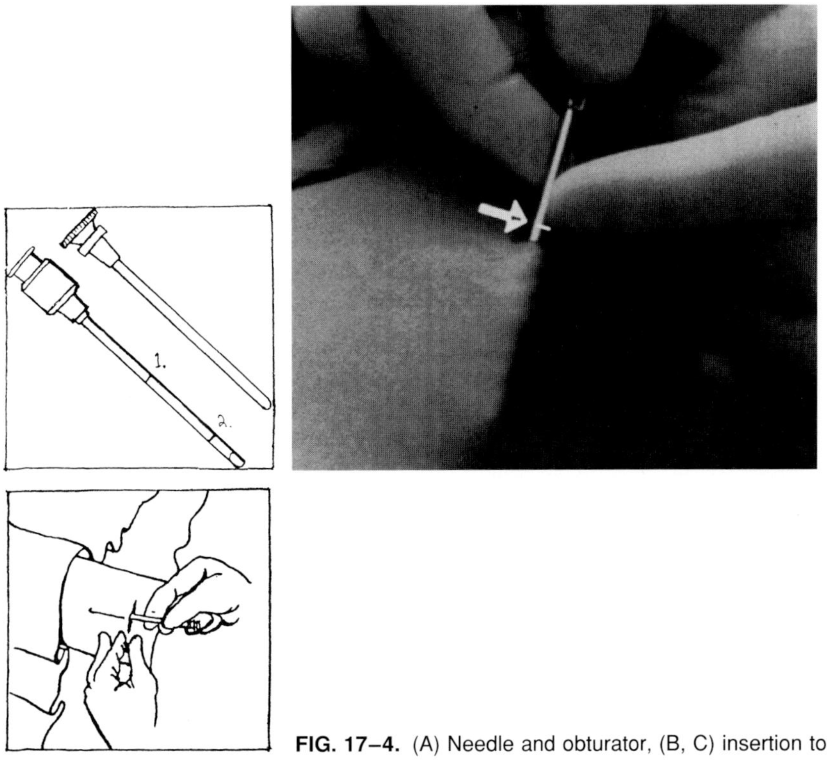


A B C

FIG. 17–4. (A) Needle and obturator, (B, C) insertion to point #1.

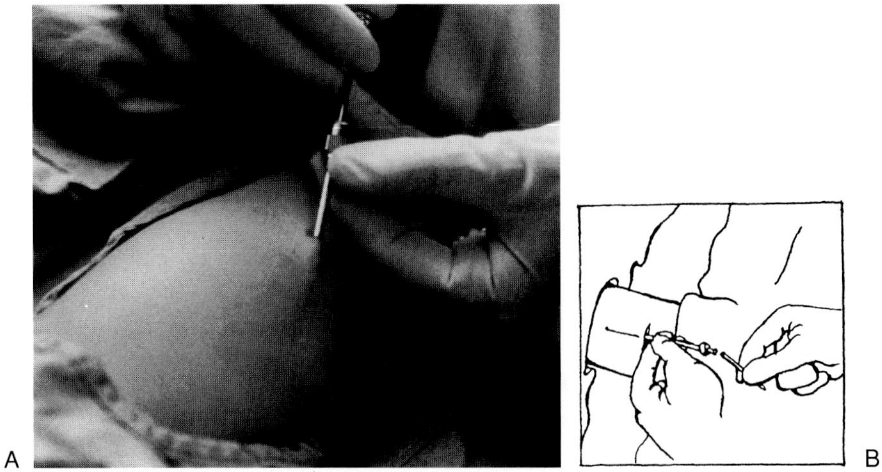


**FIG. 17–5.** (A, B) Retraction of hub of the device.

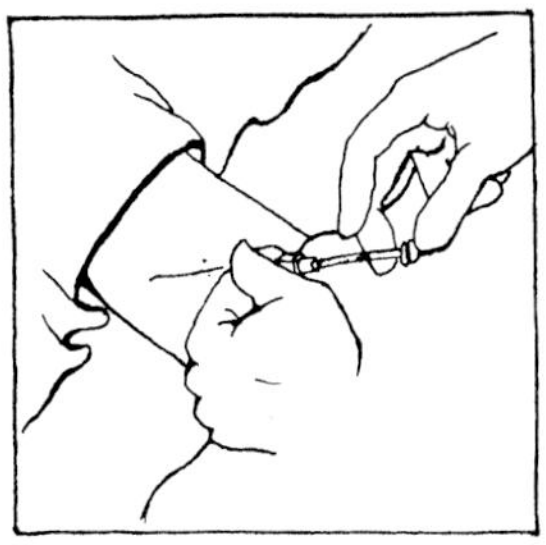

**FIG. 17–6.** Loading Norplant capsule.

causes a fibrous reaction to take place, and sometimes the powder can increase this fibrous reaction. The obturator is then reinserted into the needle and advanced with light pressure until resistance is met, which is when the obturator has reached the proximal portion of the Norplant device (Fig. 17–7). Grasp the hub of the needle and retract it with one hand while holding the knurled end of the obturator steady with the other (Fig. 17–8). Do not press on the obturator or advance it in any fashion. Do not attempt to hold the obturator with one hand while withdrawing the needle with the other. Both of these procedures can result in extrusion of the Norplant capsule, causing the capsule to be deformed in a "J" or "U" shape. Advancing the obturator can result in a stair-step placement of the devices. The sleeve of the needle is withdrawn to the more distal indentation, which is 1.0 cm from the needle tip (Fig. 17–9). This mark should clear the incision site, but the needle should not be removed from the incision site. When the second indentation is apparent there should be a slight change in the feel of the needle, indicating that the Norplant capsule has been released from the needle sleeve. If the Norplant is not totally released from the sleeve, it can pull the proximal portion of the first capsule up, again

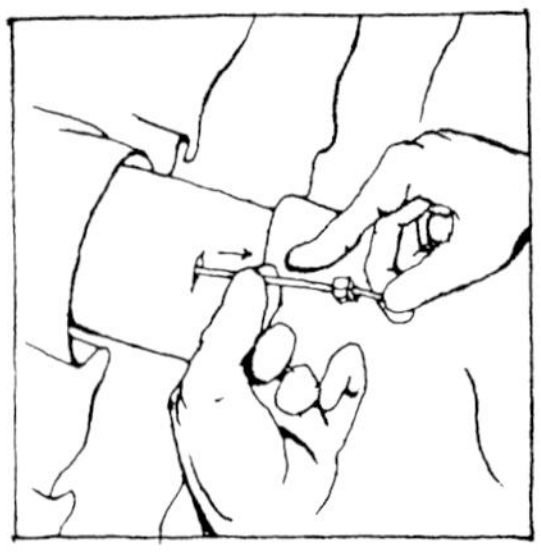

**FIG. 17–7.** Obturator being advanced.

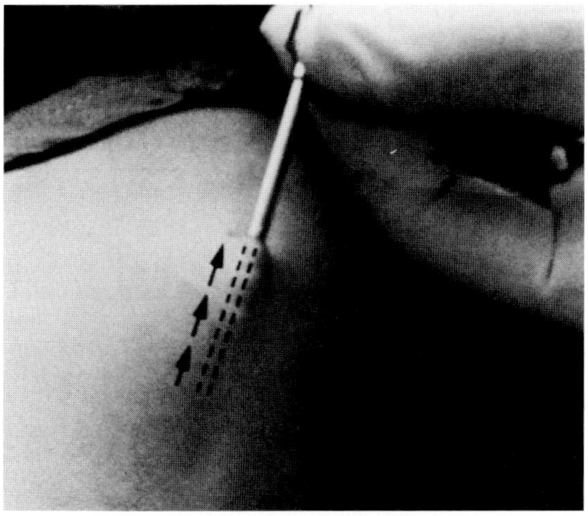

A

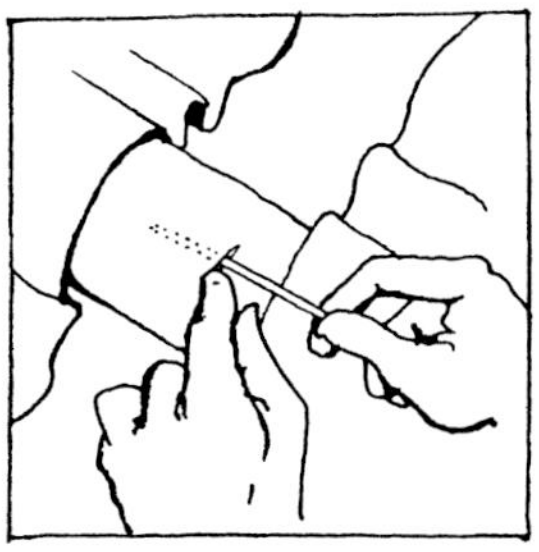

B

**FIG. 17–8.** (A, B) Retraction of needle.

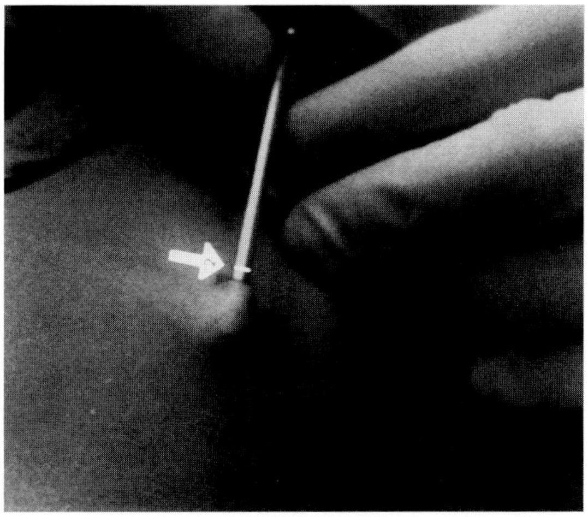

**FIG. 17–9.** Retraction to distant notch.

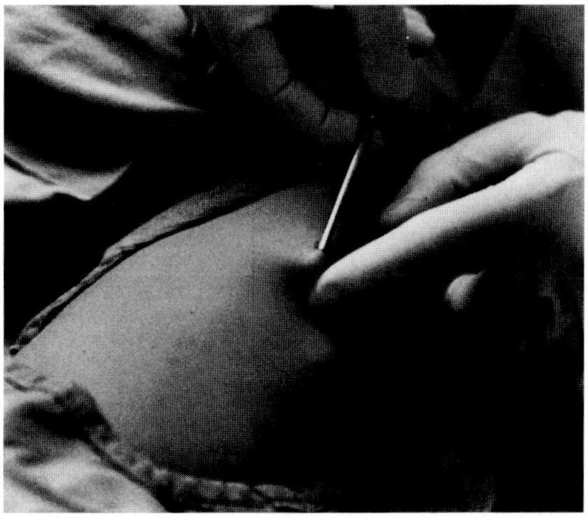

**FIG. 17–10.** Picking direction for second capsule.

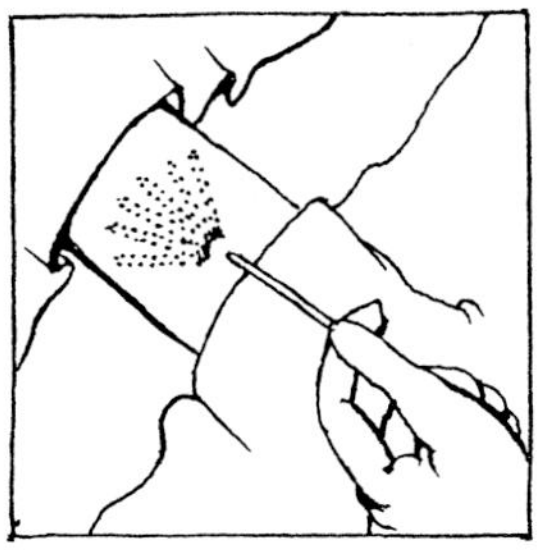

**FIG. 17–11.** Distribution of Norplant capsules and removal of device.

resulting in an abnormal shape or a twisting of the capsule when the next advance of the needle is made. By the time the second indentation is visible, the obturator should be fully reinserted.

Stabilize the previously inserted Norplant capsule using the forefinger of one hand and guide the needle forward again just beneath the dermis and at approximately 15° from the first insertion capsule (Fig. 17–10). Repeat this procedure for each subsequent insertion.

After all 6 capsules are inserted, remove the needle with its obturator (Fig. 17–11).

Press down on the proximal portion of the capsules just above the incision site, which should result in elevation of the more distal ends of the capsules, and palpate these ends to ensure that all six capsules are in place.

Clean the incision area by using alcohol to remove the betadine. Then close the incision with steristrips. Apply a light pressure bandage to minimize bleeding using $4 \times 4$ gauze and roller gauze (Fig. 17–12). Excessive pressure can result in numbness or tingling of the fingers, and when this occurs the roller gauze should be removed and reapplied.

Postinsertion instructions should include the following:

- Ice pack may be applied to the area to reduce swelling.
- Analgesics such as aspirin or Tylenol can be used every 3–4 hours for pain or discomfort.
- Keep the dressing dry, wrap it in a saran wrap for bathing.
- Remove the dressing in 24 hours and the steristrips in 72 hours.
- Call if there is any sign of infection with redness or induration at the incision site.

The insertion of Norplant is relatively easy and should usually take somewhere between 10–15 minutes. It is important to maintain sterility throughout the insertion. If any of the capsules fall off the field, they should not be replaced. No attempt should be made to clean the capsules and use them; the unused capsules should be returned to the manufacturer for replacement of further sterile capsules, which then can be inserted at a second sitting.

### *COMPLICATIONS*

Infection has been reported to occur in 0.5% of insertions. Local infections should be managed with hot soaks and appropriate antibiotics. Expulsion of the capsules through the insertion site

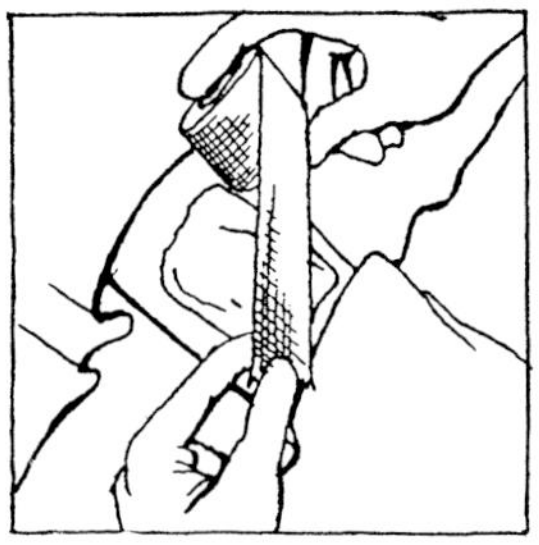

**FIG. 17–12.** Application of bandages.

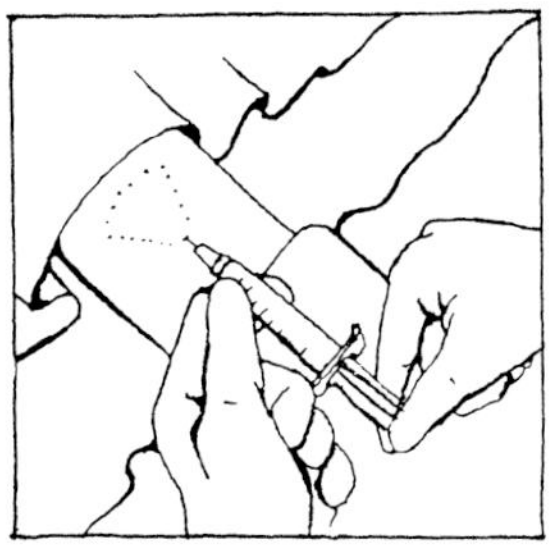

**FIG. 17–13.** Anesthetizing the area.

or tract may occur in <0.3% of all insertions. If a capsule is expelled, with or without associated infection, it is best to wait 4–6 weeks until further healing has occurred. At this juncture, the appropriate number of capsules that need to be replaced can be inserted using the techniques described above.

## REMOVAL TECHNIQUE

### *EQUIPMENT*

Equipment for removal is similar to that for insertion.

### *PROCEDURE*

The removal of the Norplant capsules appears to be relatively simple and there is a very rapid learning curve for most physicians.[3] It should be pointed out that each capsule takes approximately 5–6 minutes to remove; thus the total removal time is approximately 25–30 minutes. This time can decrease with increasing familiarity and competence of the operator. Each Norplant capsule is enclosed in a fibrous tissue that is the body's normal reaction to a foreign body. For this reason, the overlying fibrous tissue must be incised by either sharp or blunt dissection in order to grasp the Norplant capsule itself for removal.

The following approach is suggested. Palpate the position of all 6 capsules. Be sure that you can identify that there are 6 capsules present and locate their relative positions. This is important because the capsules may have moved, be sitting on top of the other, be in an abnormal shape, or be in a stair-step fashion. Mark the location of the capsules if necessary with indelible ink and then apply betadine to the area.

Using 1–2 mL of 1% xylocaine without epinephrine, create a wheal at the incision site (Fig. 17–13). This site does not have to be the same used for insertion; it can be modified based on the location of the capsules. The incision can be placed in such a position that the capsules are of equal distance from the incision site, particularly if they are in a stair-step arrangement. Use approximately 0.5 mL of the local anesthetic inserted beneath the proximal tip of each capsule. This will cause the capsule to be elevated and remain palpable. It is important to stress the fact that the anesthetic should go under the capsule rather than on top. Excessive anesthetic can enhance bleeding and result in local tissue swelling. A vertical incision rather than horizontal is preferred since this is in the body line (Fig. 17–14). Approximately

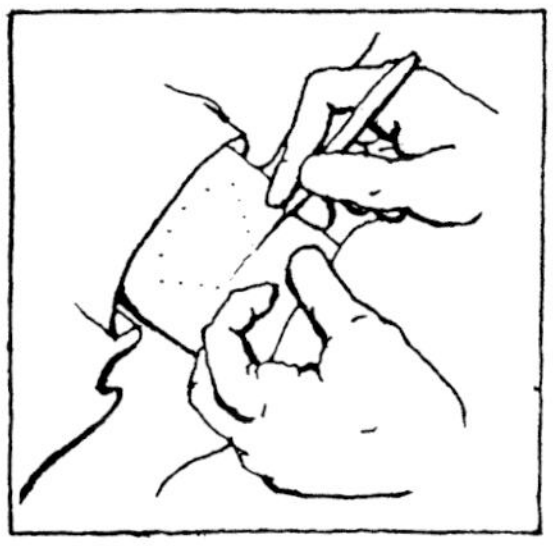

**FIG. 17–14.** Incision.

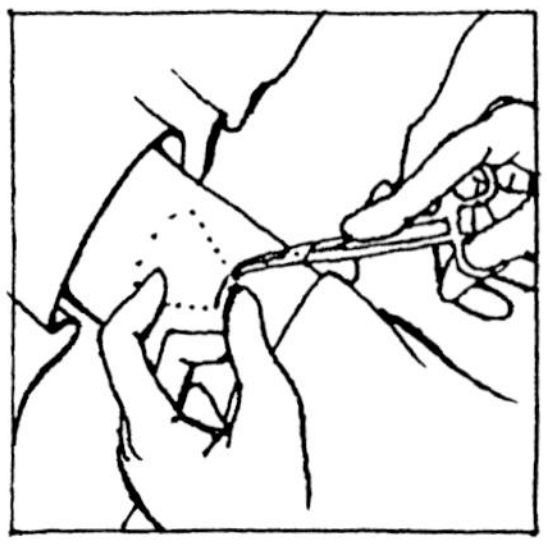

**FIG. 17–15.** Hemostat dissection around capsule.

a ¼-inch incision is made roughly in the middle of the proximal ends of the Norplant capsules. The skin is further opened with a mosquito forceps, either straight or curved.

Using a hemostat, bluntly dissect around the proximal tips of the capsule (Fig. 17–15). Each capsule is encased in a fibrous tissue adherent to the surrounding subcutaneous material; it helps if this is broken down. This can be done either by the use of the hemostat or, in some instances, by rubbing or rotating the capsules externally. Using the free hand of the operator, stabilize the capsule to be removed by applying downward pressure from the distal end while holding vertical pressure on the proximal portion of the capsule with forefinger (Fig. 17–16). Using a hemostat, either curved or straight, grasp the capsule and its covering by opening the tips of the clamp and pushing with the external finger directing the capsule into the jaws of the clamp (Fig. 17–17). At this juncture, with the capsule and fibrous tissue grasped, the hemostat is pulled into the incision site or sometimes it is best to take the hemostat and direct the finger grips cephalad, rotating the end of the capsule into the incision site (Fig. 17–18). Identify the proximal end of the capsule either visually or by palpation. Then incise the fibrous connective tissue using sharp dissection with a knife or by blunt dissection using a second hemostat. Once the fibrous capsule is open, the end of the Norplant should be immediately visible as white, in contrast to the gray, fibrous covering. Grasp the white capsule using a second hemostat, release the holding hemostat, and withdraw the capsule. Repeat this procedure for each subsequent capsule for removal.

An alternative removal method has been described using a modified vasectomy clamp instead of a hemostat. With this procedure, the Norplant capsule and its covering fibrous tissue are held in the vasectomy clamp, which is circular, and the fibrous tissue is not grasped. The proximal ends of the Norplant capsule are bluntly dissected using the hemostat or the vasectomy clamp. Stabilizing the Norplant rod as described above is done with the free hand and the vasectomy clamp, which is then used to grip the Norplant capsule through the skin incision. The Norplant capsule is commonly grasped approximately ¼ inch or more from its proximal end. Thus, when the Norplant capsule is brought into the incision, there can be a slight bend in the capsule. Holding the capsule in the incision, an incision is then made in the fibrous sheath. The Norplant capsule is then recognized since it is white rather than gray. The capsule is removed by grasping with the hemostat or inserting the hemostat bluntly underneath the curve of the Norplant capsule, flipping out the more proximal end. The reason for this is that

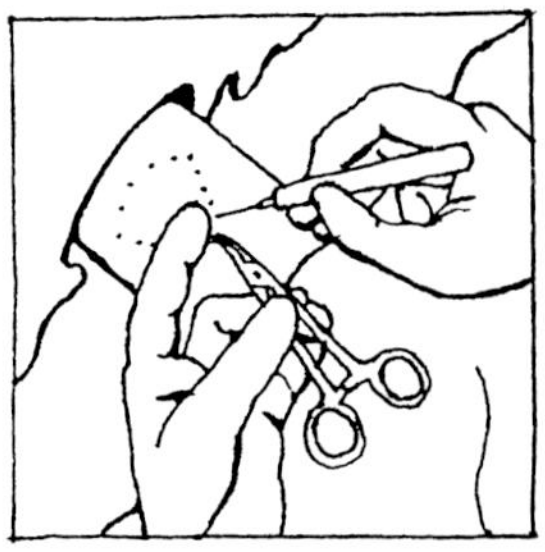

**FIG. 17–16.** Freeing adhesions with scalpel.

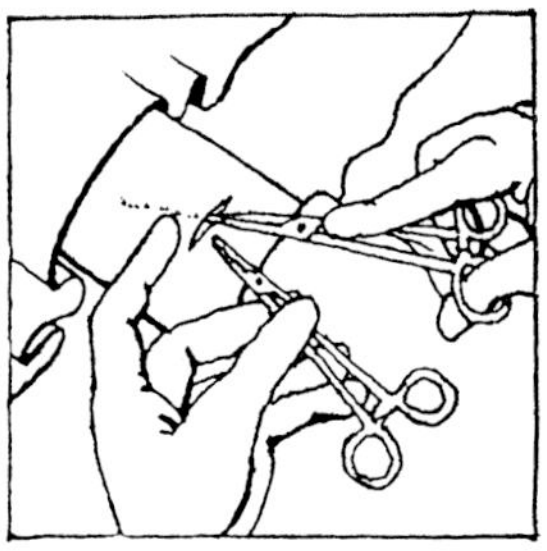

**FIG. 17–17.** Grasping capsule with hemostat.

the capsule is usually not held at its most dependent end. Then the incision is made away from the end of the fibrous capsule, over the capsule.

A no-clamp technique has also been described.[3] In this technique, the capsules are bluntly dissected, again using a hemostat, from the surrounding connective tissue or by externally rolling the capsules back and forth with the finger. This will serve to break down the connection between the fibrous tissue and the surrounding subcutaneous tissue. An incision is made in the appropriate place through the skin. Each capsule is then bluntly dissected free of the surrounding tissue using the hemostat or the rolling technique. The distal end of the capsule is pushed down, resulting in the proximal end of the capsule being brought into the incision site. Counterpressure is made at the incision site with the opposite hand or, in some instances, with the thumb of the hand that is pressing down from above on the capsule. The proximal end of the capsule is identified by visual inspection or palpation. The capsule is held in place with one hand and the fibrous tissue is sharply or bluntly opened with further identification of the Norplant capsule. The Norplant capsule is then removed by continued pressure on the distal end of the Norplant or with a hemostat.

### COMPLICATIONS

Removal difficulties may be encountered when the implants were inserted too deep; placed either in the muscle or subcutaneous fat. If the capsules cannot be palpated, locating them with x-ray or ultrasound may be required. Once the location of the implants has been identified, the skin overlying the capsules should be marked to facilitate their removal. Placement of the devices in a stair-step fashion rather than in a fan-shaped manner can result in having to use more anesthetic to reach the further devices. Alternatively, extension of the incision may be required and, in some instances, a second incision to reach the capsules further away may also be necessary. When the proximal ends of the capsules cannot be located at the time of removal, identify the more distal end, placing more anesthetic at this end of each device, and use a second or third incision for removal. The capsules are then removed from the distal rather than from the proximal end of the fan. The patient can experience pain, particularly on grasping and pulling down on the encapsulated Norplant devices. The reason for this is that the fibrous tissue adheres to the subcutaneous tissue, and with traction there is discomfort or pain. The solution to this is to use more anesthetic at the more distal end of the devices. Alternatively,

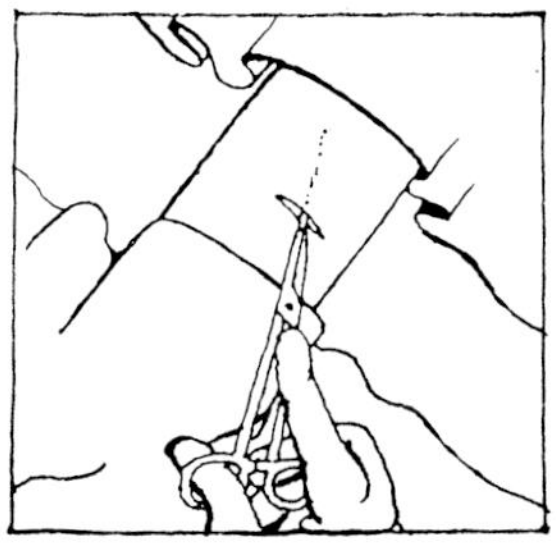

**FIG. 17–18.** Removal of capsule.

the discomfort experienced by the individual can be used by the operator to indicate that the appropriate capsule has been grasped and is being mobilized in an appropriate fashion. Inability to identify, grasp, or remove all of the capsules can occur at any time. This can result from initial poor placement or swelling due to prolonged time or multiple attempts to identify or remove the capsule. If this occurs, in some instances it is best to stop the procedure for 5–10 minutes. This will allow both the patient and the operator a break. The situation is then reassessed and, if the capsules are not readily identified and located, the procedure should be stopped. The patient should then be rescheduled for a second attempt in 4–6 weeks. This allows for wound healing and reduced swelling. During this interim, a check on the remaining capsules is indicated to determine whether or not they can be felt or if the use of x-ray or ultrasound is necessary.

In the event of problems in removal or in the need to refer a patient for removal, a national 1–800 number has been made available from the sponsor of Norplant. This number can be used for accessing a national network of individuals who would be helpful in removing the Norplant.

## SIDE EFFECTS

***Changes in Menstrual Pattern.*** Use of Norplant profoundly changes menstrual bleeding pattern. Usually, lighter women tend to develop oligomenorrhea or amenorrhea, whereas women who weigh more than 60 kg are likely to experience irregular or acyclic bleeding. Bleeding and spotting episodes usually decrease after the first year.[2] Women should be informed regarding the occurrence of oligomenorrhea and, more importantly, counseled about irregular bleeding and spotting. Specifically, Norplant users should be given assurances that neither one of these events compromises their future fertility.

Clearly, irregularity of menses is troublesome to many women and is a major cause of discontinuation of this form of contraception. For those women who experience frequent episodes of excessive bleeding or spotting, the following approach is recommended.[4,5]

- Record bleeding or spotting on a diary card
- Ibuprofen 800 mg tid for 5 days
- A course of ethinyl estradiol 0.02–0.05 mg daily for 10 days, which could be repeated at least once if effective and necessary.
- If above treatments are not effective, a course of oral contraceptive for a full 21-day period

Above all, counseling and assurance should be provided by a caring and informed physician. If there is persistent bleeding despite above treatment regimen, an endometrial biopsy should be obtained to exclude an organic cause of bleeding.

***Nonmenstrual Side Effects.*** These side effects are related to levonorgestrel released into the circulation and are much less prevalent than menstrual disturbances. These include progestational and androgenic effects such as headache, skin and hair problems, mood changes, weight gain, and gastrointestinal complaints.[2] Fortunately, the majority of these complaints resolve spontaneously after the first year of use. Ovarian enlargement due to persistent enlarged follicle may be observed in some women (0.5% of cases) and may be associated with pelvic pain. These women should be observed for 6–10 weeks, during which time follicular regression will generally occur. More aggressive management is not usually required.

***Recovery of Fertility.*** Levonorgestrel quickly disappears from the body after implants are removed, and by the end of 1 week the drug is no longer detectable. Several studies have documented that the rates of conception following removal of the implants and outcome of pregnancy are normal.

## ACCEPTABILITY AND CONTINUATION RATE

Norplant contraception is generally well-accepted among properly selected, motivated women. In developing countries, the continuation rate for the first year has been generally greater than 90%.[6,7] In the United States, 74% of the current users have indicated that they would use implants again.[6]

## REFERENCES


1. Moghissi KS, Marks C. Effects of microdose norgestrel on endogenous gonadotropic and steroid hormones, cervical mucus properties, vaginal cytology and endometrium. Fertil Steril 1971;22:424.
2. Sivin I. Contraception with Norplant implants. Hum Reprod 1994;9:1818–1826.
3. Hatcher R. Insertion and removal of levonorgestrel subdermal implants. Contraception report 1994;5(5):3–14.
4. Archer DF. Management of bleeding in women using subdermal implants. Contemp Ob Gyn July 1995:11–25.
5. Diaz S, Croxatto H, Pavez M, et al. Clinical assessment of treatment for prolonged bleeding in users of Norplant implant. Contraception 1990;42:97–109.
6. Sivin I. International experience with Norplant and Norplant-2 contraceptives. Stud Family Plann 1988;19:81–94.
7. Darney PD, Atkinson E, Tanner S, et al. Acceptance and perceptions of Norplant among users in San Francisco, U.S.A. Stud Family Plann 1990;21:152–160.

# Index

Note: Page numbers followed by *f* refer to figures; page numbers followed by *t* refer to tables.